IMMUNOLOGY

2nd EDITION

B.M. Hannigan, C.B.T. Moore and D.G. Quinn

*Biomedical Sciences Research Institute, School of Biomedical Sciences,
University of Ulster, Coleraine, UK*

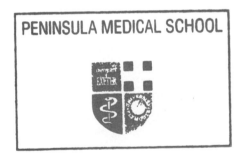

PENINSULA MEDICAL SCHOOL

Scion

Second edition © Scion Publishing Ltd, 2009

ISBN 978 1904842 56 9

First edition published in 2000 by Arnold (ISBN 0 340 76381 7)

A CIP catalogue record for this book is available from the British Library.

Scion Publishing Limited
Bloxham Mill, Barford Road, Bloxham, Oxfordshire OX15 4FF
www.scionpublishing.com

Important Note from the Publisher

The information contained within this book was obtained by Scion Publishing Limited from sources believed by us to be reliable. However, while every effort has been made to ensure its accuracy, no responsibility for loss or injury whatsoever occasioned to any person acting or refraining from action as a result of information contained herein can be accepted by the authors or publishers.

Typeset by Phoenix Photosetting, Chatham, Kent, UK
Printed by Gutenberg Press Ltd, Malta

Contents

Preface

This second edition of *Immunology* has been written eight years after the first. During this time our understanding of the mechanisms of action of immunological processes has advanced enormously. These advances are evidenced by the large number of innovative new businesses that have been enabled by using naturally derived or synthesized reagents that are based upon components of the immune system. Much of our current understanding of immunology has been achieved by the widespread application of molecular biology techniques to probe and interpret the genetic basis of immunity. Likewise, the practice of diagnostic immunology has been greatly enriched by the inclusion of laboratory techniques that rely on molecular biology approaches. Manipulation of the immune system as a means of treating human diseases has been a goal of scientists and clinicians for well over a century. We now know that the complexity of immunity was significantly underestimated, so the goal has proven to be very elusive. It is only now that patients are beginning to derive real benefit from therapeutic interventions that can modify immune processes. These successes indicate that many more therapeutic advances may be achieved in the relatively near future.

To take account of the expansion in our knowledge of immunology, every chapter in the second edition has been substantially updated or rewritten. Separate chapters on lymphocyte development, immune regulation, immunotherapy, and transplantation and tumour immunology have been included to reflect scientific advances in these areas. In terms of organization, in the first half of the book we have attempted to provide an overview of how an immune response is generated and controlled, while in the second half of the book we discuss the role of the immune system in infections and diseases as well as the application of immunological reagents to diagnostics and therapy.

The expansion in our knowledge of immunology is reflected not only in the content of the second edition but also in its authorship. Although there was a sole author of the first edition (BH), there are three co-authors of the second edition. This was necessary to bring the cutting-edge knowledge and understanding that were essential to have this immunology textbook right up to date. We also hope that the textbook has benefited from our experience in teaching immunology in the various campus-based and online programmes offered by the School of Biomedical Sciences at the University of Ulster.

The authors would like to thank Killian McDaid and Lisa Rodgers, cartographers in the Faculty of Life and Health Sciences at the University of

Ulster, for their assistance with some of the figures. We are also indebted to Jonathan Ray at Scion Publishing who suggested that we produce this second edition. His helpful advice, feedback and patience were invaluable during the preparation of this book. Finally, we would like to thank our students, past and current, whose desire to understand immunology has helped shape the content of this textbook. We hope it proves to be a useful aid to learning, particularly to Biomedical Science undergraduate and postgraduate students.

Bernie Hannigan, Tara Moore, Daniel Quinn
January 2009

Abbreviations

ACAD	activated cell autonomous death
ADCC	antibody-dependent cell-mediated cytotoxicity
AICD	activation-induced cell death
AID	activation-induced cytidine deaminase
AIDS	acquired immune deficiency syndrome
ALPS	autoimmune lymphoproliferative syndromes
ANA	antinuclear antibody
APC	antigen-presenting cell
APECED	autoimmune polyendocrinopathy-candidiasis-ectodermal dystrophy
APP	acute phase protein
BAFF	B cell activating factor of the TNF family
BCG	Bacillus Calmette-Guerin
BCR	B cell receptor
BLS	bare lymphocyte syndrome
Btk	Bruton's tyrosine kinase
CAD	caspase-activated DNase
CAMs	cellular adhesion molecules
CCR	CC-chemokine receptor
CD	cluster of differentiation
CEC	cortical epithelial cell
CID	combined immunodeficiencies
CLIP	class II-associated invariant chain peptide
C_M	central memory
CPEs	cytopathic effects
CRP	C-reactive protein
CSR	class switch recombination
CTL	cytotoxic T lymphocyte
CVID	common variable immunodeficiency
CXCR	CXC chemokine receptor
DAF	decay accelerating factor
DC	dendritic cell
DISC	death-inducing signalling complex
DMARDs	disease-modifying anti-rheumatic drugs
DN	double negative
DP	double positive
DTH	delayed-type hypersensitivity
EAE	experimental allergic encephalomyelitis
EBV	Epstein–Barr virus

ELISA	enzyme-linked immunosorbent assay
E_M	effector memory
ER	endoplasmic reticulum
ERAAP	ER-associated aminopeptidase
FADD	Fas-associated death domain
FDC	follicular dendritic cells
FHL2	type 2 familial haemophagocytic lymphohistiocytosis
FMLP	formylmethionyl-leucyl-phenylalanine
GALT	gut-associated lymphoid tissue
GM-CSF	granulocyte–macrophage colony stimulating factor
GvHD	graft-versus-host disease
HAART	highly active antiretroviral therapy
HDN	haemolytic disease of the newborn
HEV	high endothelial venule
HIV	human immunodeficiency virus
HLA	human leukocyte antigens
HSC	haematopoietic stem cell
HSP	heat shock protein
IDO	indoleamine 2,3-dioxygenase
IFN	interferon
Ig	immunoglobulin
IL	interleukin
ITAM	immunoreceptor tyrosine-based activation motif
ITIM	immunoreceptor tyrosine-based inhibitory motif
iT_{REG}	inducible regulatory T cells
IVIG	intravenous injection of gammaglobulin
JAK	Janus kinase
KAR	killer activator receptor
KIR	killer inhibitory receptor
LAD	leukocyte adhesion deficiency
LAK	lymphokine-activated killer
LGL	large granular lymphocyte
LPS	lipopolysaccharide
LT	lymphotoxin
MAC	membrane attack complex
MALT	mucosa-associated lymphoid tissue
MASP	MBL-associated serine protease
MBL	mannan-binding lectin
MCP	membrane cofactor of proteolysis
MEC	medullary epithelial cell
MHC	major histocompatibility complex
MIIC	MHC class II loading compartment
MRSA	multi-drug resistant *Staphylococcus aureus*
M-tropic	macrophage-tropic
MZ	marginal zone
NK	natural killer
NO	nitric oxide

NRTI	nucleoside analogue RT inhibitor
NSAIDs	non-steroidal anti-inflammatory drugs
PAF	platelet activating factor
PALS	peri-arteriolar lymphoid sheath
PAMPs	pathogen-associated molecular patterns
PCR	polymerase chain reaction
pDC	plasmacytoid dentritic cell
PLC	peptide loading complex
PMN	polymorphonuclear
PRA	panel reactive antibody test
PRR	pattern recognition receptor
RAST	radioallergosorbent test
RBC	red blood cell
RCA	regulators of complement activity
RSSs	recombination signal sequences
RT–PCR	reverse transcriptase PCR
scFv	single chain variable fragment
SCID	severe combined immunodeficiency
SHM	somatic hypermutation
SLE	systemic lupus erythematosus
SMAC	supramolecular activation cluster
SOCS	suppressor of cytokine signalling
SP	single positive
SRS-A	slow reacting substance of anaphylaxis
Stat	signal transducer and activator of transcription
TAA	tumour-associated antigen
TAP	transporter of antigen presentation
TCR	T cell receptor
T_{FH}	follicular helper T cells
Th	helper T cell
TIL	tumour infiltrating lymphocytes
TLR	toll-like receptor
TNF	tumour necrosis factor
TSH	thyroid stimulating hormone
TSLP	thymic stromal lymphopoietin
TST	tuberculin skin test
WAS	Wiskott–Aldrich syndrome
WHO	World Health Organization
XHIM	X-linked hyper-IgM syndrome
XLA	X-linked agammaglobulinaemia
XLP	X-linked lymphoproliferative disease

The immune response explained

Learning objectives

After studying this chapter you should confidently be able to:

- **State the overall function of the immune response**
  Ultimately the function of the immune system and the various tissues, cells and proteins involved is to provide protection against anything that would be harmful to the host.

- **State the two principal types of human immune response**
  Immune responses have historically been classified as innate or adaptive. Innate (or natural) responses are inborn, unchanging and relatively non-specific, while the adaptive (or acquired) responses display memory, specificity and include both cell-mediated and antibody-mediated responses. Appreciation of the complex cooperative interactions between the innate and adaptive responses has grown and the concept of distinction into innate or adaptive is diminishing.

- **Discuss the evolution of immune responses**
  All animals display some element of an immune system that has evolved from very simple systems some 600 million years ago. Even the simplest immune systems provide the protection that the hosts need. Invertebrates mount only innate immune responses. The development of more efficient immune responses coincides with the evolution of warm-bloodedness.

- **Describe the principal components of the human immune system**
  Organs, tissues, cells, signalling and effector molecules distributed throughout the body, contribute to the immune system

- **Understand that immune responses may be implicated in disease processes**
  The term immunopathology can be used to describe the disease processes resultant as a consequence of immune responses. Hypersensitivities and autoimmune diseases cause damage to the host while immune deficiencies lead to multiple infections in the host

1.1 WHAT IS IMMUNOLOGY?

Immunology is the study of how the human body can remain intact and unharmed in the midst of a vast universe of other life-forms and inanimate objects which might otherwise threaten our survival. Immunologists study the immune system to understand how humans can live healthy lives in environments that contain millions of other organisms and chemicals. This involves understanding how infection can be resisted, how the body recovers from illness, and why sometimes things go wrong. A familiarity with biochemistry, cell biology and microbiology as well as human anatomy and physiology is of great benefit to the study of immunology. Recent advances in techniques and new hypotheses in the biological and biomedical sciences have been used to reveal some of the more complex components of immune responses. This improved understanding of the components of immune responses has also provided many technologies for diagnosing human diseases that are used in modern healthcare laboratories. In the twenty-first century this knowledge is providing innovative new disease treatments such as monoclonal antibody therapies for rheumatoid arthritis and there is real promise that immunology will deliver even more exciting, effective treatments in the future.

Since multi-cellular organisms evolved it has become necessary for each organism to contain cells and molecules capable of defending it. These cells and molecules comprise the organism's immune system and they work together to generate immune responses. Through immunology, biomedical science students, clinicians and researchers can discover the components of the immune system, how it functions and how communication takes place between the immune system and the rest of the body which is being protected. Current knowledge and understanding reveals a complex but highly organized immune system; indeed, as in many aspects of science, the more we learn, the more clearly the organization becomes apparent.

The immune system is a series of cells, some of which are organized as discrete components within tissues, and molecules that work together to allow immune responses to occur. All of the important components are in place but in a non-responsive or resting state until the host is exposed to something that they must defend against. Thus the function of immune responses may be defined as: to provide protection against anything that would be harmful to the host.

Not everything that the host comes in contact with is potentially harmful so an immune system must be able to decide when to mount a response. The decision to respond or not to respond is, without doubt, one of the most critical functions of an immune system and it has proved extremely difficult for scientists to reach agreement on how this decision is made. The state of non-responsiveness is known as immunological tolerance, which is the opposite of an immune response.

Today, just over a century since the first useful application of immunology, understanding of how immune responsiveness and tolerance are controlled remains incomplete. Immunologists continue to undertake experiments to test hypotheses on the mechanisms of regulation within immune systems.

It is useful to have a generic name that can be used to refer to all the agents that may be the targets of immune responses. Targets may be:

■ infectious organisms (bacteria, viruses, fungi, parasites)

- macromolecules (foods, drugs or chemicals)
- cells (tumour cells or cells in mis-matched transfusions or transplants)

The collective term traditionally used for these targets is 'non-self', i.e. that which is not part of the host.

1.2 TYPES OF IMMUNE RESPONSE

The most basic type of defence is that provided by the human body's range of physical and chemical barriers. These barriers exist whether or not a threat is present; therefore the concepts of response or tolerance are irrelevant to these defences. The barriers regulate the initial interactions between host and non-self and so exist at the interfaces between the individual and the environment. It must be remembered that for human bodies the 'environment' is not just external but also internal. At the external interface skin, tears and sweat are effective physical and chemical barriers to non-self.

- Layers of tightly packed epidermal cells in the skin prevent the entry of most pathogens.
- In addition, the sebaceous glands in the dermis secrete on to the skin an oily substance called sebum, which is composed primarily of fatty acids and lactic acid. The low pH of sebum (pH 3–5) inhibits the growth of most pathogens.
- Tears and sweat contain anti-bacterial substances, most notably the enzyme lysozyme in tears, and the normal bacterial flora of the skin can compete with any newly encountered bacteria and so inhibit their growth.

At the point where the internal environment meets the host the range of defences is greater.

- The gastrointestinal, respiratory and genito-urinary tracts are lined by mucous membranes consisting of an outer epithelial cell layer underlaid by connective tissue. These epithelial cells secrete a viscous substance called mucus which traps invading microbes.
- The ciliated epithelia of the gastrointestinal tract and lower respiratory tract 'sweep' the trapped microbes from these sites.
- Saliva and urinary flow wash away potential invading microbes.
- Invasion by potential pathogens at mucosal surfaces also can be inhibited by non-pathogenic resident or commensal flora which can successfully compete with pathogens for survival in these niches.

Humans are able to exert some control over both their internal and external environments. Externally, we use disinfectants and antiseptics which reduce the numbers of micro-organisms; for the same purpose we practice good hygiene and we have innate, physiological senses that allow us to avoid contact with potentially harmful substances, physical injuries or sources of infection. Internally, we again try to reduce the load of micro-organisms by taking antibiotic or antiviral drugs and we try to avoid consuming products that would be harmful, either through their chemical nature or the presence of contamination. We also try to avoid the introduction of potential hazards into other internal spaces by, for example, avoiding unsafe sexual practices with potentially infected partners or not inhaling apparently noxious fumes. It is interesting to note that the total external surface area over which host and non-self can interact is many times smaller than that of the internal interface. The average total adult skin surface is 2 m^2, while there are approximately 400 m^2 of mucosal surface including the gut, respiratory and genito-urinary tracts. It is clearly vital that our internal interfaces are well defended.

Despite the obvious effectiveness of physical barriers, they are routinely overcome by cuts or abrasions to the skin, whether occurring accidentally or deliberately, such as during surgery. This permits potentially harmful products to enter host tissues. The elimination of gut bacteria through over-use of antibiotics allows potentially harmful bacteria to colonize the gut, and lesions of the gastrointestinal tract wall permit micro-organisms that normally would be excreted to enter the tissues. Once the physical barriers are breached the body normally begins to mount an immune response.

The first wave of responses constitutes innate, or natural, immune responses for which the collective term acute inflammation is commonly used (see *Chapter 4*). It is important to remember that these rapid inflammatory responses are intended to be beneficial. In later chapters instances will be presented of inflammation that is associated with pathological situations, i.e. long-lasting, chronic inflammation (see *Section 9.10*). In contrast, an acute inflammatory response which takes place in an appropriate location and is resolved at the appropriate time is not harmful; it is an effective immune response.

The key features of innate responses are that they are:

- inborn
- unchanging
- relatively non-specific

This means that, provided the individual is healthy and not immunosuppressed in any way (e.g. through immune deficiency diseases or therapies to prevent transplant rejection), innate immune responses are always the same regardless of the type of agent which is invading. Acute inflammation is a highly effective process which can result in the elimination of the harmful agent. However, this innate response is not capable of ensuring that the individual can respond even more effectively in the future, i.e. the body retains no immunological memory of the encounter with that particular harmful agent. A useful analogy for an organism that has only natural responses in its defensive arsenal is a person who attends school every day of life from age 5 to 25 but who is unable to remember any of the material taught. This person would then have to be re-exposed to exactly the same information on each day of the 20 years of schooling and would emerge no more competent than on day 1. This is obviously wasteful and contrary to biological systems which we know to undergo constant adaptation and change in order to cope better with their environment. The immune system is no exception and mammals have evolved immune responses (see *Chapter 6*), which have the following key features:

- memory – this causes the immune system to be permanently altered on every encounter with harmful material
- specificity – allows each response to be tailored so as to be the most appropriate for dealing with the particular type of threat being confronted at a particular point in time or location

Hence, learning, in the context of the immune system, means acquiring the ability to respond with greater efficiency each time the system is called upon to deal with a threat.

Adaptive immune responses are further sub-divided into cell-mediated responses and humoral responses (see *Box 1.1*). Cell-mediated responses are critically dependent on the actions of a type of cell called the T lymphocyte. In contrast, humoral responses, also called antibody responses, rely on the activities of a protein called an antibody that is secreted by B lymphocytes. There is much interaction between these two types of responses and, in most cases, optimal production of an antibody requires assistance from T lymphocytes.

Box 1.1 Humoral responses

Antibody-mediated immune responses are sometimes termed 'humoral' responses. This name reflects the archaic term 'humor' which meant a body of fluid. Antibodies were originally described purely as soluble proteins within the fluid phases of the circulation, i.e. in the lymph or blood plasma.

1.3 THE EVOLUTION OF IMMUNE RESPONSES

At the beginning of the twentieth century the work of two great pioneers of immunology was recognized with the award of the 1908 Nobel Prize in Medicine to Ilya Metchnikoff and Paul Ehrlich (see *Table 1.1* for other significant work). Many other Nobel Prizes have been awarded to immunologists since that time and details of their achievements are peppered throughout this book. Much of the early work was performed on very simple animal species that also need to defend against components of their environments.

Alongside the knowledge that animals possessed a defence system made up of cells and molecules, came the realization that this ability had been present in simple creatures such as starfish since the time they originally evolved, some 600 million years ago. Elements of the human immune system that we know today are detectable in virtually all living organisms, and comparative immunology tells us how the immune system differs in different species. By observing what aspects of immune responses are present in simple animals, we can conclude that those responses are of the most ancient origin. For example, many invertebrates only produce innate responses and so we can conclude that the adaptive response is probably of

Table 1.1 Significant discoveries in immunology

Who or Where?	What discovery?	When?
Greece, Rome, Far East, Middle East	Disease transmission and immunity Immunization	3000BC–100AD
Edward Jenner	Vaccination	1798
Robert Koch	Rational identification of organisms causing infectious diseases, Type IV hypersensitivity	1880s–1890s
Ilya Metchnikoff	Phagocytosis; cellular immunity	
Louis Pasteur	Active immunization	
Emil von Behring	Antibodies	1890s
Paul Ehrlich	Theory of antibody formation	
G.H.F. Nuttall	Antisera for diagnosis	1895–1910
Jules Bordet	Complement	1900–1910
Theobald Smith	Transplacental transmission of antibodies	
Karl Landsteiner	Antigen–antibody reactions Blood groups	1900–1930
Peter Medawar	Graft rejection/tolerance	1945–1955
George Snell	Genetics of histocompatibility	1940s
Niels K. Jerne	Numerous contributions including: antibody formation and immune regulation	1950–1980
F. Macfarlane Burnet	Clonal selection theory	1959
Rodney Porter	Structure–function relationships in antibodies	1960s
Gerald Edelman		
R.M. Zinkernagel	MHC restriction	1974
P.C. Doherty		
C. Milstein	Monoclonal antibodies	1975
G. Köhler		
S. Tonegawa	Immunoglobulin gene rearrangement	1980s
L. Montagnier	HIV virus	
Tim Mosmann and Robert Coffman	Th1 and Th2 cells	
Polly Matzinger	Danger model of immunological tolerance	1994
S. Sakaguchi	Regulatory T cells	1995
Charles Janeway III and others	Characterization of toll-like receptors	1996–1998

more recent origin. Responses that are possible only in higher animals, such as mammals, probably evolved more recently – the production of specific antibodies is an example of a more recently evolved response.

Clearly, however, the ability to recognize potential threats is well developed in most species. Some of the very simplest creatures, for example protozoans such as paramoecia, consist of only a single cell. Nonetheless that one cell can defend itself in a way that is remarkably similar to phagocytosis performed by specialized immune cells in humans (see *Section 4.6*). Multicellular animals of increasing complexity gradually diversified their immune responses. Phagocytic cells (cells that can engulf and destroy organisms) are present in invertebrates together with the ability to produce soluble mediators that resemble the cytokines of higher animals (see *Section 2.6* and *Appendix II*). These soluble mediators ensure that communication can take place between different components of an animal so that the defence response can be appropriate, coordinated, effective, and initiated when required. Cytotoxic cells (cells that can directly kill other cells) are present in animals such as sponges, corals and annelids (earthworms). In general, the comparatively simple defence system of each species of lower animal must be sufficient to deal with the potential threats to that species. As further additions were made to the arsenal of the immune system over time, the complexity of responses increased. New components added to the immune system included both a range of cell types and a greater diversity of molecules involved in the immune response. The molecules are present both as components of cells, especially the outer cell surfaces, and as molecules secreted into extracellular fluids and the circulatory system. In mammalian immune systems, large families of molecules have been discovered which have structural and / or functional similarities, to other members of their family. For example, the immunoglobulin gene superfamily (see *Box 1.2*) comprises molecules that participate in immune responses and are found predominantly on cell surfaces. It is thought that such families arose through gene duplication events and subsequent mutation of each family member.

Box 1.2 The immunoglobulin gene superfamily

The principal structural feature of proteins encoded by the immunoglobulin gene superfamily is a sequence of approximately 110 amino acid residues known as an immunoglobulin domain. The secondary structure of the domain consists of two anti-parallel β sheets stabilized by disulphide bonding.

The pattern of changes that led to the evolution of mammalian immune systems may well have been spurred by changes in the environment. One such change is thought to have been the evolution of warm-bloodedness that allowed bacteria and other micro-organisms to proliferate more rapidly within their hosts. The hosts that survived to reproduce were the ones best able to halt the growth of their aspiring colonists, i.e. those with the most effective immune responses. At that time point it is likely that germinal centres evolved in a number of tissues throughout the body. Germinal centres are specialized areas of tissues such as lymph nodes where large numbers of immune cells are found clustered together. They permit the rapid expansion and differentiation of B lymphocytes and are essential for the generation of high affinity antibody responses (see *Section 6.9*).

1.4 LOCATION OF THE IMMUNE RESPONSE

The immune system is everywhere in the body. There are, of course, specialized cells and molecules which are the only ones able to carry out particular functions but the actions of these special cells cannot take place in isolation. There must be constant cross-talk and interaction between these cells and other cells and tissues throughout the body. In particular, the immune cells must be able to exchange messages with components of the other major regulatory systems: the brain, nervous systems and endocrine system. The idea that the components of circulatory systems, i.e. the blood, lymph and tissue fluids, are the major sites of immune responses is certainly not appropriate. However, these circulatory systems are vital as transport systems that ensure that the cells and molecules of the immune response can reach their correct destinations. The most significant immune responses occur within tissues.

In recent years immunologists have begun to understand the cellular and molecular features that actually allow, indeed encourage, immune cells to leave the circulation and enter the tissues in response to a variety of stimuli. For this reason the vascular endothelial cells that line the blood and lymphatic vessels are considered to be key regulators of immune and inflammatory responses (see *Section 4.5*). They provide a dynamic interface between tissues and the circulating fluids, cells and molecules.

1.5 REGULATION OF IMMUNE RESPONSES

The past decade has seen an explosion in our understanding of the complex cellular and molecular biology that allows initiation, regulation and termination of immune responses. A very sizeable part of this book (see *Chapters 2–7*) introduces and explains current knowledge of the cells, molecules and processes that work together to regulate responses.

1.6 RESPONSES TO DIFFERENT HARMFUL AGENTS

Responsiveness to combat infectious micro-organisms is essential for human life, although sometimes the 'bugs' bite back. The ongoing battle between the human immune system and the microbial world is explained in *Chapter 8*, together with an explanation of how procedures such as immunization give the host a real advantage. On occasions, agents considered to be non-self, will be introduced deliberately into our bodies, for example, transfused blood or transplanted tissues. To enable patients to benefit from these potentially life-saving procedures, it is essential to understand the immune responses in these situations. *Chapter 11* introduces the intriguing and exciting world of tumour immunology, and raises an important question: can immune responses protect against cancer?

1.7 CONTRIBUTION OF IMMUNE RESPONSES TO DISEASE PROCESSES

Under certain circumstances the responses generated by the immune system may cause harm to the body. For example, when responses are directed against infectious micro-organisms, damage to normal healthy cells may occur either because the host and the harmful target share some features in common, or responses to non-self are exaggerated. The disease processes observed when infectious organisms attack may not all be caused directly by the organisms but sometimes by the host's response to the organism. Other immune responses may be excessively strong, for example, in the case of hypersensitivities such as allergy (see *Section 9.2*). Our current understanding of the range of diseases known as autoimmune diseases, suggests that defects may occur in the immune system causing it to destroy parts of the host itself, for example, in rheumatoid arthritis, multiple sclerosis or diabetes (see *Chapter 10*).

Despite these severe, and sometimes fatal, consequences of immune responses, nature has also provided us with some unfortunate examples of how difficult it is to survive in the absence of a functional immune system. One or more components of the immune system may be defective or absent in immunodeficiency diseases (see *Chapter 12*). People with these conditions suffer recurrent infections, with the type of infection depending on which component of the immune system is defective. Some deficiencies may be so severe that the person dies from overwhelming infection, for example, if a baby is born with a severe immune deficiency, death from infection is likely to occur before the second birthday. Our observations on people infected with the human immunodeficiency virus (HIV) show clearly how a progressive decline in immune function goes hand-in-hand with an increasing burden of infections and other diseases such as specific cancers. The ultimate destruction of the immune system by the virus leads to acquired immune deficiency syndrome (AIDS), which is fatal (see *Section 12.7*).

1.8 APPLICATIONS OF IMMUNOLOGY

Improved understanding of immunology has led to the development of many of the most sensitive and specific techniques used in research and diagnostic biomedical science laboratories (see *Chapter 13*). Many of these make use of the highly specific antibody proteins that are generated during immune responses because their specificity is retained when employed in the laboratory. A preparation of antibodies directed against a particular molecule of interest, e.g. a hormone, can be labelled with a marker that can be visualized. The appearance of the marker indicates that the hormone of interest is present in a test sample. This straightforward technology is the basis of modern pregnancy tests for use at home.

An understanding of immune systems has revolutionized ideas on many aspects of the aetiology, pathogenesis, diagnosis and treatment of a wide range of human diseases. In addition, immune cells such as T and B cells, dendritic cells and natural killer cells can also play a central role in immunotherapy. The manipulation of immune responses or components of the immune system (see *Chapter 14*), is now providing novel treatments for human diseases. There were some initial disappointments where products failed to live up to their apparent potential, e.g. the use of interferons and antibodies to treat cancer, although there is no doubt that the use of various immune mediators as therapeutic agents has revolutionized the treatment of rheumatoid arthritis and various autoimmune diseases. Nonetheless, it is critical that perceived failures are viewed against the excessively optimistic initial hopes that were based upon incomplete understanding of the processes involved. A thorough understanding of the molecular bases of activation and trafficking of immune cells and characterization of the mechanisms involved in immune regulation and tolerance will allow further advances to be made. More research, clinical trials and careful matching of therapies to patients' needs, in a personalized medicine-based approach, will result in real clinical benefits in the future.

SELF-ASSESSMENT QUESTIONS

1.   Distinguish between acute and chronic inflammation.
2.   List three physical/chemical barriers that protect the host from potential threats.
3.   List three ways in which innate immune responses differ from adaptive responses.
4.   What is the opposite of immunological tolerance?
5.   State one type of defence mechanism that is present in simple, unicellular animals.
6.   What are autoimmune diseases?
7.   What do the acronyms 'HIV' and 'AIDS' stand for?
8.   What contribution to the development of immunology was made by Edward Jenner?
9.   What is the location of the immune system in the body?
10. What is your understanding of the term non-self?

Components of the immune system

Learning objectives

After studying this chapter you should confidently be able to:

■ **Describe the functions of primary lymphoid tissues**
Primary lymphoid tissues are generative tissues in which lymphocytes develop. In man the primary lymphoid tissues are bone marrow and thymus. B lymphocytes differentiate to the immature B cell stage before leaving the bone marrow to complete their maturation in the spleen. T lymphocytes develop in the thymus from pro-thymocytes that exit the bone marrow and migrate to the thymus. In addition to being a primary lymphoid tissue, the bone marrow is also the main site of haematopoiesis after birth.

■ **Describe the structure and functions of secondary lymphoid tissues**
Secondary lymphoid tissues, such as the spleen and lymph nodes, contain discrete T cell and B cell areas. In lymph nodes, T cells are localized to the paracortex, whereas B cells are found in the cortex primarily in clusters of cells called follicles. Lymph nodes are situated along lymphatic vessels and allow foreign material present in tissues to be presented there for examination by lymphocytes. Mucosa-associated lymphoid tissues are secondary lymphoid tissues adapted to acquire material at mucosal surfaces. The spleen is a highly vascular organ and is suited for filtering substances from the circulation. Splenic white pulp has discrete T cell areas, called the peri-arteriolar lymphoid sheath, with adjacent B cell follicles.

■ **Describe the function of the main classes of immune cells**
Leukocytes consist of mononuclear cells and granulocytes, which are the main effector cells of innate immunity.
Granulocytes include three different cell types called neutrophils, eosinophils, and basophils. Neutrophils are the first cells to arrive at sites of infection and are the predominant constituents of the acute inflammatory infiltrate. They engulf and destroy infectious agents via oxygen-dependent and independent mechanisms. Eosinophils are also phagocytic and they are important for control of parasitic infections. Basophils are thought to be involved in allergic reactions.
Mast cells are important for regulating cellular infiltration at sites of inflammation and are referred to as the gatekeepers of the inflammatory response.
Mononuclear cells consist of lymphocytes (T and B cells), the primary effector cells of adaptive immunity, as well as monocytes, natural killer (NK) cells and dendritic cells. B cells are responsible for secretion of

antibodies. CD4$^+$ T cells are crucial for providing help to B cells and for regulating the immune response, and they are rich sources of cytokines, the proteins that help cells of the immune system communicate. CD8$^+$ T cells are killer T cells and are important in defence against viral infections. T cells require antigen to be presented to them by cells such as dendritic cells which are known as professional antigen-presenting cells. Monocytes are precursors of tissue macrophages and dendritic cells and they infiltrate the tissue at sites of infection, helping to eliminate debris and senescent neutrophils. Natural killer cells are cytotoxic cells and are important for the elimination of tumours and certain viral infections, while NK T cells share some characteristics of T cells and NK cells.

■ **Explain the terms antigen, immunogen and epitope**
An antigen is any substance that can be recognized by the immune system. Antigens can be proteins, lipids, nucleic acids or carbohydrate. Not all antigens can induce an immune response; those that do are called immunogens and are said to be immunogenic. An epitope is a discrete portion of an antigen that is recognized by a given lymphocyte. Antigens usually contain many epitopes.

■ **Discuss the roles of secreted factors and cell surface molecules in the immune response**
These factors play key roles in communication and could very much be considered to be the mobile phones of the immune system. They allow the vital cross-talk and signalling to occur between all the cells of the immune system, and also between the immune cells and other cells of the body. Such signals are essential for communication of instructions and to facilitate the movement of cells and regulation of the proteins cells express. Communication is essential to a successful immune response.

■ **Describe the structure and function of immunoglobulin**
Immunoglobulins are protein molecules that are secreted by cells of the B lymphocyte lineage. A B cell differentiates into a plasma cell and becomes a high level immunoglobulin secreting factory. Immunoglobulins can also be called antibodies and in humans five different classes of immunoglobulin exist called: IgM, IgA, IgD, IgG and IgE. Each type carries out different biological functions but they all have a similar structure consisting of two heavy (H) chains of approximately 50 kDa each, and two light (L) chains of approximately 25 kDa each. The different immunoglobulin classes contain different H chains. Immunoglobulins/antibodies bind to antigens and facilitate their elimination.

2.1 INTRODUCTION TO COMPONENTS OF THE IMMUNE SYSTEM

The immune system uses three strategies, of increasing complexity, to protect the integrity of the body. The first strategy is to prevent harmful material from gaining access to the body. Any threats that breach the physical and chemical barriers are subjected to the second strategy, a rapid, albeit relatively non-specific, innate immune attack that is primarily mediated by neutrophils. The third, and most sophisticated, approach is a highly specific adaptive immune response designed to eliminate the invaders without damaging host tissues.

Communication is essential to a successful immune response. For example, during infection or trauma, affected cells and tissues send out signals to alert the immune system to the danger. Cells of the immune system must be able to interpret such warning signals from all other cells of the body and communicate instructions to these cells.

Substances that can be recognized by the immune system are called antigens (see *Box 2.1*). Not all antigens are harmful, so the immune system must be able to modulate its response to match the threat posed by the antigen. This chapter will discuss the tissues and cells of the immune system that facilitate this coordinated approach to immune defence.

Box 2.1 Antitoxins and antibodies

In 1890, Emil von Behring and Shibasaburo Kitasato demonstrated that animals immunized with diphtheria or tetanus toxins produced antitoxins that neutralized the effect of the toxins. These antitoxins were later termed antibodies, and substances used to induce their production were called antigens (for antibody generating). Nowadays the term antigen is used to describe anything that can be recognized by the adaptive immune response. Von Behring received the Nobel Prize in 1901.

2.2 THE LYMPHATIC SYSTEM

The lymphatic system represents an important part of the immune system and comprises a complex network of tissues (lymphoid tissues), connecting vessels (lymphatic vessels) and circulating cells that are important in generation of immune responses. All of the important cells of the immune system spend at least part of their lifespan circulating in the bloodstream and, consequently, often are called blood cells. Unlike the more abundant red blood cells, the immune cells are known as white blood cells or leukocytes (see *Table 2.1*). Leukocytes consist of granulocytes, which are the main effector cells of innate immunity, and mononuclear cells. Mononuclear cells consist of lymphocytes, the primary effector cells of adaptive immunity, as well as monocytes, natural killer (NK) cells and dendritic cells.

The lymphatic system is closely associated with the cardiovascular system. Oxygenated blood is pumped around the body to supply nutrients and oxygen to the tissues and as it does, fluid seeps out of the blood at the capillary beds due to hydrostatic pressure from the heart. This fluid, which fills the interstitial spaces, is called lymph. The composition of lymph, therefore, resembles that of blood plasma. To ensure that fluid does not accumulate within tissues, the lymph is collected in lymphatic vessels which drain every cubic millimetre of the body. Movement of lymph is exceedingly slow compared to that of the blood due to its location which is remote from the pumping action of the heart. Flow of lymph occurs due to peristalsis, semilunar (one-way) valves, and the contraction of adjacent skeletal muscles which squeeze lymph through the lymphatic vessels. The lymph is collected

Table 2.1. The main cellular constituents of peripheral blood

Cell type leukocytes	Normal range per μl blood	% of total
Erythrocytes	Males: 4.2–5.4 x 10⁶	
	Females: 3.6–5.0 x 10⁶	
Platelets	1.5–4.0 x 10⁵	
Leukocytes (total)	5.0–10.0 x 10³	
Neutrophils	3.0–6.0 x 10³	70%
Eosinophils	50–300	1–2%
Basophils	50	1%
Lymphocytes	1.25–3.5 x 10³	25–35%
Monocytes	0.30–0.60 x 10³	6%

in successively larger vessels which ultimately empty into the right lymphatic duct (for fluid collected from the right upper body) and the thoracic duct (for fluid collected from the rest of the body). The right lymphatic duct and the thoracic duct drain into the right and left subclavian veins, respectively. In this way fluid that seeps out into the tissues is returned via lymphatic vessels to the circulation.

Tissues of the lymphatic system, referred to as lymphoid tissues, can be subdivided into primary lymphoid tissues and secondary lymphoid tissues. Primary lymphoid tissues are the site of development of cells involved in the immune response.

2.3   PRIMARY LYMPHOID TISSUES

In humans, the thymus and the bone marrow are primary lymphoid tissues and are the sites of lymphocyte production (see *Figure 2.1*). The bone marrow is also the primary site of production of all other blood cells. The process whereby blood cells develop is called haematopoiesis. During the first trimester of fetal life, the liver is the main site of haematopoiesis. By 32 weeks of gestation, the bone marrow has almost totally taken over this function and by birth the liver is no longer haematopoietically active. In the neonate, haematopoietically active bone marrow is found in the central cavities of many bones, including the long bones of the upper and lower limbs. As the child grows this bone marrow function declines such that, by about the time of puberty, haematopoietically active bone marrow is present only in the pelvis and sternum (breast-bone). In adults the marrow cavities of long bones are filled with adipose (fatty) tissue.

Haematopoietically active bone marrow contains stem cells, termed pluripotent or totipotent haematopoietic stem cells (HSC). These HSCs are necessary for the production of blood cells of all types and they have a self-maintenance and self-renewal capacity that allows them to persist through-

(a)

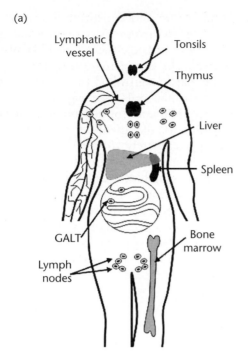

(b)

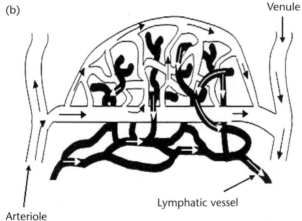

Figure 2.1

(a) The primary lymphoid tissues, bone marrow and thymus, are the sites of development of lymphocytes. Secondary lymphoid tissues include gut-associated lymphoid tissue (GALT), spleen, tonsils and lymph nodes. Lymph nodes are particularly numerous adjacent to the respiratory, gastrointestinal and genito-urinary tracts. Lymphatic vessels collect fluid (lymph) that has seeped from the bloodstream into peripheral tissues and return it to the circulation. En route the lymph passes through lymph nodes which are dotted along lymphatic vessels. For clarity, the lymphatic drainage of the right arm only is shown. (b) The fluid that seeps out of blood vessels at capillary beds is collected by lymphatic capillaries. The direction of flow of blood is indicated by the black arrows whereas the direction of flow of the collected fluid is indicated by the white arrows.

out adult life. HSCs are quite rare and constitute approximately 1 in 10^5 normal bone marrow cells. They in turn produce other progenitor cells, each of which can give rise to a more restricted range of blood cells which lose their capacity for self-renewal. The differentiation of HSCs into the different lineages of blood cells is partly controlled by cytokines that are largely produced by bone marrow stromal cells (see *Figure 2.2*). There is much interest in elucidating the requirements for self-renewal of HSCs to facilitate *in vitro* expansion of HSCs for therapeutic use (see *Box 2.2*).

During haematopoiesis, approximately 10^{11}–10^{12} blood cells are produced per day. Following their development, mature blood cells exit the bone marrow via the circulation. Loss of blood cells caused, for example, by a variety of disease processes, infections, or treatment with cytotoxic drugs, can be compensated for by an increase in production of these cells. This process is called *induced* haematopoiesis. Increased production of cells is largely restricted to the specific cell type that is required in the particular

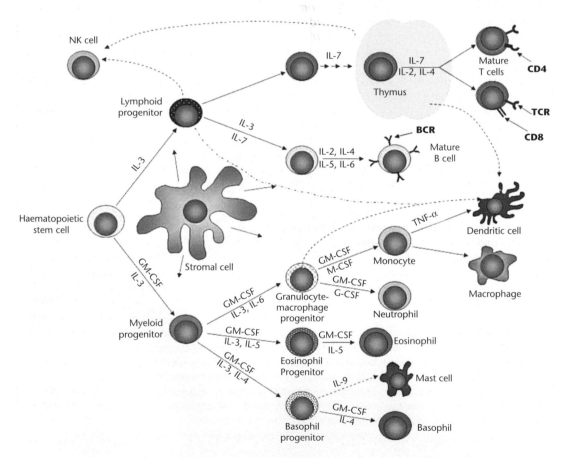

Figure 2.2
Development of leukocytes from haematopoietic stem cells. Cytokines that promote development of the various cell types are indicated. Dotted lines represent postulated pathways of development.

Box 2.2 Stem cells

Stem cells might be considered as a repair system for the body due to their ability to divide and develop into many different cell types, without limit, and replenish other cells. When a stem cell divides, the new cells can either remain as stem cells or become another type of cell with a more specialized function, such as a red blood cell or a brain cell. Stem cells can be classified as embryonic or adult.

Embryonic stem cells are those that are isolated from the eight-cell stage of an embryo, known as a blastocyst. These cells are currently the topic of much debate as governing bodies try to decide on regulations regarding their use in research.

Human embryonic stem cell research holds much promise for the development of innovative therapies for conditions such as spinal cord injuries, diabetes, heart disease, or Parkinson's disease. It may also elucidate how organisms, including humans, develop, enabling further understanding of how the body might repair itself. In addition, such stem cells would be useful as a surrogate system for testing new drugs.

Pluripotent or totipotent haematopoietic stem cells are present in haematopoietically active bone marrow. These are adult stem cells and they give rise to the different types of blood cells (red blood cells, white blood cells and platelets). Due to their plasticity, i.e. ability to become different cell types, they are also thought to be able to give rise to nerve cells in the brain or heart muscle cells. Their stem cell properties, of self-maintenance and self-renewal, ensure they persist throughout adult life. They are relatively rare and constitute approximately 1 in 10^5 normal bone marrow cells. Their differentiation into the different lineages of blood cells is thought to be controlled in part by cytokines. Specific growth factors or cytokines may well encourage differentiation toward a certain type of cell, but it is now known these factors play a small role in a larger network of events that guides cells toward different destinies. There is much interest in elucidating the requirements for self-renewal of these stem cells to facilitate their *in vitro* expansion for therapeutic use. The potential to use adult stem cells for cell-based therapies holds much promise for numerous conditions.

During their lifetime, when an adult stem cell is dividing, a decision must be made as to whether the progenitor cell takes on a new specialized cell identity or remains a stem cell. Perhaps quite a simplistic view would be that the cells are instructed to progress along prearranged pathways.

A recent study showed how cell populations maintain a built-in variability that nature can allow to change under the right conditions, allowing blood stem cells to make a decision to become white blood cell progenitors or red blood cell progenitors[1,2]. This is known as phenotypic cell to cell variability. This individuality between cells within the same clone is not genetically encoded but rather occurs due to slow fluctuations in protein levels which result in a heterogeneous clone. The authors proposed that a protein called Sca-1, a cell marker of 'stemness' occurs in highly variable amounts (a 1000-fold range) between different stem cells. This range of Sca-1 expression was associated with a range of biological activities. Blood stem cells with low levels of Sca-1 differentiated into red blood cell progenitors seven times more often than cells high in Sca-1, when exposed to erythropoietin, a growth factor that promotes red blood cell production. Conversely, stem cells with more Sca-1, stimulated with granulocyte–macrophage colony-stimulating factor, which stimulates white blood cell formation, were more likely to become white cells than those with less Sca-1. In addition, microarray analysis of gene expression found great variability within the apparently uniform stem cell population, with more than 3900 genes differentially expressed.

Together, these findings suggest that a slow fluctuation or cycling of gene activity tends to maintain cells in a stable state, while also priming them to differentiate when conditions are right. These findings have significant implications for stem cell researchers as stem cell differentiation can be made dramatically more efficient by choosing the right subpopulation of stem cells and stimulating them correctly, at the right time.

[1] Chang, H.H., Hemberg, M., Barahona, M., Ingber, D.E. and Huang, S. (2008) Transcriptome-wide noise controls lineage choice in mammalian progenitor cells. *Nature.* **453**: 544–547.

[2] Children's Hospital Boston (2008) Many Paths, Few Destinations: How Stem Cells Decide What They'll Become. *Science Daily,* www.sciencedaily.com/releases/2008/05/080521131552.htm

stress situation; for example, haemolysis (the abnormal breakdown of red blood cells) induces erythropoiesis – the process by which red blood cells (erythrocytes) are produced.

All immune cells develop to maturity in the bone marrow with the exception of mast cells and lymphocytes. Mast cell precursors are released from the bone marrow and enter tissues where they complete their differentiation. B lymphocytes, or B cells, exit the bone marrow as differentiated transitional B cells and complete their maturation in secondary lymphoid tissues. By contrast, T lymphocytes, or T cells, leave the bone marrow as immature pro-thymocytes and migrate to the thymus to complete their differentiation programme.

The thymus, or thymus gland, is a bi-lobed, multi-lobulated, lympho-epithelial tissue that derives from the endoderm of the third and fourth pharyngeal pouches during fetal development. It is situated in the upper anterior region of the chest, partially overlying the heart (see *Figure 2.1*). Similar to the bone marrow, the thymus also degenerates during childhood. Its size and function are greatest in young children but, by about the time of puberty only a thymic rudiment remains. Nonetheless, thymic output of T cells, although diminished, continues throughout adult life.

Pro-thymocytes enter the cortex of the thymus and percolate through the tissue, interacting with many different cell types including thymic epithelial cells. Thymocyte maturation and differentiation occur during this passage through the thymus (see *Section 3.6*). Mature T cells exit the thymus at the medulla and migrate to secondary lymphoid tissues.

2.4 SECONDARY LYMPHOID TISSUES

Secondary lymphoid tissues (see *Table 2.2*) are organized sites where mature lymphocytes congregate in close proximity with other specialized cells. The structural organization and localization of secondary lymphoid tissues allows antigens to be brought to lymphocytes in an environment that is conducive for the generation of immune responses. Adaptive immune responses are initiated in secondary lymphoid tissues. The site of entry of antigen into the body determines the predominant site at which the adaptive immune response against that antigen will be initiated.

Table 2.2. Major secondary lymphoid tissues in man

Secondary lymphoid tissue
Tonsils, adenoids and associated lymph nodes – Waldeyer's ring
Spleen (white pulp)
Gut-associated lymphoid tissues (GALT) including Peyer's patches
Mesenteric lymph nodes
Appendix

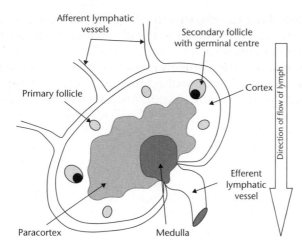

Figure 2.3
Diagram of a lymph node indicating the T cell area (paracortex) and the B cell area (follicles in the cortex). Lymph enters the node via afferent lymphatic vessels and leaves via the efferent lymphatic vessel.

If antigen is introduced into a tissue it will be picked up in the lymph that bathes the cells of that tissue and be collected by a lymphatic vessel. The lymph ultimately will be returned to the circulation, but en route it will pass through small nodules of lymphoid tissue, called lymph nodes, that are located at various points along the lymphatic vessels in a manner often likened to beads on a string. A lymph node is a kidney-shaped structure made up largely of lymphocytes, with some macrophages and dendritic cells. A lymph node acts as an immunological filter, allowing antigenic material to come into close contact with these immune cells. In this way, an adaptive immune response is initiated in lymph nodes against antigenic material present in peripheral tissues.

Like all secondary lymphoid tissue, lymph nodes have distinct areas that are rich in T cells and areas that are rich in B cells (see *Figure 2.3*). T cell areas are found towards the central portion, or paracortex, of lymph nodes. B cells in lymph nodes are largely confined to the outer portion of the node, the cortex. Within the cortex, many of the B cells are organized into clusters. These clusters are called B cell follicles. During an immune response, these follicles increase in size due to rapid proliferation of responding B cells. The larger follicles ultimately become germinal centres, which are crucial structures for antibody-mediated immune responses (see *Section 6.9*).

The lymph node through which the lymph from a particular tissue, or area, passes is termed the draining lymph node for that tissue. It is also sometimes called the regional lymph node. The immune response against an infection in a particular tissue is initiated in the draining lymph node for that tissue. For example, the immune response against influenza virus infection is initiated in the lymph nodes proximal to the respiratory tract.

Lymph nodes are particularly numerous adjacent to the gastrointestinal and respiratory tracts as these are major portals of entry of pathogens into the body. They are the sites where the body is most likely to encounter non-self. The specialized lymphoid tissues closely associated with mucosal surfaces are collectively termed mucosa-associated lymphoid tissue (MALT).

When situated along the digestive tract, MALT is known as gut-associated lymphoid tissue (GALT). These lymphoid tissues are very similar to lymph nodes but are specialized to pick up foreign substances at these sites. An important aspect of GALT function is to ensure that an inappropriate immune response is not mounted against dietary antigens. Sometimes this process breaks down, resulting in conditions such as coeliac disease (see *Box 2.3*).

Box 2.3 Coeliac disease

Also called gluten-sensitive enteropathy, coeliac disease is characterized by an immune response against the α-gliadin component of gluten. The inflammatory response leads to flattening of the lining of the small intestine which impairs nutrient absorption.

Blockage or disruption of the flow of lymph through lymphatic vessels results in lymphoedema – the accumulation of lymph in tissue. Surgical removal of regional lymph nodes is sometimes performed following removal of a tumour (e.g. mastectomy for breast cancer) to prevent metastatic spread of cancerous cells via the lymphatic system. This disrupts the lymphatic drainage at that site resulting in secondary lymphoedema.

The spleen is the largest of the secondary lymphoid organs. It is where senescent (old and imperfect) erythrocytes are destroyed. The spleen is

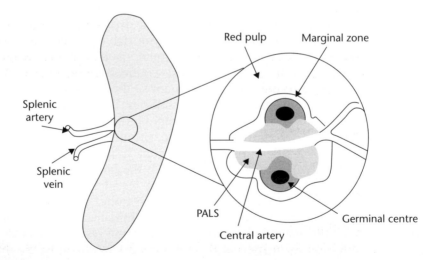

Figure 2.4
Structure of the spleen showing the T cell-rich periarteriolar lymphoid sheath (PALS) with associated B cell follicles containing germinal centres. Together these areas constitute the white pulp. The white pulp is separated from the red pulp by the marginal zone.

made up of red pulp and white pulp. The red pulp is composed primarily of sinuses, erythrocytes and macrophages. The white pulp constitutes the lymphoid tissue and contains a T cell area, the peri-arteriolar lymphoid sheath (PALS), which is localized around arterioles, B cell follicles adjacent to the PALS, and a marginal zone that separates the red and white pulp (see *Figure 2.4*). The spleen is a highly vascular organ and is ideally suited to filter out and concentrate antigenic material from the circulation. It is the main site of initiation of immune responses against systemic infections found in peripheral blood, i.e. septicaemia.

Tertiary lymphoid tissue

A third class of lymphoid tissue, termed tertiary lymphoid tissue, is sometimes formed at sites of chronic inflammation or chronic infection. As outlined above, secondary lymphoid tissue is developmentally programmed and characterized by well ordered compartments of lymphocyte subsets and tissue architecture. In contrast, tertiary lymphoid tissue is defined as that induced in ectopic sites by inflammation, and its immunological role is incompletely understood.

2.5 CELLS OF THE IMMUNE SYSTEM

Effective immune-mediated defence requires the coordinated actions of a variety of cells (see *Figure 2.5*). These cells are usually characterized by flow cytometry (see *Section 13.10*) based on their expression of particular cell surface markers called cluster of differentiation (CD) molecules (see *Appendix I*). Immune system cells are frequently classified based on whether they participate in the innate immune response or in the adaptive immune response. However, as appreciation of the complex cooperative interactions between the innate and adaptive responses has grown, this distinction seems increasingly contrived.

Granulocytes

Granulocytes include three different cell types called neutrophils, eosinophils and basophils. There are differentiated based on their staining characteristics with particular histological dyes.

Neutrophils

Neutrophils, or polymorphonuclear (PMN) leukocytes, are the predominant leukocyte in peripheral blood, accounting for 50–60% of the circulating white blood cells. They constitute the body's initial defence against substances that breach the physical and chemical barriers. A mature neutrophil takes about 2 weeks to develop in the bone marrow. Neutrophils have a half-life of only 4–10 hours in the circulation before they enter tissues

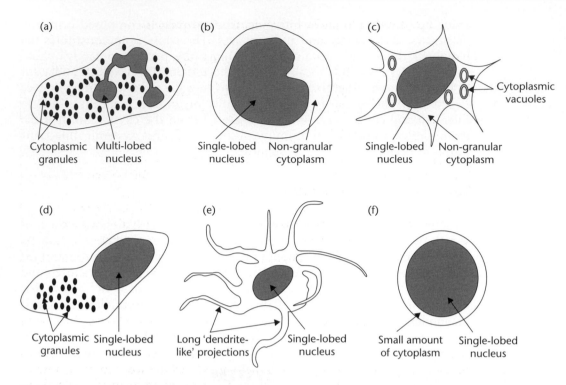

Figure 2.5
Diagram comparing characteristics of immune cells. (a) Neutrophil; (b) monocyte; (c) macrophage; (d) mast cell; (e) dendritic cell; (f) lymphocyte.

where they survive for 1–2 days. They are the first cells to arrive at sites of infection and are the predominant constituents of the acute inflammatory infiltrate. The major role of neutrophils is to engulf and destroy infectious agents via oxygen-dependent and -independent mechanisms. Neutrophils have three main types of granules in their cytoplasm: azurophilic; specific; and small storage granules. These granules contain enzymes that attack and kill ingested micro-organisms (see *Table 2.3*). In addition, neutrophils generate free radicals which attack ingested micro-organisms. As well as their role in host defence, neutrophils have also been implicated in the pathogenesis of many chronic inflammatory diseases, such as rheumatoid arthritis (see *Section 10.7*). Senescent neutrophils are thought to undergo apoptosis (see *Box 2.4*) prior to final elimination by macrophages.

Box 2.4 Apoptosis

This is a form of programmed cell death. It involves a series of biochemical events leading to characteristic morphological changes and, ultimately, cell death.

Table 2.3. Selected granule constituents of neutrophils

| | Granule type | | |
Category	Azurophilic	Specific	Small storage
Antimicrobial	Myeloperoxidase Lysozyme Defensins	Lysozyme Lactoferrin	
Neutral proteinases	Elastase Cathepsin G Proteinase 3	Collagenase	Gelatinase Plasminogen activator
Acid hydrolases	Phospholipase A_2 β-D-glucuronidase Cathepsins	Phospholipase A_2	Phospholipase A_2 β-D-glucuronidase Cathepsins

Eosinophils

Eosinophils, so named because of their intense colour when stained with eosin, are motile phagocytic cells. They have a bi-lobed nucleus and contain many basic cytoplasmic granules. The granules contain mediators such as major basic protein and eosinophil peroxidase that are toxic to many micro-organisms. Eosinophils are important for control of parasitic infections. They also play a prominent role in the pathogenesis of allergic diseases such as asthma (see *Section 9.2*).

Basophils

Basophils are a minor cell population in peripheral blood. Their functions are poorly understood but they are known to be involved in promoting allergic responses. Stimulation of basophils causes them to release pharmacologically active mediators such as histamine and various cytokines. Basophils share many features with mast cells and both cell types arise from a common progenitor cell (see *Figure 2.2*).

Mast cells

Mast cells are found only in tissues where they develop from undifferentiated precursor cells that have been released from the bone marrow. Mast cells do not re-enter the circulation. There are two types of mast cells: connective tissue mast cells and mucosal mast cells. Mast cells contain numerous granules containing preformed mediators, including histamine and various cytokines, which can be released following stimulation of the mast cells. Mast cell stimulation also leads to the production of newly formed mediators such as eicosanoids (see *Section 2.6*). Activation of mast cells is a pivotal event in allergic reactions (see *Section 9.2*) and in acute inflammatory responses (see *Section 4.4*). The activities of mast cells are so important for regulating cellular infiltration at sites of inflammation that they are sometimes called the gatekeepers of the inflammatory response.

Mononuclear cells

The second class of leukocytes is called mononuclear cells. Unlike granulo-cytes, mononuclear cells do not have multi-lobed nuclei. Mononuclear cells include: lymphocytes; monocytes; macrophages; dendritic cells; and natural killer (NK) cells.

Lymphocytes

Lymphocytes are the most numerous of the mononuclear cells and are the key effector cells of adaptive immune responses. There are two major classes of lymphocytes, B and T lymphocytes also known as B and T cells.

B cells are the immune cells that are responsible for producing antibod-ies, the secreted protein molecules that bind to antigens and facilitate their elimination from the body. B cells are named after the bursa of Fabricius, the lymphoid tissue where these cells develop in birds (see *Box 2.5*). Humans do not have a bursa and B cells develop from stem cells in the bone marrow. Immature B cells exit the bone marrow and migrate to the spleen where they complete their differentiation into mature B cells. These mature B cells either remain in the spleen, as marginal zone B cells, or migrate to the B cell areas of lymphoid organs as follicular B cells. Prior to encounter with antigen, B cells are called naïve or virgin B cells. B cells that do not encounter antigen die within 7–10 days and this fate accounts for greater than 90% of the B cells. Those B cells that do encounter antigen are stimu-lated to proliferate and develop into cells called plasma cells that produce high levels of antibodies which bind specifically to the stimulating antigen. In most cases, production of antigen by B cells requires help from the other class of lymphocytes, T cells.

Box 2.5 B cells

In 1956 two students, Bruce Glick and Timothy Chang, made the serendipitous discovery that birds who had their bursa removed just after they had hatched, failed to produce antibodies. The cells responsible for producing the antibody were called Bursa-derived cells, or B cells.

T cells are so called because they develop in the thymus (see *Box 2.6*). T cells are further categorized into two main subgroups based on whether they express the CD4 or the CD8 molecule on their surface. $CD4^+$ T cells are frequently referred to as helper T (Th) cells and are crucial for provid-ing help to B cells and for regulating the immune response. $CD4^+$ T cells are a particularly rich source of cytokines, secreted polypeptides that allow cells of the immune system to communicate with each other and with other cells of the body. The importance to the immune system of $CD4^+$ T cells is evidenced by acquired immune deficiency syndrome (AIDS) which devel-ops as a result of depletion of $CD4^+$ T cells following infection with the human immunodeficiency virus (HIV). The other subset of T cells, $CD8^+$

T cells are cytotoxic T lymphocytes (CTLs) that are crucial for defence against most viral infections and tumours. T cells respond to antigen by virtue of a surface receptor called the T cell receptor. Unlike B cells, however, T cells require that antigen be presented to them by another cell, called an antigen-presenting cell (APC), before they can respond to it.

Box 2.6 The role of the thymus

The role of the thymus as a primary lymphoid tissue was elucidated in 1961 by Jacques Miller. He found that neonatal thymectomy of mice led to deficiency of a class of lymphocytes that were subsequently called T cells after their tissue of origin.

Monocytes

Monocytes comprise approximately 3–8% of peripheral blood leukocytes and are precursors of tissue macrophages and dendritic cells. Before they enter the tissues, monocytes circulate in the blood for 1–3 days after leaving the bone marrow. Monocytes migrate quickly and are usually the second cell type, after neutrophils, to infiltrate the tissue at sites of infection. In tissues they play an important role in eliminating debris and senescent neutrophils.

Macrophages

When monocytes enter the tissues and become macrophages they greatly increase in size. Macrophages are highly phagocytic, long-lived cells which, like mast cells, do not normally re-enter the circulation. Macrophages are found in tissues throughout the body but their appearance and functions differ depending on the tissue in which they occur (see *Table 2.4*). Together monocytes and tissue macrophages may be grouped under the collective term the mononuclear phagocyte system.

Macrophages usually exist as resting cells unless they are activated during an immune response. Activated macrophages engulf and remove unwanted particulate matter, including senescent neutrophils and invading micro-

Table 2.4 Tissue distribution of macrophages

Cell type	Location within the body
Histiocytes	Connective tissue
Kupffer cells	Liver
Alveolar macrophages	Lungs
Glomerular mesangial cells	Kidney
Osteoclasts	Bone
Splenic macrophages	Spleen
Synovial macrophages	Synovial joints

organisms. Macrophages also function as APCs and present antigens to T cells, a crucial step in the initiation of an adaptive immune response.

Dendritic cells

Dendritic cells are a heterogeneous class of phagocytic cell. They are called dendritic cells (DCs) because they have long cellular projections, or dendrites, that allow them to interact with multiple cells simultaneously. They constitute the most efficient APCs in the body and are crucial for initiation of most adaptive immune responses. In this capacity they acquire antigen in peripheral tissues and carry it to the T cell areas of secondary lymphoid organs. The two major classes of DCs are myeloid DCs, which develop from the monocytic lineage, and plasmacytoid DCs which develop from lymphoid progenitor cells.

Natural killer cells

Natural killer (NK) cells are sometimes called large granular lymphocytes (LGLs). This minor cell population is characterized by the cell surface expression of CD16 and CD56 molecules. Like $CD8^+$ CTLs, NK cells are cytotoxic cells and are important for the elimination of tumours and certain viral infections.

NK T cells

NK T cells share some characteristics of T cells and NK cells. They have a T cell receptor and are thought to react specifically against microbial glycolipid antigens.

2.6 NON-CELLULAR COMPONENTS OF THE IMMUNE SYSTEM

In order to protect the integrity of the body effectively, cells of the immune system must be able to communicate with each other and with cells of other tissues. A wide variety of cell surface molecules are critical to the functioning of the immune system (see *Appendix I*). Surface receptors determine the range of substances that immune cells can respond to and alteration of receptor expression during the course of an immune reaction is a common mechanism to control cellular responses. Cell surface adhesion molecules determine the migratory pathways of immune cells and allow leukocytes to exit from the circulation into tissues at the sites of infections (see *Section 4.5*) and generation of adaptive immune responses is also dependent on cell–cell interactions mediated by specific cell surface molecules (see *Sections 6.3* and *6.8*). In addition, the immune system relies heavily on secreted factors to control the generation (see *Figure 2.2*), migration and activities of immune cells. Most of these immunoregulatory secreted factors are either lipid mediators or polypeptide factors.

Lipid mediators

The major class of secreted lipid-derived immunoregulatory molecules is the eicosanoids. Eicosanoids are generated by the oxidation of omega-3 (ω-3) or omega-6 (ω-6) 20-carbon essential fatty acids (see *Figure 2.6*). The four classes of eicosanoids are prostaglandins, prostacyclins, leukotrienes and thromboxanes. Eicosanoids exert a wide variety of effects throughout the body, including the induction of platelet aggregation, smooth muscle contraction, pain, and sleep.

Platelet activating factor (PAF) is another lipid mediator involved in platelet aggregation and inflammation. It is synthesized from lysophosphatidylcholine and acetyl coenzyme A by the enzyme lysophosphatidylcholine acetyltransferase.

Eicosanoids and PAF are secreted following stimulation by a variety of cell types including neutrophils, monocytes, and the cells that line the luminal surfaces of blood vessels, the vascular endothelial cells.

Polypeptide factors

The activities of the immune system are regulated by a wide variety of secreted polypeptide factors. Three major families of secreted polypeptide factors are cytokines, complement, and acute phase proteins.

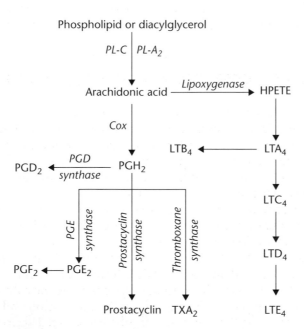

Figure 2.6
Membrane phospholipids or diacylglycerol are cleaved by phospholipase A_2 (*PL-A$_2$*) and phospholipase C (*PL-C*), respectively, to generate arachidonic acid. The lipoxygenase enzyme complex converts arachidonic acid into hydroperoxyeicosatetraenoic acid (HPETE), the precursor of leukotrienes (LT). The cyclooxygenase (*Cox*) enzyme complex converts arachidonic acid into prostaglandin (PG)H_2, the precursor of the other prostaglandins as well as of the thromboxanes (TX) and prostacyclin.

Cytokines

Cytokines are crucial elements of the immune response. They act as messengers between the cells which secrete them and their cellular targets. An almost bewildering array of cytokines have been discovered, many of them with multiple and overlapping functions (see *Appendix II*). Cytokines with more than one function are said to be pleiotropic. It is important to note that although cytokines are crucial for communication within the immune system, they are not restricted to function in this manner and can exert their effects throughout the body. In this way, cytokines provide the major mechanism whereby the immune system communicates with other systems in the body.

The major classification of cytokines is the interleukin (IL) system. The term interleukin was originally used to describe cytokines whose principal targets were leukocytes. It is now accepted that interleukins exert effects on cells other than leukocytes. Cytokines can also be classified into cytokine families that share structural motifs (see *Table 2.5*). Chemokines are chemotactic cytokines that are crucial for controlling migration of immune cells.

Concentrations of cytokines found *in vivo* are extremely low: 10^{-6}–10^{-15} M. Abnormally high levels can have detrimental effects, in some cases resulting in death, for example, septic shock resulting from excessive production of

Table 2.5. Selected cytokine family members and their functions[a]

Family	Cytokine	Producer cells	Actions
Haematopoietins	IL-2	T cells	T cell proliferation
	IL-4	T cells, mast cells	B cell activation, switch to IgE, Th2 differentiation
	IL-7	Stromal cells	Growth of pre-B cells and pre-T cells
Interferons	IFN-α	Leukocytes	Antiviral state
	IFN-β	Fibroblasts	Antiviral state
	IFN-γ	T cells, NK cells	Macrophage activation, Ig class switching
TNF family	TNF-α	Macrophages, NK cells, T cells	Inflammation
	LT-α	T cells, B cells	Cytocidal
	CD154 (CD40L)	T cells, mast cells	B cell activation
	FasL	T cells	Apoptosis
IL-12 family	IL-12	Macrophages, dendritic cells	Th1 differentiation
	IL-23	Dendritic cells	Th17 expansion

[a]**Abbreviations**: IFN, interferon; Ig, immunoglobulin; IL, interleukin; LT, lymphotoxin; TNF, tumour necrosis factor.

Table 2.6. Selected cytokine receptor family members[a]

Type	Example	Shared feature
Type I cytokine receptor	Type 1 IL receptors Erythropoietin receptor GM-CSF receptor Prolactin receptor	Conserved motifs in extracellular domain. JAK-Stat-dependent signal transduction.
Type II cytokine receptor	Type II IL receptors IFN-α/β receptor IFN-γ receptor	
TNF family	CD30 CD40 CD120	Cysteine-rich extracellular domain.
Chemokine receptors	IL-8 receptor CCR1 CCR5 CXCR4	Seven transmembrane helix, G-protein coupled receptors.

[a]**Abbreviations**: CCR, CC-chemokine receptor; CXCR, CXC chemokine receptor, GM-CSF, granulocyte–macrophage colony stimulating factor; IFN, interferon; IL, interleukin; JAK, Janus kinase; Stat, signal transducer and activator of transcription; TNF, tumour necrosis factor.

TNF-α. The disastrous human trial of the drug TGN1412 further demonstrates the catastrophic effects of overproduction of cytokines *in vivo*. The subjects in the trial developed systemic cytokine release syndrome, with several of them succumbing to multiple organ dysfunction.

The extent of action of any given cytokine will depend on the expression of appropriate receptors on the cell membranes of target cells. Like cytokines, cytokine receptors can also be grouped into families based on shared structural features (see *Table 2.6*). Cytokines act via three main mechanisms:

- autocrine signalling, in which the cytokine binds to receptors on the cell that secretes the cytokine
- paracrine signalling, in which the cytokine binds to receptors on cells adjacent to the cell that secretes the cytokine
- juxtacrine signalling, in which cell membrane-associated cytokine molecules interact with their cognate receptors on other cells during cell–cell interaction

The effects of a cytokine can be reduced by antagonists. Many antagonists act by preventing the cytokine from binding to its receptor on the target cell. These antagonists have an immunoregulatory effect and can dampen immune responses. Several cytokine antagonists have been developed and are being used clinically to treat autoimmune diseases (see *Sections 10.9* and *14.5*).

Complement

Complement consists of a series of plasma proteins that are secreted, predominantly by the liver, as inactive precursors. The components of the pathway are sequentially activated by proteolytic cleavage, leading to the generation of several immunologically active molecules (see *Section 4.3*). Complement factors are important in attracting cells to sites of infections, enhancing the ability of immune cells to engulf foreign material, and also directly killing micro-organisms.

Acute phase proteins

Acute phase proteins (APPs) are a group of mediators that are synthesized predominantly by hepatocytes, but also by macrophages. Production of APPs is induced by the cytokines IL-1, IL-6, and TNF-α. Plasma concentrations of APPs are elevated within 2 days of infection, a reaction that is called the acute phase response. APPs play important roles in immune responses. APPs include:

■ complement proteins
■ haemostatic proteins which induce blood clotting
■ C-reactive protein (CRP) and mannan-binding lectin which can activate the complement system
■ protease inhibitors such as α_1-proteinase inhibitor which inhibits neutrophil elastase to prevent tissue damage
■ metal-binding proteins which have antibacterial properties

Monitoring APP levels can provide assistance in patient treatment, for example, high levels of CRP are commonly seen after serious trauma. Thus increased concentrations noted during recovery are an indication of infection or further complications.

The soluble mediators described above are crucial for controlling the immune response against antigens. Another important factor, however, is the nature of the antigen itself.

2.7 THE NATURE OF ANTIGENS

The nature and extent of an immune response is determined primarily by antigen. At the most basic level, the presence of antigen may be regarded as the 'on-off' switch. Without antigen there can be no immune response.

Many antigens are large molecules, although not all parts of an antigen molecule will be recognized by the immune system. Those parts that are recognized are called epitopes and large antigens can have many epitopes. Importantly, any given lymphocyte will recognize only one epitope.

Although antigens are capable of being recognized by the immune system, not all antigens are capable of generating an immune response. Antigens that can generate an immune response are called immunogens and they are said to be immunogenic. Several factors contribute to the immunogenicity of antigens.

Degree of difference from self

Self antigens normally do not elicit an immune response whereas non-self antigens do. This is because our immune systems are self-tolerant (see *Section 10.2*). Some foreign (non-self) antigens may, however, resemble self, so the response may be weak.

Antigen size

Larger antigens will usually contain more epitopes than smaller antigens and are therefore more likely to stimulate responses. In general, larger antigens are more immunogenic. Antigens with molecular weights less than 1 kDa are generally not immunogenic and such small non-immunogenic molecules are called haptens. Generation of hapten-specific immune responses generally requires that the haptens be chemically coupled to larger molecules called carriers.

Antigen dose

Below a threshold dose, antigens do not induce an immune response (low zone tolerance). Very high concentrations of antigen may also predispose to less effective responses. This is thought to be because very high doses of antigen exhaust the immune response and induce high zone tolerance.

Classes of antigens

Carbohydrates, lipids, nucleic acids and proteins all are antigenic; however, their relative immunogenicity differs substantially. Carbohydrates are usually only immunogenic when they are complexed with proteins, for example, as glycoproteins. The ABO blood group antigens are carbohydrate antigens on the surface of red blood cells. Similarly, lipids and nucleic acids are rarely immunogenic on their own but can become so if conjugated to proteins. Proteins tend to be large molecules with multiple epitopes and because of this, most proteins are immunogenic.

2.8 THE NATURE OF ANTIBODY

One of the major functions of the immune system is the production of antibodies. Antibodies, or immunoglobulins, are soluble proteins that bind specifically, and with high affinity, to antigens. Immunoglobulins also exist as a membrane-bound form on B cells where they function as the B cell receptor for antigen. The structure of immunoglobulin molecules will be introduced prior to discussing the generation and function of the B cell receptor.

Basic structure of immunoglobulins

Immunoglobulins are the secreted products of B lymphocytes. When a B cell differentiates into a cell called a plasma cell, it becomes a high level immunoglobulin-secreting factory. Importantly, all of the immunoglobulin molecules secreted by a given B cell are identical.

There are different types, or classes, of immunoglobulin molecules, each of which is adapted to carry out a different biological function. All immunoglobulins, however, have a similar structure (see *Figure 2.7*).

The basic immunoglobulin molecule has a four-chain structure (see *Box 2.7*). It comprises two heavy (H) chains of approximately 50 kDa each, and two light (L) chains of approximately 25 kDa each. H and L chains are made up of immunoglobulin domains – linear sequences of approximately 110 amino acids that fold into a characteristic conformation and that are homologous between different members of the immunoglobulin gene superfamily. Each immunoglobulin domain consists of two ß-sheets folded together to form an anti-parallel ß-barrel. Immunoglobulin domains each contain one intrachain disulphide bond.

Each L chain is made up of one constant immunoglobulin domain, C_L, and one variable immunoglobulin domain, V_L. These two domains are connected by a short stretch of amino acids called a switch region. The H

Box 2.7 Immunoglobulin structure

The basic structure of immunoglobulin molecules was determined independently in the 1960s by Rodney Porter and Gerald Edelman. They shared the Nobel Prize for this work in 1972.

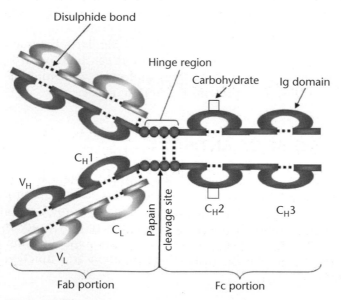

Figure 2.7

Basic structure of an immunoglobulin molecule showing the constant (C) and variable (V) regions of the heavy (H) and light (L) chains. Intrachain and interchain disulphide bonds are indicated by the dashed lines. The enzyme papain cleaves the structure in the hinge region to give the Fc and Fab portions indicated.

chains are made up of three or four constant domains, depending on the class of immunoglobulin, called C_H1, C_H2, C_H3, and C_H4, and one variable domain, V_H. V_H is connected to C_H1 by a switch region similar to that found in the L chain.

C_H1 is connected to C_H2 by a sequence of cysteine- and proline-rich amino acids called the hinge region. The cysteine residues in this region allow the formation of disulphide bonds between the two H chains. The proline residues disrupt folding of the molecule in this region and confer a high degree of rotational flexibility on the antigen-binding arms of the immunoglobulin molecule. The H chain is coupled to the L chain by disulphide bonding between C_H1 and C_L. In addition to disulphide bonding, the immunoglobulin molecule is held together by extensive non-covalent interactions between the H and L chains.

The basic Y-shaped immunoglobulin structure can be split into three parts using the enzyme papain, which cleaves the molecule at the hinge region, just above the disulphide bonds between the two H chains (see *Figure 2.7*). The part called the Fc portion comprises the lower stem of the molecule. This contains the portion of the immunoglobulin molecule (C_H2) that is responsible for activating complement via the classical pathway (see *Section 4.3*). It is also the part of the molecule that binds to surface receptors (Fc receptors) on phagocytes to enhance phagocytosis of antibody-coated material. The other two parts generated by papain digestion are the two arms of the Y-shaped structure. These are the fragments that have antigen binding activity and are called Fab fragments (both together are called $F(ab)_2$). Binding of immunoglobulin molecules to specific antigens are a result of non-covalent interactions, such as hydrogen-bonding and hydrophobic interactions.

2.9 IMMUNOGLOBULIN ISOTYPES

There are five different classes (isotypes) of immunoglobulin that are variations of this basic four chain unit. They are called IgM, IgA, IgD, IgG, and IgE (MADGE). These different immunoglobulin classes contain different H chains (see *Table 2.7*). Consequently, the different isotypes have different effector functions; for example, IgE binds to mast cells and IgG crosses the placenta. In addition, there are two different types of L chains, called κ (kappa) and λ (lambda) that can pair with any of the heavy chains. Note that any given antibody molecule will contain either κ or λ light chains, but not both. The heavy chains of antibodies of a particular isotype are different from those of other isotypes. Within one isotype, all subtypes have similar heavy chains.

IgG

IgG is the most abundant immunoglobulin in serum and extravascular spaces. Approximately 75% of total serum immunoglobulin is IgG. It is

Table 2.7. Characteristics of immunoglobulin classes and subclasses

Immunoglobulin	Heavy chain	Size (kDa)	Serum concentration (mg ml⁻¹)
IgM	μ	800	0.5–2.0
IgG1	γ1	150	5.0–12.0
IgG2	γ2	150	2.0–6.0
IgG3	γ3	165	0.5–1.0
IgG4	γ4	150	0.1–1.0
IgA1	α1	160	0.5–3.0
IgA2	α2	385	0–0.5
IgD	δ	170	0–0.5
IgE	ε	190	<0.001

made up of two γ H chains, each of approximately 50 kDa, and two L chains (either κ or λ), each of approximately 25 kDa. The H chain is made up of three constant Ig domains, $C_\gamma 1$, $C_\gamma 2$ and $C_\gamma 3$, and one variable domain, V_γ.

There are four IgG subclasses in humans. These are IgG1, IgG2, IgG3 and IgG4, comprising approximately 66%, 23%, 7% and 4% of total serum IgG, respectively. Except for IgG3, which has a half-life of only 7 days, the half-life of IgG in the circulation is 23–28 days. Apart from the variable regions, which are diverse, the IgG subclasses share approximately 90% homology in their amino acid sequences. The general structural features of IgG1 and IgG3 are shown in *Figure 2.8*.

Compared with IgG1, IgG3 has an extended hinge region. In contrast, IgG4 has a very short hinge region. As a consequence of this shortened hinge region, IgG4 is unable to activate complement via the classical pathway (see *Section 4.3*) due to steric hindrance caused by the proximity of the $C_H 1$ and $C_H 2$ domains.

IgG1   IgG3

Figure 2.8
Structural comparison of IgG1 and IgG3 illustrating the extended hinge region in IgG3.

Functions of IgG

Transplacental transfer. IgG is the only Ig isotype that can cross the placenta. IgG binds to the receptor FcRn, expressed by placental cells, and is actively transported across the placenta into the fetus. Consequently, IgG is crucial for transferring immunity from the mother to the developing fetus. FcRn is also expressed in the intestine of neonates up until 2 weeks after birth, allowing infants to absorb IgG present in the milk of nursing mothers. It is only when serum levels of maternal IgG drop at 4–6 weeks after birth that the infant begins to make its own IgG.

Although transplacental transfer of IgG is generally beneficial to the developing fetus, transplacental transfer of pathogenic antibodies can cause a disease called haemolytic disease of the newborn (see *Section 9.8*).

Agglutination. When IgG binds to antigens such as bacteria or viruses, it causes them to clump, or agglutinate. The resulting insoluble antigen–antibody complexes are efficiently eliminated from the body by phagocytes, in particular by splenic macrophages and by Kupffer cells in the liver.

Activation of complement. When bound to antigens, IgG1 and IgG3 can activate the classical complement pathway. IgG2 is poor at activating this pathway and, as noted earlier, IgG4 cannot activate the classical pathway of complement at all.

Opsonization. When IgG binds to an antigen, it can greatly enhance the ability of a phagocyte to engulf that antigen. This is because phagocytes such as neutrophils have Fcγ receptors on their surfaces that bind with high affinity to the Fc portion of IgG molecules. This 'coating' of antigen is called opsonization. Opsonization greatly increases the efficiency of phagocytosis and IgG1 and IgG3 are the most efficient opsonins.

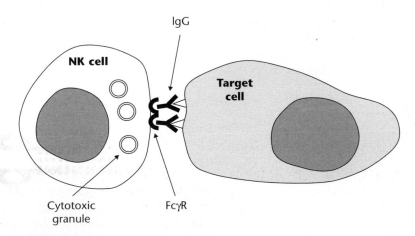

Figure 2.9
NK cells express membrane receptors that bind to the Fc portion of IgG (FcγR). When target cell-associated IgG binds to FcγRs on NK cells it stimulates the NK cells to release the contents of their cytotoxic granules towards the point of contact, resulting in death of the target cell.

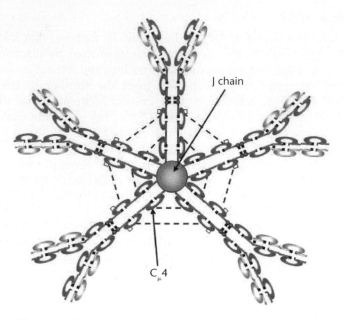

Figure 2.10
The majority of serum IgM is a pentamer held together by disulphide bonds (dashed lines) and the J chain. Unlike IgG, IgM has an additional domain in the heavy chain called $C_\mu 4$.

Antibody-dependent cell-mediated cytotoxicity (ADCC). NK cells express on their surfaces Fc receptors that can bind to the Fc portion of IgG1 or IgG3. Consequently, NK cells can bind to IgG1 or IgG3 molecules that have bound to a target cell and can kill that target cell (see *Figure 2.9*).
Neutralization. IgG can bind to the active site of toxins, such as tetanus toxin, and inhibit their action. Similarly, IgG can bind to surface molecules of viruses and block the viruses from infecting host cells. Such antibodies are called neutralizing antibodies. Induction of neutralizing antibodies is a characteristic of many successful vaccines.

IgM

IgM makes up approximately 7% of total serum immunoglobulin, and has a half-life in serum of approximately 10 days. In contrast to IgG, which consists of just one of the four-chain immunoglobulin units, IgM is a multimer made up of five such units, with a total molecular mass of >800 kDa (see *Figure 2.10*). Unlike IgG, IgM monomers do not have a classic hinge region. However, conformational flexibility is conferred by a short sequence of amino acids between $C_\mu 2$ and $C_\mu 3$ which has hinge-like properties. In addition, each µ heavy chain contains an additional constant domain, $C_\mu 4$. The IgM pentamer is held together by additional disulphide bonds between adjacent $C_\mu 3$ and $C_\mu 4$ domains, as well as by a covalently attached polypeptide chain called the J chain (~15 kDa). The pentameric IgM molecule is assembled, together with its associated J chain, in the endoplasmic reticulum of the cell prior to secretion. The pentameric nature of IgM gives it up to 10 antigen-binding sites. Due to its size, IgM is largely excluded from extravascular spaces.

Of the five antibody classes, IgM is usually the one that is made first during an immune response. This initial response to antigen is called the primary response. The next time that same antigen is encountered (during a secondary response), a switch from making IgM to making one of the other immunoglobulin classes or subclasses occurs. This is called immunoglobulin class switching. The class of antibody that is made during the secondary response is largely determined by cytokines made by T cells. These, in turn, are largely determined by the nature of the antigen and the site of entry of the antigen. In this way the immune system tries to adapt and generate the most appropriate antibody response. For example, T cells respond to respiratory pathogens by making cytokines that tell B cells to switch to making IgA, the class of antibody that is most effective at protecting mucosal surfaces.

Functions of IgM

Fetal protection. Although IgM cannot cross the placenta, it is the only class of immunoglobulin that can be made by the fetus. Production of fetal IgM begins at about 22 weeks of gestation.

Agglutination. The valency of an IgM pentamer makes IgM very efficient at binding to and aggregating microbes and other antigens.

Activation of complement. IgM is the most efficient immunoglobulin at activating complement. This, coupled with the fact that IgM is the first immunoglobulin made following infection, makes IgM an important first line of defence against infectious pathogens.

B cell receptor. Unlike the pentameric form found in serum, IgM also exists as a monomer on the surface of mature B cells, where it is referred to as surface IgM (sIgM). Together with its associated signalling molecules, sIgM functions as the B cell receptor (BCR) for antigen.

IgA

IgA accounts for approximately 15% of total serum immunoglobulin. In human serum, >80% of IgA consists of monomeric IgA of approximately 165 kDa. The half-life of IgA in serum is approximately 6 days. The majority of IgA, however, is not found in serum, but rather in secretions such as saliva, tears, sweat, and mucus. This form of IgA, termed secretory IgA, exists as a dimer of two four-chain units linked together by a J chain (as described above for IgM) and is approximately 400 kDa (see *Figure 2.11*). Dimeric IgA also contains a polypeptide called the secretory piece. The origin of this polypeptide will be discussed below. There are two subclasses of IgA in humans: IgA1, making up about 90% of total IgA, and IgA2, comprising the remaining 10%. An exception to this is in the colon where IgA2 is the predominant IgA subclass, accounting for about 60% of total IgA in this

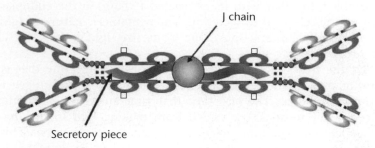

Figure 2.11
Secretory IgA is an 'end-to-end' dimer held together by the J chain. The associated secretory piece is important for transcytosis of IgA across epithelial cells (see *Figure 2.12*) and also provides protection against proteolytic degradation.

tissue. The secretory piece, together with the extensive glycosylation of the α heavy chains, protects IgA from proteolytic degradation by enzymes in the gut.

Unlike IgG and IgM, IgA is usually unable to activate complement. Secretory IgA is the most important immunoglobulin isotype conferring protection at mucosal surfaces. The function of serum IgA remains unclear.

Functions of IgA

Neonatal protection. Secretory IgA is the main immunoglobulin found in colostrum and during the first weeks after birth it plays an important role in protecting newborn infants from enteric pathogens.

Mucosal protection. Secretory IgA is the major antibody found in secretions such as tears and sweat, and is secreted on to the respiratory and gastrointestinal mucosa. Its main function is to block the entry of pathogens at these surfaces. Dimeric IgA is secreted by plasma cells in the lamina propria underlying epithelial cells. The dimeric IgA binds to the polymeric-Ig (poly-Ig) receptor on the basal surfaces of adjacent epithelial cells. The poly-Ig receptor/dimeric IgA complex is endocytosed and transported through the cytoplasm of the epithelial cell by a process termed transcytosis (see *Figure 2.12*). At the apical side of the epithelial cell the poly-Ig receptor is cleaved, releasing the dimeric IgA complexed with a 70 kDa fragment of the receptor. The fragment of the poly-Ig receptor that remains associated with the dimeric IgA is called the secretory piece. Small amounts of pentameric IgM can also be transported across epithelial cells by binding to the poly-Ig receptor.

IgE

IgE has a basic four chain structure somewhat similar to that of IgG except that the ε heavy chain contains an additional domain, $C_\varepsilon 4$. The molecular weight of IgE is approximately 190 kDa. Of all immunoglobulins, IgE is

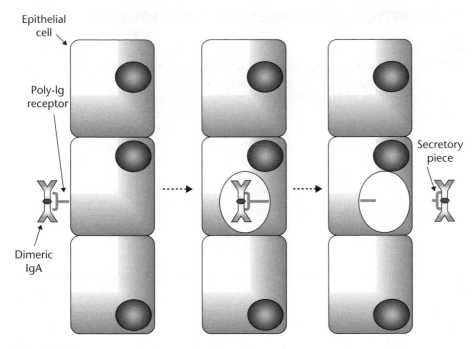

Figure 2.12
Transcytosis of secretory IgA across epithelial cells. Dimeric IgA binds to the polymeric immunoglobulin (poly-Ig) receptor on the basal surface of epithelial cells. The IgA–poly-Ig receptor complex is endocytosed and transported across the cell. IgA is released at the apical surface of the epithelial cell following cleavage of the poly-Ig receptor. The portion of the poly-Ig receptor that remains associated with the dimeric IgA molecule is called the secretory piece.

present at the lowest concentration in serum and has a half-life of only 2 days.

In developing countries, IgE plays an important role in protection against parasitic infections, especially against helminth infections. In developed countries, we are more familiar with the role of IgE in allergic diseases. In this context, IgE binds to Fcε receptors on mast cells and causes them to degranulate. Approximately 50% of total IgE is bound to the surfaces of mast cells and basophils.

IgD

IgD also has a basic four chain structure similar to that of IgG. It has a molecular weight of about 170 kDa and has a half-life in serum of only 3 days. It is not secreted by plasma cells and the low levels of IgD in serum may reflect IgD molecules that have been shed from the surface of mature B cells. Like monomeric IgM, a transmembrane form of IgD, together with associated signalling molecules, functions as an antigen receptor on mature B cells. Co-expression of IgD and IgM on the B cell surface serves as a marker for mature B cells.

2.10 RECOGNITION OF ANTIGEN BY LYMPHOCYTES

The generation of adaptive immune responses relies on the ability of B cells and T cells to react specifically against antigens. The ability of lymphocytes to recognize antigens is determined by their surface antigen receptors. When an antigen binds to the antigen receptor on a lymphocyte, this causes the lymphocyte to proliferate and give rise to many progeny cells. All of these progeny cells will express the same antigen receptor as the parental cell and will therefore recognize the same antigen as the parental cell.

The antigen receptor of B cells, the BCR, is a membrane-associated form of an immunoglobulin molecule together with a non-covalently associated signalling complex. When B cells become activated by antigen they proliferate and differentiate into plasma cells that secrete large amounts of antibody. The antigen specificity of the antibody that is secreted by the B cells is the same as the antigen specificity of the BCR.

The antigen receptor on T cells, the T cell receptor (TCR), resembles a Fab fragment of an antibody molecule. This is expressed on the T cell

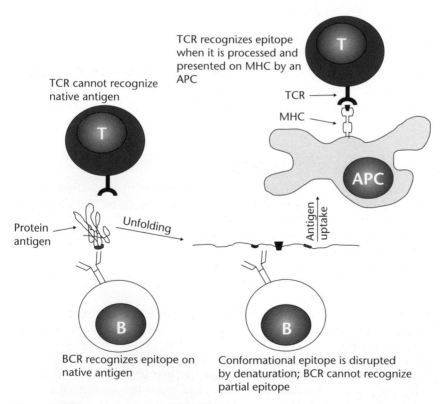

Figure 2.13
Unlike B cells, T cells are unable to recognize native antigens but require those antigens to be taken up by antigen presenting cells (APC), processed, and presented on major histocompatibility complex (MHC) molecules.

surface together with the signalling complex CD3. When $CD4^+$ T cells become activated by antigen they proliferate and differentiate into cells that secrete large amounts of cytokines. When $CD8^+$ T cells become activated by antigen they proliferate and differentiate into cytotoxic cells.

T cells and B cells recognize different forms of antigens. The BCR can bind to antigens, either soluble or cell-associated, in their native conformation. As a consequence, the epitopes that B cells recognize are conformational epitopes. The term 'conformational' describes epitopes that depend on the three-dimensional shape of the antigen. In contrast, T cells cannot recognize native antigen. T cells can only respond against protein antigens after they have been broken down and presented to them by APCs (see *Figure 2.13*).

Each day our bodies encounter a wide range of disparate agents that are capable of causing disease and the immune system has to respond to these threats and eliminate them. To do this effectively the immune system must be able to generate B cells and T cells that have specific receptors that can recognize these diverse agents. In the next chapter the mechanisms which allow the immune system to generate such a large number of BCRs and TCRs will be discussed.

SUGGESTED FURTHER READING

Crivellato, E., Vacca, A. and Ribatti, D. (2004) Setting the stage: an anatomist's view of the immune system. *Trends Immunol.* **25**: 210–217.
LaRosa, D.F. and Orange, J.S. (2008) Lymphocytes. *J. Allergy Clin. Immunol.* **121**: S364–S369.

SELF-ASSESSMENT QUESTIONS

1. What is primary lymphoid tissue?
2. What is secondary lymphoid tissue?
3. List six cell types involved in the immune system and give a brief description of their function.
4. What is your understanding of the term epitope?
5. How do the cells of the immune system communicate instructions to each other?
6. Describe what an immunoglobulin is and name five different types.
7. Discuss the three defence strategies an invading agent may be confronted with.
8. What does low zone tolerance refer to?
9. Discuss the role of acute phase proteins in the immune system and name 5 types.
10. What are haematopoietic stem cells?

Lymphocyte development

Learning objectives

After studying this chapter you should confidently be able to:

■ **Understand the concept of lymphocyte development and be aware of the stages involved**
During development and maturation within lymphoid tissues, T cells and B cells change their surface molecule expression. Lymphocytes capable of reacting against self are destroyed to establish tolerance.

■ **Appreciate the need for a mechanism such as gene rearrangement within the immune system**
Antigen-specific recognition in the adaptive immune response ensures specific responses to a wide and varied range of pathogens. Immune cell receptor genes undergo a process known as gene rearrangement to generate a large number of different antigen receptors so a great diversity of antigens can be recognized.

■ **Describe the organization and rearrangement of immunoglobulin receptor (B cell receptor, BCR) and T cell receptor (TCR) genes**
The variable regions of immunoglobulin, or BCR, heavy and light chains are encoded by smaller gene segments – V, D and J segments for heavy chains, V and J gene segments for light chains. The gene segments are cut, rearranged randomly and joined imprecisely to form the wide array of genes to be expressed. The possible number of antigen binding sites may be greater than 10^{11}. The process of TCR gene rearrangement follows the same processes as for BCR gene rearrangement.

■ **Discuss the development of mature lymphocytes and the mechanisms whereby they are rendered tolerant to self antigens during development**
Rearrangement of immunoglobulin heavy and light chain genes, as well as surface expression of BCR, occurs as B cells develop in the bone marrow. Developing B cells make extensive contacts with bone marrow stromal cells and soluble factors. If the BCR binds to cell surface-associated self antigen, a signal is transmitted into the immature B cell causing it to die by apoptosis. If the BCR binds to soluble self antigen, a signal causes the B cell to become non-responsive. Signalling via a self-recognizing BCR may also cause further rearrangement of gene segments. Rearrangement of TCR genes occurs as the immature T cells, called thymocytes, develop in the thymus. As a result of interaction with thymic cells and signalling via CD3, thymocytes begin to express both CD4 and CD8; they are then selected positively if they express functional TCRs and negatively, i.e. destroyed by apoptosis, if they bind strongly to self-

antigen. Signalling via CD8 causes thymocytes to lose CD4; signalling via CD4 causes them to lose CD8. Mature T cells express TCR, CD3, and CD4 or CD8 and do not recognize self antigen. The presence in the thymus of the Aire gene product allows tolerance against self antigens to be established.

■ **Be aware of the consequences of dysfunction in T cell and B cell maturation**
Dysregulation of immune responses can occur when T or B cell maturation does not proceed normally and can result in autoimmune diseases and conditions such as immune dysregulation, polyendocrinopathy, enteropathy X-linked (IPEX) syndrome.

3.1 INTRODUCTION TO LYMPHOCYTE DEVELOPMENT

Antigen specificity is one of the defining characteristics of acquired immune responses. This antigen-specific recognition is made possible by the receptors expressed by T cells and B cells. Within a lifetime the myriad pathogens encountered requires the immune system to have the ability to generate large numbers of diverse B cell receptors (BCRs) and T cell receptors (TCRs). It has been estimated that each individual has the capacity to generate more than 10^{15} different BCRs and TCRs. This would greatly exceed the coding capacity of the human genome if each of these antigen receptors needed to be encoded by a separate gene.

To solve this problem, B cells and T cells generate their antigen-specific receptors by a process called gene rearrangement (see *Box 3.1*) during their development in the bone marrow and thymus, respectively. During this process the developing lymphocytes actually alter their genomic DNA by moving gene segments around and deleting DNA sequences. During their development, T cells and B cells also are rendered tolerant to self antigens, a process called central tolerance. This is a critical process and is essential to stop the development of immune responses against self antigens.

This chapter will discuss the mechanisms responsible for the generation of the wide variety of TCRs and BCRs and how lymphocytes are selected against self antigens during development.

Box 3.1 Somatic gene rearrangement

Susumu Tonegawa received the Nobel Prize in 1987 for demonstrating that immunoglobulin diversity is generated by a process of somatic gene rearrangement.

3.2 ORGANIZATION AND REARRANGEMENT OF IMMUNOGLOBULIN GENES

The variable regions of the immunoglobulin heavy and light chains are encoded by smaller gene segments. The heavy (H) chains are encoded by V,

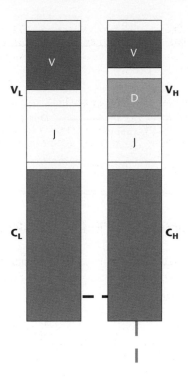

Figure 3.1
Diagram of a Fab portion of an immunoglobulin molecule. The V_L portion is encoded by V and J gene segments whereas the V_H portion is encoded by V, D and J gene segments.

D and J gene segments whereas the light (L) chains are encoded only by V and J gene segments (see *Figure 3.1*). These are brought together through a process of gene rearrangement during development. It is the random rearrangement and imprecise joining of a relatively small number of these gene segments that allow the generation of a diverse repertoire of BCRs.

Rearrangement of immunoglobulin heavy chain genes

The immunoglobulin heavy chain locus is situated on chromosome 14. The locus contains approximately 50 V_H gene segments, 20–25 D_H gene segments and 6 J_H gene segments, situated upstream of the constant region gene segments (see *Figure 3.2*). During immunoglobulin heavy chain gene rearrangement, the first event to occur is rearrangement of a randomly chosen D_H gene segment so that it lies next to a randomly selected J_H gene segment. The intervening sequence between the two gene segments is looped out and is excised from the genome. The result is a rearranged DJ downstream of the V_H gene segments. Next, a randomly selected V_H gene segment is rearranged so that it lies next to the already rearranged DJ portion, resulting in a rearranged VDJ, that is positioned upstream of the constant region gene segments. It is important to note that the constant gene segments do not participate in gene rearrangement.

The next step in generation of the heavy chain is transcription of the rearranged gene. Transcription yields a primary RNA transcript in which

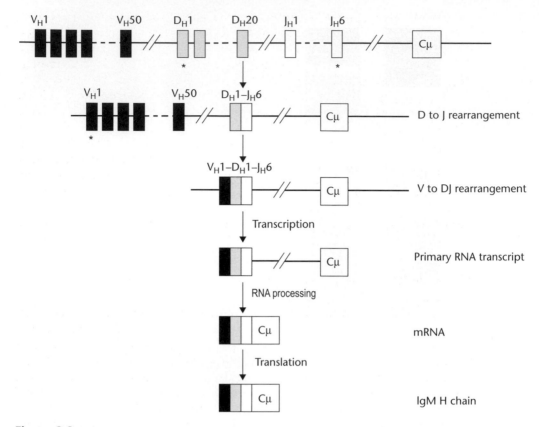

Figure 3.2
Organization and rearrangement of immunoglobulin heavy (H) chain gene segments. In the example shown, D_H1 rearranges to J_H6, and this is followed by rearrangement of V_H1 to the rearranged D_H1-J_H6. The intervening sequences are excised from the chromosome. The rearranged locus is transcribed into a primary RNA transcript which is processed into mRNA and translated into the IgM H chain polypeptide.

the rearranged VDJ is situated upstream from C_μ, which encodes the constant region of IgM. This primary RNA transcript is processed so that the intervening sequence between the rearranged VDJ and C_μ is deleted so that the VDJ and $C\mu$ are now continuous. This is the mRNA for the IgM heavy chain.

Mechanism of gene rearrangement

The V, D and J gene segments are flanked by short sequences known as recombination signal sequences (RSSs). These sequences are recognized by an enzyme complex called V(D)J recombinase which is responsible for gene rearrangement. One component of V(D)J recombinase is a dimeric complex of the products of recombination activating gene-1 (*RAG-1*) and *RAG-2*. This complex recognizes and cleaves the DNA at the RSSs of the gene segments to be rearranged and enables the formation of closed hairpin structures at each RSS. Recombination between the selected gene segments requires that the hairpins are cleaved and that the recombining segments are ligated together. Cleavage of the hairpins is thought to be mediated by the ARTEMIS nuclease enzyme which forms a complex with DNA-protein kinase. Following cleavage of the hairpins, nucleotides may be added to the cleaved ends of DNA by the enzyme terminal deoxynucleotidyl transferase or removed by exonuclease activity. The ends of the DNA strands are then joined together by the enzymes DNA ligase IV and XRCC4.

Since the process of gene rearrangement is random it is possible that the synthesized heavy chain might be non-functional. This could happen due to the introduction of a stop codon or nonsense codon in the DNA sequence during recombination. The process of gene rearrangement is also energy intensive. Because of this it is essential to test the heavy chain to see if it is functional before the cell is committed to rearranging the immunoglobulin light chain genes.

Formation of the pre-BCR

The mRNA for the heavy chain is translated into polypeptide by ribosomes on the rough endoplasmic reticulum (ER). The polypeptide chains are then translocated across the membrane of the ER, where they fold. For the heavy chain to be functional it must be able to 'pair' with the light chain and form a functional immunoglobulin molecule. At this stage though, the cell has not yet rearranged the light chain genes. However, the developing B cell expresses two proteins called V_{preB} (CD179a) and λ_5 (CD179b). V_{preB} resembles the variable region of a light chain whereas λ_5 resembles the constant region of the light chain. These two proteins non-covalently associate with each other and form a complex called the surrogate light chain. V_{preB} and λ_5 genes do not rearrange so the surrogate light chain molecules expressed in all developing B cells are identical. The surrogate light chain acts as a template to test whether the rearranged heavy chain has the correct overall conformation and is, therefore, likely to be able to pair with an immunoglobulin light chain. If the complete heavy chain protein cannot be made (e.g. contains a nonsense or premature stop codon) or cannot pair with surrogate light chain, then the immunoglobulin heavy chain locus on the homologous chromosome will undergo rearrangement. If the heavy chain is successfully rearranged and binds to the surrogate light chain then this complex is expressed on the surface of the cell (see *Figure 3.3*). On the cell surface, the heavy chain–surrogate light chain complex is non-covalently associated with two other molecules, CD79a and CD79b. Together the heavy chain–surrogate light chain–CD79a–CD79b complex is called the pre-BCR. If the pre-BCR is expressed on the cell surface then a signal is transmitted via CD79a–CD79b into the developing B cell. This signal allows the developing B cell to survive and proliferate to give many daughter cells that have a functional heavy chain rearrangement. Any B cell that fails to successfully rearrange its heavy chain genes and form a pre-BCR will not get this survival signal and will die by apoptosis.

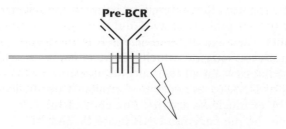

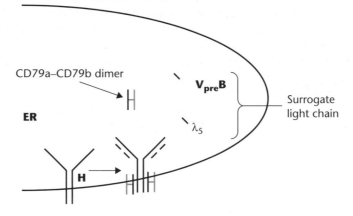

1. Stop rearranging H chain – **Allelic exclusion**
2. Proliferate
3. Start rearranging L chain
4. Stop expressing surrogate L chain

Figure 3.3
In the endoplasmic reticulum (ER), the IgM heavy chain (H) associates with the surrogate light chain and with the CD79a–CD79b signalling complex. The resultant multimolecular complex, the pre-BCR, is expressed on the surface of the pre-B cell and transmits a signal into the cell that allows B cell development to continue.

If rearrangement was successful at the first heavy chain locus, the signal transmitted via the pre-BCR will stop rearrangement at the heavy chain locus on the homologous chromosome. This is termed allelic exclusion (see *Box 3.2*) and it ensures that the developing B cell will express only one type of heavy chain. The signal delivered via the pre-BCR also will inhibit expression of V_{preB} and λ_5 and will induce rearrangement at the immunoglobulin light chain locus. This makes sense because the surrogate light chain has done its job and is no longer needed. The next step in making a functional immunoglobulin molecule is to rearrange the light chain genes.

Rearrangement of immunoglobulin light chain genes

The loci encoding the two different types of light chain are on different chromosomes. The κ locus is on chromosome 2 whereas the λ locus is on chromosome 22. The process of rearrangement of the light chain genes is identical to that for the heavy chain genes except that the light chain loci do not contain D gene segments. This means that there is a single recombination event during light chain gene rearrangement, V to J. As in heavy chain gene rearrangement, rearrangement of light chain gene segments is RSS-dependent and is mediated by V(D)J recombinase.

During light chain gene rearrangement, the κ locus rearranges first. If the κ loci on both copies of chromosome 2 fail to rearrange successfully then the λ locus rearranges.

The κ locus contains approximately 40 V_κ gene segments and 5 J_κ gene segments (see *Figure 3.4*). During light chain gene rearrangement, one of the V_κ gene segments is selected randomly and rearranged so that it lies next

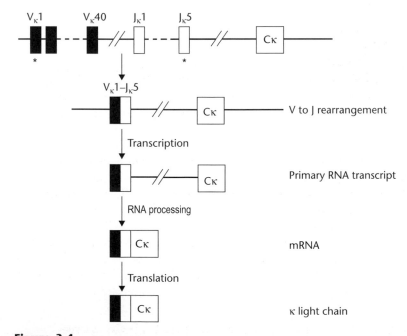

Figure 3.4

Organization and rearrangement of immunoglobulin chain gene segments. In the example shown, V1 rearranges to J5. The intervening sequences are excised from the chromosome. The rearranged locus is transcribed into a primary RNA transcript which is processed into mRNA and translated into the light chain polypeptide.

to a randomly selected J_κ gene segment. As in heavy chain gene rearrangement, the intervening sequence between the recombining gene segments is looped out and is excised from the genome. The result is a rearranged VJ located upstream of C_κ. Transcription and processing of the primary RNA transcript occurs as described for the heavy chain gene. The mRNA for the κ light chain is translated by ribosomes on the rough ER and the polypeptide chains are translocated into the lumen of the ER where they fold.

Successful rearrangement at the immunoglobulin κ chain locus results in a light chain that will pair with the heavy chain and be expressed on the cell surface. If neither κ locus successfully rearranges, however, then the cell will attempt to rearrange the λ light chain loci. The process of rearrangement at the λ loci happens as described above for κ rearrangement except that the λ locus contains approximately 30 V_λ gene segments and 4 J_λ gene segments. If rearrangement at both λ loci is unsuccessful then the cell will die. However, if the cell does successfully rearrange one of its light chain genes then the light chain polypeptide will associate with the heavy chain and will be expressed on the surface of the cell. The immunoglobulin heavy chain–light chain complex is non-covalently associated with the signalling molecules CD79a and CD79b to form the BCR complex. Expression of the BCR on the cell surface transmits a survival signal into the cell via CD79a–CD79b (see *Figure 3.5*).

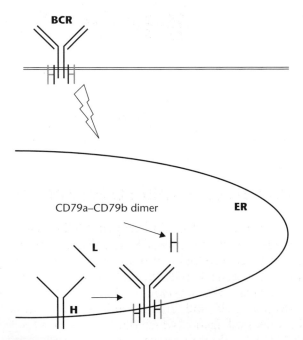

Figure 3.5
In the endoplasmic reticulum (ER), the IgM heavy chain (H) associates with the light chain and with the CD79a–CD79b signalling complex. The resultant multimolecular complex, the BCR, is expressed on the surface of the immature B cell and transmits a survival signal into the cell.

Diversity generated by gene rearrangement

The random rearrangement of V, D and J gene segments is capable of generating greater than two million different antigen binding sites (see *Table 3.1*). As this diversity results from the different possible combinations of these gene segments, it is referred to as combinatorial diversity. There is also an additional source of diversity, termed junctional diversity, which results from the mechanism of gene rearrangement itself. When the gene segments are joined together there is frequently addition of nucleotides by the enzyme terminal deoxyribonucleotidyl transferase. Alternatively, exonuclease activity may remove nucleotides at the joins between the recombining gene segments. Together, this increases the potential diversity by several orders of magnitude and the possible number of antigen binding sites has been estimated to be greater than 10^{11}.

Table 3.1. Combinatorial diversity generated by gene rearrangement

Gene segment	Estimated number of gene segments		
	Heavy chain	Light chain	
		κ	λ
V	50	40	30
D	25		
J	6	5	4
Possible combinations of V–D–J or V–J	$50 \times 25 \times 6 = 7500$	$40 \times 5 = 200$	$30 \times 4 = 120$
Possible associations of H and L chains	$7500 \times (200 + 120) = 2.4 \times 10^6$		

3.3 B CELL DEVELOPMENT AND SELECTION

Rearrangement of immunoglobulin heavy and light chain genes, as well as surface expression of the pre-BCR and BCR complexes, occurs at defined stages of B cell development in the bone marrow (see *Figure 3.6*). Progression of developing B cells through these stages is dependent on bone marrow stromal cells. Developing B cells make extensive contacts with these stromal cells and are dependent on stromal cell-derived factors, such as stem cell factor (which binds to *c-kit* on the B cell progenitor cells) and IL-7 for their differentiation.

At the pro-B cell stage the heavy chain loci on both copies of chromosome 14 undergo D to J rearrangement. The locus that successfully rearranges D to J will then go on to rearrange V to DJ. The V to DJ rearrangement occurs at the pre-B cell stage. If the V to DJ rearrange-

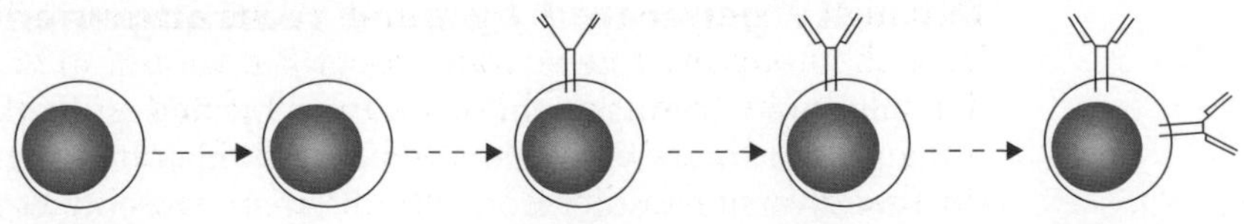

	Lymphoid progenitor	Pro-B cell	Pre-B cell	Immature B cell	Mature B cell
V(D)J rearrangement	–	D_H–J_H	V_H–D_H–J_H	V_L (κ or λ)	–
Membrane Ig expression	–	–	μ + surrogate light chains	IgM	IgM + IgD

Figure 3.6
B cell developmental scheme illustrating the ordered rearrangement of immunoglobulin genes and expression of BCR and pre-BCR complexes. For clarity, the CD79a–CD79b signalling complex has been omitted.

ment is successful then the pre-B cell will make a heavy chain and attempt to express this heavy chain on the surface as part of the pre-BCR. Signalling via the pre-BCR promotes transition to the immature B cell stage. The signal for progression to the immature B cell stage also requires the enzyme Bruton's tyrosine kinase (Btk). Light chain gene rearrangement occurs at the immature B cell stage. If the immature B cell successfully rearranges a light chain then it will attempt to express this light chain on the surface as part of the BCR. If the cell fails to express a BCR it will die.

Importantly, at this immature stage B cells are also tested for their reactivity to self antigens (see *Figure 3.7*). This process identifies and removes potentially auto-reactive B cells, which could attack the host (self) and cause autoimmune disease.

There are three possible fates for an immature B cell if its BCR binds with high affinity to self antigen. If the BCR binds to cell surface-associated self-antigen this can effectively crosslink the BCRs on the surface of the immature B cell. The resultant signal transmitted into the immature B cell causes death of the cell by apoptosis. If the BCR binds to soluble self-antigen, the resultant signal transmitted into the immature B cell causes it to become non-responsive, or anergic. There is, however, another option open to immature B cells that express an autoreactive BCR. Signalling via the BCR can reactivate the V(D)J recombinase in these cells, allowing them to replace their rearranged V_H gene segment with another genomic V_H gene segment, or to replace their rearranged light chain VJ sequence with an alternative VJ rearrangement. These processes are called receptor editing. Immature B cells that have 'edited' their BCRs will again be tested to determine if they bind to self-antigens. Collectively, these mechanisms of purging autoreactive B cells in the bone marrow are referred to as central tolerance.

The majority of developing B cells (>90%) do not survive selection in the bone marrow. Only those immature B cells whose BCRs do not bind with high affinity to self antigen in the bone marrow will survive. These cells leave the bone marrow as transitional B cells and migrate to the spleen. In the spleen the transitional B cells are subjected to further selection against self antigens. Transitional B cells with a BCR which binds to self antigen in the spleen are either deleted or rendered non-responsive, whereas those with a BCR that does not bind self antigen survive. Survival of transitional B cells is dependent on the cytokine BAFF (**B** cell **a**ctivating **f**actor of the TNF **f**amily). BAFF is produced by a variety of cells, including splenic macrophages and DCs. When BAFF binds to its receptor on transitional B cells it stimulates paracrine or juxtacrine (see *Section 2.6*) proliferation of these cells. There are three known receptors for BAFF, BAFF-R (or BR3), APRIL (**a pr**oliferation **i**nducing **l**igand), and TACI (**t**ransmembrane **a**ctivator and **C**AML **i**nteractor), of which BAFF-R is thought to be the most important for promoting survival of transitional B cells. Dysregulated expression of BAFF or its receptors may lead to survival of autoreactive B cells and contribute to the pathogenesis of diseases like rheumatoid arthritis (see *Section 10.7*) and systemic lupus erythematosus (see *Section 10.8*).

Transitional B cells with a BCR that does not bind to self antigen in the spleen undergo alternative splicing of their rearranged heavy chain RNA to allow the co-expression of IgM and IgD on their cell surfaces. At this stage of development the B cells are referred to as mature B cells. Some of these mature B cells will localize to the marginal zone of the spleen. Marginal zone B cells are specialized for picking up antigen from the circulation. The rest of the mature B cell pool will localize to the B cell areas of secondary lymphoid tissues and become follicular B cells. These mature B cells are now ready to respond to foreign antigen.

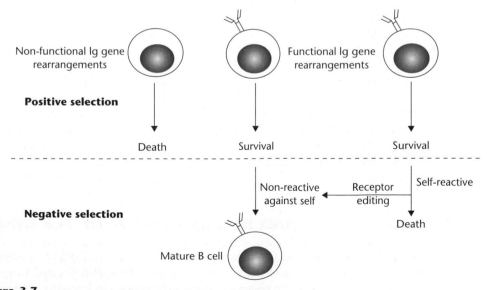

Figure 3.7
B cells must express a BCR in order to receive a survival signal. BCR-expressing immature, and transitional, B cells are tested for their reactivity against self antigens. Cells that express an autoreactive BCR may undergo receptor editing to generate a non-self-reactive BCR.

3.4   CELL SURFACE MOLECULES OF MATURE B CELLS

In addition to the BCR, mature B cells express many other cell surface molecules that can modulate B cell responses (see *Figure 3.8*). CD19, CD21 and CD81 form a non-covalently associated complex called the B cell co-receptor. Stimulation of the B cell co-receptor promotes B cell responses by reducing the level of antigen required to achieve B cell activation. This is because the complement receptor CD21 binds to antigens opsonized with C3d (see *Section 4.3*) and causes a stimulatory signal to be transmitted via CD19. B cells also express receptors that serve to dampen B cell responses. The inhibitory receptor CD22 opposes the stimulatory activity of the B cell co-receptor and CD32, a low affinity receptor for the Fc portion of IgG, can also dampen B cell responses. Ligand binding to cell surface cytokine and chemokine receptors regulate B cell function and trafficking patterns, and expression of a variety of adhesion molecules regulates B cell migration into tissues, in particular into lymphoid tissues. Additionally, B cells express surface molecules that are essential for T cell–B cell interaction. These include CD40, CD80/CD86 and MHC class II (see *Section 6.8*).

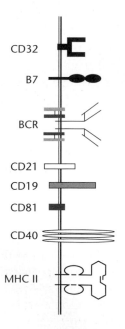

Figure 3.8
In addition to the BCR, mature B cells express a variety of other surface molecules that are crucial for B cell function. Of these, B7, CD40 and MHC II allow B cells to interact with T cells. The B cell co-receptor complex, consisting of CD19, CD21 and CD81, allows B cells to become activated at lower antigen concentrations. CD32 is a low affinity Fc receptor which can inhibit B cell responses.

3.5   ORGANIZATION AND REARRANGEMENT OF TCR GENES

There are two types of TCR, denoted TCRα/β and TCRγ/δ, respectively. TCRα/β is expressed on >95% of all T cells and these α/β T cells comprise the major type of T cell involved in immune responses in humans. Any given T cell will express either TCRα/β or TCRγ/δ, but never both. This is because the TCRα and TCRδ genes are closely linked, and rearrangement of the TCRα genes results in deletion of the TCRδ locus (see *Figure 3.9*). At present

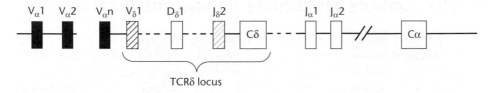

$V_\alpha 1$ $V_\alpha 2$ $V_\alpha n$ $V_\delta 1$ $D_\delta 1$ $J_\delta 2$ $J_\alpha 1$ $J_\alpha 2$

Cδ Cα

TCRδ locus

Figure 3.9
The TCRδ locus is situated between the Vα and Jα gene segments. Consequently, rearrangement of the TCRα genes will result in excision of the TCRδ locus.

the function of γ/δ T cells remains unclear. In general, they do not recognize peptide antigen bound to MHC molecules. Some γ/δ T cells have been shown to recognize mycobacterial antigens and glycolipids. This section will focus on the generation and functions of α/β T cells.

The process of TCR gene rearrangement is the same as that described for immunoglobulin BCR gene rearrangement. TCR genes are organized in a manner similar to immunoglobulin genes, and also undergo random rearrangement to generate, ultimately, TCR polypeptides. The recombination process is also mediated by the V(D)J recombinase in an RSS-dependent manner.

Schematically, the α/β TCR resembles a Fab fragment of an immunoglobulin molecule (see *Figure 3.10*). Similar to the variable region of the immunoglobulin heavy chain, the variable region of TCRβ chain is encoded by V, D and J gene segments. The TCRα chain resembles the immunoglobulin light chain in that the variable region is encoded by V and J gene segments only.

Rearrangement of TCR genes occurs as the immature T cells are developing in the thymus. At this stage of their development the immature T cells are called thymocytes.

Rearrangement of TCR genes

The first locus to rearrange is the TCRβ chain locus. As with immunoglobulin heavy chain rearrangement, TCRβ gene rearrangement is an ordered process, starting with D_β to J_β rearrangement and followed by rearrangement of a randomly selected V_β gene segment to the rearranged DJ. The end result of this process is a rearranged VDJ positioned upstream of C_β. Transcription and processing of the primary RNA transcript occur as described for the immunoglobulin heavy chain gene (see *Section 3.3*). The TCRβ chain mRNA is translated by ribosomes on the rough ER and the polypeptide chains are translocated into the lumen of the ER where they fold.

The next step is to determine whether or not the rearranged TCRβ chain is functional. To be functional, the TCRβ chain must pair with the TCRα chain to form the TCR. At this stage the cell has not yet rearranged the TCRα chain genes. Instead, the rearranged TCRβ chain must form a

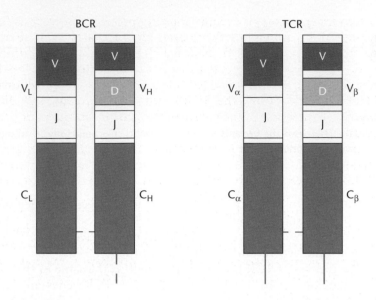

Figure 3.10
The structural organization of an α/β TCR resembles that of an immunoglobulin Fab fragment.

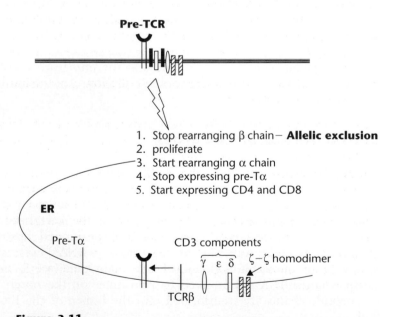

Figure 3.11
In the endoplasmic reticulum (ER), the TCRβ chain associates with pre-Tα and with the CD3 signalling complex. The resultant multimolecular complex, the pre-TCR, is expressed on the surface of the double negative thymocyte and transmits a signal into the cell that allows T cell development to proceed.

heterodimeric complex with another protein, called pre-Tα, which is expressed by immature thymocytes. Pre-Tα acts as a template to test whether the rearranged β chain has the correct overall conformation, and is therefore likely to be able to pair with a TCRα chain. Pre-Tα genes do not rearrange so the pre-Tα molecules expressed in all thymocytes are identical. In contrast, the TCRβ and TCRα chains will differ between thymocytes because of the nature of the gene rearrangement process utilized to generate these molecules.

If the first attempt at rearrangement does not generate a functional TCRβ chain (e.g. if it contains a nonsense or premature stop codon), or if the TCRβ chain cannot pair with pre-Tα, then the β chain locus on the homologous chromosome will undergo rearrangement. If this second rearrangement is also unsuccessful then the thymocyte will die by apoptosis. If the TCRβ gene rearrangement is functional then the TCRβ chain is expressed on the cell surface together with pre-Tα. The TCRβ chain–pre-Tα complex is non-covalently associated with the multi-chain signalling complex, CD3, on the cell surface. The resultant multi-molecular complex is known as the pre-TCR (see *Figure 3.11*).

Expression of the pre-TCR on the cell surface results in transmission of a signal, via CD3, into the developing thymocyte. This pre-TCR-dependent signal has several effects:

■ it will allow the thymocyte to survive and proliferate
■ if rearrangement was successful at the first TCRβ locus, the signal via the pre-TCR will prevent rearrangement at the homologous locus (allelic exclusion); this ensures that T cells express only one TCRβ chain
■ it will induce expression of both CD4 and CD8 molecules on the developing thymocytes; the resultant thymocytes are called double positive (DP) thymocytes
■ it will induce rearrangement at the TCRα chain locus and prevent expression of pre-Tα

Rearrangement of the TCRα chain genes occurs essentially as described above for TCRβ chain genes; however, there are no D gene segments in the TCRα locus so the rearrangement process is a one-step V_α to J_α recombination. Following synthesis, the TCRα chain must pair with the TCRβ chain. If the chains cannot pair then the cell attempts to rearrange the TCRα chain genes on the homologous chromosome. If this rearrangement is also unsuccessful then the cell dies by apoptosis. If the cell makes a functional TCRα chain, the TCRα/β heterodimer is expressed on the surface of the thymocyte together with CD3. In mature T cells CD3 is responsible for transmitting signals to the interior of a T cell following recognition of antigen by the TCR.

3.6 T CELL DEVELOPMENT

In the bone marrow, common lymphoid progenitor cells give rise to cells that will become B cells and also cells that will become T cells (pro-thymocytes). Pro-thymocytes leave the bone marrow and migrate to the thymus to complete their development. Although T cell development proceeds throughout life, the thymus greatly decreases in size at puberty, with a concomitant decrease in thymic output.

Pro-thymocytes enter the subcapsular cortex of the thymus and undergo several rounds of proliferation. As the thymocytes mature they transit through the cortex to the medulla from where mature T cells will exit the thymus and migrate to secondary lymphoid tissues. During their development, thymocytes make extensive contacts with thymic stromal cells. These contacts, together with stromal cell-derived factors such as IL-7, are essential for T cell development.

Immature thymocytes express neither CD4 nor CD8 molecules on their surfaces, and are called double negative (DN) thymocytes. The next event to occur is the rearrangement of TCR genes (see *Section 3.5*) to generate a functional TCR. Since T cell selection is based on TCR reactivity, TCR gene rearrangement is a prerequisite for thymic selection. Following TCR gene rearrangement the TCR-expressing cells also express both CD4 and CD8 and are called DP thymocytes. CD4 and CD8 are often called co-receptors because when they bind to MHC class II or class I molecules, respectively, they not only stabilize the interaction between the TCR and the MHC molecule but they also transmit a signal into the T cell. When CD4 and CD8 are expressed on its surface the DP thymocyte then undergoes a process known as selection (see *Figure 3.12*).

Thymic selection is a two-stage process. The first stage is positive selection. Positive selection takes place in the cortex of the thymus. The purpose of positive selection is to select any thymocyte that expresses a TCR that is potentially useful. The only way a T cell can recognize antigen is when MHC molecules present antigen to it. Therefore TCRs must be able to bind to MHC molecules to be potentially useful. During positive selection, the DP thymocytes encounter cells called thymic cortical epithelial cells (CECs). The CECs express both MHC class I and II molecules on their surfaces. Thymocytes with TCRs that bind to either class of MHC molecule receive a survival signal via their TCRs. Thymocytes with TCRs which do not bind to MHC class I or II molecules, will never be able to respond to antigen (immunologically they are useless), so they do not receive a survival signal and die by apoptosis. The surviving thymocytes are said to have been positively selected.

At this time a decision is also made regarding a thymocyte becoming a CD4$^+$ T cell or a CD8$^+$ T cell. The current model of how this decision is made proposes that the strength of the signal the thymocyte receives via its TCR and co-receptors determines whether the cell will continue to express CD4 or continue to express CD8. If the TCR binds to MHC class II, then the strong signal that is transmitted via CD4 together with the TCR–CD3 complex will shut off expression of CD8 and the thymocyte will become a CD4$^+$ single positive (SP) cell. If, however, the TCR binds to MHC I molecules on the CECs then the weaker signal transmitted via CD8 together with the TCR–CD3 complex will shut off expression of CD4 and the cell will become an SP CD8$^+$ cell. The SP thymocytes are now subjected to negative selection.

Negative selection occurs at the boundary between the cortex and the medulla (the cortico-medullary boundary) and in the medulla of the thymus. The cells that carry out the negative selection are medullary epithelial cells (MEC) and thymic dendritic cells. Positive selection allows all cells that are potentially useful to survive, while negative selection attempts to eliminate all thymocytes that are potentially harmful. Potentially harmful thymocytes are those which have TCRs that bind with high affinity to self antigens. This can be a difficult process as all cells whose TCRs bind with high affinity to all self antigens, and not just to antigens that are only expressed in the thymus, must be eliminated. Therefore this process must test the thymocyte to see if its TCR binds to an antigen which may, for

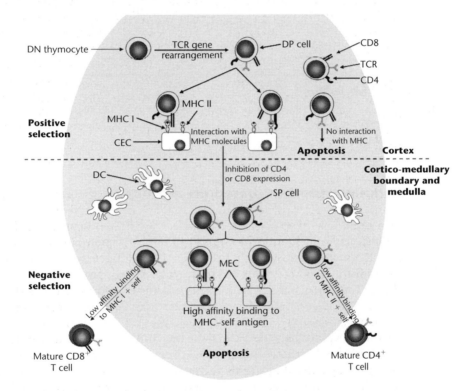

Figure 3.12

Pro-thymocytes that migrate to the thymus from the bone marrow do not express either CD4 or CD8 molecules on their surfaces. These double negative (DN) thymocytes rearrange their TCR genes and are induced to express both CD4 and CD8 and, therefore, become double positive (DP) cells. The DP cells are tested for their ability to bind to MHC molecules on thymic cortical epithelial cells (CEC). This process is termed positive selection and only those thymocytes whose TCRs bind to MHC molecules will receive a survival signal. DP thymocytes that fail to bind to MHC die by apoptosis. The surviving DP thymocytes then extinguish expression of either CD4 or CD8 and become single positive (SP) thymocytes. At the cortico-medullary boundary and in the medulla the SP thymocytes are subjected to negative selection. Any SP thymocytes that bind with high affinity to MHC + self antigen presented by medullary epithelial cells (MEC), or dendritic cells (DC), receive a signal to undergo apoptosis. Those SP thymocytes that bind with low affinity to MHC I + self peptide or to MHC II + self peptide survive and leave the thymus as mature CD8+ T cells or mature CD4+ T cells, respectively.

example, normally only be present in the pancreas. The gene called *Aire*, expressed in MECs in the thymus, makes this possible.

Function of Aire

Aire stands for autoimmune regulator. The *Aire* gene product is a transcriptional activator (see *Box 3.3*) that allows ectopic gene expression in MECs. This means that it induces the transcription, in the MECs, of genes that are not normally expressed there. Therefore the presence of Aire allows expression in the thymus of proteins that are normally only expressed in other tissues. This function of Aire is essential for negative selection. The rare multi-organ autoimmune disease <u>a</u>utoimmune <u>p</u>oly<u>e</u>ndocrinopathy–<u>c</u>andidiasis–<u>e</u>ctodermal <u>d</u>ystrophy (APECED) is a result of a mutated *Aire* gene.

Box 3.3 Transcription factors

Transcription factors are proteins that bind to specific regions of DNA via DNA-binding domains to control the transcription of genes into mRNA. Transcriptional activators increase gene transcription while transcriptional repressors inhibit gene transcription.

Negative selection based on affinity

As a result of *Aire* expression in MECs, the SP thymocytes are exposed to a wide variety of self antigens bound to MHC molecules. Any thymocyte with a TCR which binds strongly to MHC + self antigen receives a death signal through its TCR. Deletion of self-reactive T cells in the thymus is termed central tolerance and is a major mechanism whereby autoimmune reactions are prevented. It is estimated that greater than 95% of thymocytes die in the thymus.

It has recently become clear that *Aire* function is not only important for deletion of self-reactive thymocytes but is also critical for selection of a major subset of T cells with regulatory/suppressor activity called natural regulatory T (nT_{REG}) cells. It is thought that $CD4^+$ thymocytes whose TCRs bind with intermediate affinity to self antigens presented by MECs do not die but instead develop into nT_{REG} cells (see *Figure 3.13*). nT_{REG} cells are $CD4^+CD25^+$ cells and express the X chromosome-encoded forkhead family transcription factor Foxp3.

nT_{REG} cells, and other regulatory T cells (see *Section 7.6*), are important for suppressing unwanted immune responses in the periphery. When nT_{REG} cells leave the thymus they migrate to secondary lymphoid tissues and to peripheral non-lymphoid tissues, especially to the respiratory and gastrointestinal tracts. Approximately 1–2% of human $CD4^+$ cells are thought to be T_{REG} cells. The mechanism of action of T_{REG} cells is presently an area of intense research. Current data suggest that the immunosuppressive activity exerted by nT_{REG} cells is mediated via direct cell contact. The multi-system

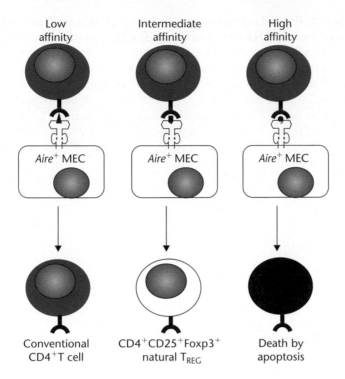

Figure 3.13
CD4$^+$ thymocytes cells that bind to self antigen, presented on thymic medullary epithelial cells (MEC), with low affinity, develop into conventional CD4$^+$ T cells. CD4$^+$ thymocytes that bind to self antigen with high affinity are eliminated by apoptosis. Current research suggests that CD4$^+$ thymocytes that bind to self antigen with intermediate affinity are induced to express the transcription factor Foxp3 and develop into CD4$^+$CD25$^+$Foxp3$^+$ nT$_{REG}$ cells.

autoimmune disease, immune dysregulation, polyendocrinopathy, enteropathy X-linked (IPEX) syndrome that occurs when *Foxp3* is mutated or deleted, illustrates the importance of T$_{REG}$ cells in maintaining self-tolerance.

SP thymocytes whose TCRs bind with low affinity to MHC + self antigen are unlikely to cause autoimmune disease and do not receive a signal to undergo apoptosis. These cells have now completed their development in primary lymphoid tissue and are ready to leave the thymus. They leave as mature T lymphocytes and migrate to secondary lymphoid tissues.

3.7 CELL SURFACE MOLECULES OF T CELLS

In addition to the TCR–CD3 and co-receptor molecules, mature T cells express many other cell surface molecules that are essential for their function (see *Figure 3.14*). CD28 binding is essential for activation of naïve

T cells (see *Box 3.4*). Following activation, T cells express CD154 (CD40L). The binding of CD154 on T cells to CD40 on B cells is essential for provision of T cell help to B cells (see *Section 6.8*). T cells also express a variety of cytokine receptors. Of particular importance are the receptors for IL-2, IL-4 and IL-12 which are important for proliferation and differentiation of T cells, and the receptors for IL-7 and IL-15 which are important for maintenance of memory T cells. Activation-associated changes in chemokine receptor expression on T cells regulate their migration to lymphoid tissues or to sites of infection. T cells also express a variety of adhesion molecules, for example, LFA-1 (lymphocyte function-associated antigen 1) and VLA-4 (very late antigen 4), which interact with blood vessel endothelial cells and enable T cells to infiltrate tissues during infections.

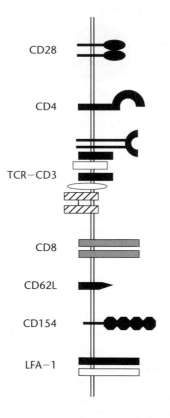

Figure 3.14
Mature T cells express a wide variety of cell surface molecules in addition to the TCR–CD3 complex and the co-receptors CD4 or CD8. These include adhesion molecules such as LFA-1 and CD62L as well as the co-stimulatory molecule CD28, and CD154 which is crucial for T cell–B cell interaction.

Box 3.4 Naïve lymphocytes

A lymphocyte is referred to as a naïve, or virgin, lymphocyte if it has not yet encountered its specific antigen. A lymphocyte that has encountered, and responded against, its specific antigen is termed an antigen-experienced lymphocyte.

3.8 LYMPHOCYTE ENCOUNTER WITH ANTIGEN

When T cells and B cells complete their differentiation they express high levels of CD62L. CD62L is a lymph node homing receptor that enables T cells, and B cells, to cross from the bloodstream into lymph nodes to await their encounter with antigen. In the case of a peripheral infection, the antigen must be brought from peripheral tissues to the secondary lymphoid tissues so that lymphocytes can respond against it. During the initial exposure to antigen, a well orchestrated innate immune response is set in motion to try to eliminate the threat and also to allow antigen to be acquired and presented, in a recognizable form, to lymphocytes. This response is called inflammation and it will be examined in the next chapter.

SUGGESTED FURTHER READING

Cambier, J.C., Gauld, S.B., Merrell, K.T. and Vilen, B.J. (2007) B-cell anergy: from transgenic models to naturally occurring anergic B cells? *Nature Rev. Immunol.* **7**: 633–643.

Germain, R.N. (2002) T cell development and the CD4$^+$-CD8$^+$ lineage decision. *Nature Rev. Immunol.* **2**: 309–322.

Jung, D., Giallourakis, C., Mostoslavsky, R. and Alt, F.W. (2006) Mechanism and control of V(D)J recombination at the immunoglobulin heavy chain locus. *Annu. Rev. Immunol.* **24**: 541–570.

Kyewski, B. and Klein, L. (2006) A central role for central tolerance. *Annu. Rev. Immunol.* **24**: 571–606.

Liston, A. and Rudensky, A.Y. (2007) Thymic development and peripheral homeostasis of regulatory T cells. *Curr. Opin. Immunol.* **19**: 176–185.

Mathis, D. and Benoist, C. (2007) A decade of Aire. *Nature Rev. Immunol.* **7**: 645–650.

Monoroe, J.G and Dorshkind, K. (2007) Fate decisions regulating bone marrow and peripheral B lymphocyte development. *Adv. Immunol.* **95**: 1–50.

Nemazee, D. (2006) Receptor editing in lymphocyte development and central tolerance. *Nature Rev. Immunol.* **6**: 728–740.

SELF-ASSESSMENT QUESTIONS

1. Why is there a need for a mechanism such as gene rearrangement within the immune system?
2. Describe briefly the process of gene rearrangement for immunoglobulin receptor (B cell receptor, BCR) and T cell receptor (TCR) genes.
3. When B cells developing in the bone marrow come in contact with bone marrow stromal cells and bind to cell surface-associated self antigen, does the signal transmitted into the immature B cell cause it to die or survive?
4. Where do thymocytes (immature T cells) undergo rearrangement of their TCR genes?

5. What cell surface molecules do mature T cells express?
6. Which product in the thymus allows self-tolerance against peripheral self antigens to be established?
7. During the process of gene rearrangement, do developing lymphocytes alter their genomic DNA by (a) moving gene segments around or (b) deleting DNA sequences?
8. How many BCRs and TCRs can one individual generate?
9. What is the fate of a developing B cell, which during development does not react with self antigen?
10. What is central tolerance?

The innate immune response

Learning objectives
After studying this chapter you should confidently be able to:

- **Describe the primary signs and symptoms of acute inflammation**
  The rapid, highly effective innate immune response to a foreign invader, known as acute inflammation is characterized by: swelling (oedema); redness (erythema); pain (noxia); heat (fever) and loss of function.

- **Explain how the functions of cells and molecules lead to the observable signs and symptoms of acute inflammation**
  Immunological processes such as cytokine secretion, endothelial gene regulation, leukocyte adherence, phagocytosis and fibroblast activation, are responsible for systemic effects of inflammation such as loss of appetite and increased heart rate. The local increase in cytokines IL-1 and TNF-α causes heat, swelling, redness and pain. The dilation of blood vessels by histamine, eicosanoids and bradykinin increases the flow of blood to the affected tissue and leads to the redness associated with acute inflammation. Increased vascular permeability allows more fluid to leave the venule and enter the tissue as inflammatory exudate, leading to swelling. The exudate contains bradykinin, which can act on local nerve endings to cause pain. Loss of function can result.

- **Describe the process of phagocytosis**
  When a neutrophil encounters a pathogen, it sends out pseudopodia to surround the pathogen and engulf and eliminate it. This process is made much more efficient if the pathogen is opsonized with complement or antibody. Neutrophils destroy ingested pathogens by activating the respiratory burst to destroy the pathogen by oxidative attack with hydrogen peroxide and hypochlorite ions, and through digestion with lysosomal enzymes.

- **Discuss the roles of complement in the immune response**
  The functions of complement are to kill target cells and to regulate inflammatory responses by enhancing phagocytosis and increasing leukocyte recruitment from the circulation.

- **Describe the role of natural killer (NK) cells and of type I interferon in immunity**
  Natural killer (NK) cells destroy virally infected cells and tumour cells using the same perforin and granzyme-dependent killing mechanism that is used by cytotoxic T lymphocytes. Type I interferon stimulates the cytocidal activity of NK cells to eliminate virus-infected cells or tumour cells with reduced MHC class I expression. Cells devoid of surface MHC

class I molecules evade CD8$^+$ T cell recognition. Killer inhibitory receptors (KIRs) and killer activator receptors (KARs) on NK cells bind to ligands on target cells and regulate signals for the NK cell to kill the target cell. If KIRs and KARs are stimulated at the same time, the inhibitory signal from the KIRs prevails and the net result is an inhibitory signal and so the target cell survives. KIRs bind to MHC class I, therefore reduced MHC I expression results in a KAR signal alone and target cell death. NK cell-deficient individuals are severely compromised in their ability to control infection by some herpes viruses.

■ **Outline the mechanisms whereby acute inflammation is resolved**
The acute inflammatory response is a highly effective and very well controlled innate immune response, terminated when the tissue is restored to the condition it was in prior to the encounter with the pathogen. This is promoted by the removal of debris by macrophages, the dissipation of chemoattractant gradients so that inflammatory cells are no longer attracted to the site, and by wound healing.

4.1   INTRODUCTION TO THE INNATE IMMUNE RESPONSE

If potentially harmful material, such as a microbial pathogen, breaches the body's natural barriers and gains access to host tissues, swift action must be taken by the host to eliminate it. The speed and magnitude of this host response will determine the extent of tissue damage or of microbial infiltration. On occasion these responses can cause damage of their own, called immunopathology, in their attempt to eliminate the initial threat. However, it is critical that this initial host response should be concerned with speed and efficacy; the short-term threat must be removed regardless of the long-term consequences of that action. Obviously, if the long-term consequences were overwhelmingly damaging to the host, evolutionary pressures would probably have produced a host response which had built-in brakes and safeguards to limit the harm to host tissues. These brakes and safeguards do in fact exist within the human immune system – the human body has an excellent system which aims to inflict the maximum damage on the foreign invader while minimizing damage to host tissues. This highly effective and very well controlled innate immune response is called acute inflammation. The acute inflammatory response is terminated when the tissue is restored to the condition it was in prior to the encounter with the pathogen.

When a site becomes infected or injured, the ensuing acute inflammatory response causes physical symptoms that are characteristic of inflammation. These symptoms are frequently referred to as the five cardinal signs of inflammation (see *Box 4.1*). They are:

1. swelling (oedema)
2. redness (erythema)
3. pain
4. heat (fever)
5. loss of function

The following sections examine how the cells and molecules of the acute inflammatory response give rise to these cardinal signs of inflammation.

4.2 INITIATION OF THE INFLAMMATORY RESPONSE

A major function of the immune system is to distinguish between harmless antigens and potentially harmful antigens, for example pathogens, and to modulate its activity accordingly. This sensing of danger (see *Box 4.2*) is carried out by molecules that are expressed on cells throughout the body, in particular on epithelial cells and on cells of the immune system. These danger-sensing molecules are called pattern recognition receptors (PRRs). The PRRs bind to molecular patterns that are common to groups of pathogens. These patterns are called pathogen-associated molecular patterns (PAMPs). PAMPs are usually microbial cell wall components, or other surface components (or nucleic acid) that are required for survival of the pathogen. PAMPs are expressed on pathogens and not on harmless antigens, therefore the immune system responds differently to pathogens than it does to harmless antigens (for example normal self cells undergoing apoptosis).

There are two main classes of PRRs: cytoplasmic PRRs and membrane-bound PRRs. Cytoplasmic PRRs include the NOD-like receptors, NOD1 and NOD2. These molecules bind to components of bacterial cell walls and, as a result, induce the production of cytokines that promote inflammation. The membrane-bound PRRs can be further subdivided into C-type lectins and toll-like receptors (TLRs).

C-type lectins recognize and bind to carbohydrates on the surfaces of pathogens. The best characterized C-type lectins are the mannose receptor and DC-SIGN, both expressed on the surfaces of macrophages and dendritic cells.

One of the most researched families of PRRs is the TLR family. Thirteen different TLRs (TLR-1–TLR-13) have been described, each of which can bind to different PAMPs of a range of viruses and bacteria and can also bind to bacterial and viral nucleic acids. Expression of TLRs can be induced on

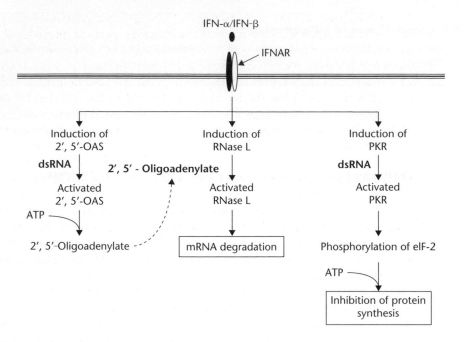

Figure 4.1
Induction of an antiviral state by type I IFN. Signalling through the IFN-α receptor (IFNAR) causes the cell to produce the enzymes protein kinase R (PKR), ribonuclease L (RNase L) and 2', 5'-oligoadenylate synthase (2', 5'-OAS). Subsequent viral infection of the cell (indicated by the presence of double-stranded (ds) RNA) activates PKR and 2', 5'-OAS. Activated PKR phosphorylates the translation initiation factor eIF-2 resulting in suppression of protein synthesis. Activated 2', 5'-OAS catalyses the synthesis of 2', 5'-oligoadenylate which activates RNase L to degrade mRNA.

a variety of cells; however, some cells constitutively express these molecules. Binding of different antigens to different TLRs and other PRRs will elicit different cellular responses. In this way the immune system is alerted not only to the presence of danger, but is also informed of the nature of the invader so that it can tailor its response to match the threat.

If a virus enters the body it must infect a host cell in order to survive. Viruses are obligate intracellular parasites and usurp the functions of host cells to make new virus particles, known as virions. Replication of many viruses results in high intracellular levels of double-stranded (ds) RNA. dsDNA binds to TLR-3 which activates the transcription factor NF-κB. Active NF-κB induces the transcription of genes for cytokines that collectively are termed type I interferon. The type I interferon, principally interferon-α (IFN-α) and IFN-β secreted by the infected cells, binds to the IFN-α receptor, IFNAR, on adjacent cells. This causes the adjacent cells to make an enzyme called protein kinase R (PKR). This 'primes' the cells adjacent to the infected cell so that they are less susceptible to viral infection (see *Figure 4.1*). Subsequent viral infection of type I IFN-primed cells activates PKR to phosphorylate the translation initiation factor eIF-2.

Phosphorylated eIF-2 is inefficient at initiating translation so protein synthesis is impaired. This reduces the number of virus particles that can be made by type I IFN-primed cells and so curtails the spread of the virus. Cells that have been primed by type I IFN also produce 2'-5' oligoadenylate which activates the enzyme RNaseL to degrade mRNA molecules within the cell. This also limits the spread of the virus within the infected tissue.

Another function of type I interferon is to stimulate the killing activity of NK cells. The cytocidal activity of NK cells is largely restricted to killing cells that have become infected with a virus, and to killing tumour cells. On their surfaces NK cells have receptors called killer inhibitory receptors (KIRs) and killer activatory receptors (KARs). When the KARs bind to their ligands on target cells they send a signal into the NK cell causing it to kill the target cell. However, if the KIRs bind to their ligands on the target cell they send a signal into the NK cell that prevents it from killing the target cell. If the KIRs and KARs are stimulated at the same time the inhibitory signal from the KIRs prevails and the net result is an inhibitory signal, i.e. no killing takes place.

The level of cell surface expression of major histocompatibility complex (MHC) class I molecules on target cells is important in controlling the reactivity of NK cells. NK cells kill virus-infected cells or tumour cells that have reduced MHC class I expression. Some viruses cause the cell that they infect to stop, or reduce, the expression of MHC class I molecules on their cell surfaces. Similarly, many tumour cells are devoid of surface MHC class I molecules. This is important because MHC class I molecules allow cytotoxic CD8$^+$ T cells to recognize and kill virus-infected cells (see *Section 5.10*). KIRs bind to MHC class I alleles. If expression of these MHC class I alleles on target cells is reduced then the NK cell will not receive an inhibitory signal via the KIRs and will only receive the activation signal via the KARs (see *Figure 4.2*). Consequently, NK cells kill cells that have decreased their cell surface expression of MHC class I molecules, so viruses and tumours do not escape the immune response. NK cells destroy virus-infected cells using the same perforin and granzyme-dependent killing mechanism that is used by cytotoxic T lymphocytes (see *Section 6.12*). NK cell-deficient individuals are severely compromised in their ability to control infections with certain herpes viruses.

Release of chemoattractants

When a virus infects a cell, that cell will release, in addition to type I IFN, an array of chemokines (see *Section 2.6*) to attract cells of the immune system to the site of infection. These chemokines bind to high affinity G protein-coupled transmembrane receptors on the surfaces of immune cells. Bacterial infection also leads to recruitment of immune cells. Cells adjacent to sites of bacterial infection respond to bacterial products by secreting chemokines. Furthermore, a secreted tripeptide peculiar to certain bacteria, called FMLP (formylmethionyl-leucyl-phenylalanine), is a highly potent chemoattractant for neutrophils. Production of chemoattractants at the site

(a)

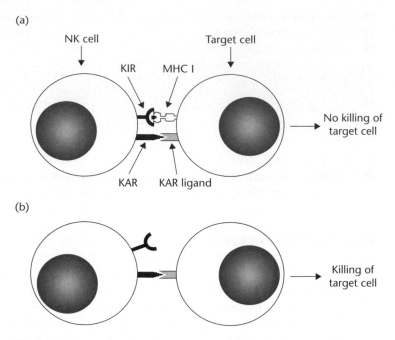

(b)

Figure 4.2
(a) When the killer inhibitory receptor (KIR) on an NK cell binds to its ligand, an MHC class I molecule (MHC I), on a target cell, a signal is transmitted into the NK cell that prevents it from killing the target cell. This inhibitory signal is dominant, so that even if a killer activatory receptor (KAR) on the same NK cell has bound to its ligand on the target cell, the NK cell still does not kill the target cell. (b) If a KAR on an NK cell binds to its ligand on a target cell in the absence of signalling via KIR, the NK cell will kill the target cell.

of infection is an important early warning system that alerts the immune system to the location of the invading pathogens. An additional chemo-attractant, called C5a, which is produced early following infection, is generated following activation of the complement pathway.

4.3 COMPLEMENT ACTIVATION

The complement system consists of a series of approximately 30 proteins including plasma proteins and membrane receptors. Many complement components are secreted as inactive precursors or proenzymes, which are activated by proteolysis. The letter C followed by a number usually indicates their name. The initial stage of complement activation is an enzyme cascade in which earlier members of the pathway activate individual components. Many of the active enzymes in the complement cascade consist of complexes of fragments of different complement components generated by proteolysis. Complement activation, or 'fixation' as it is sometimes called, can proceed by three distinct pathways:

- the classical pathway
- the alternative pathway
- the lectin pathway

The classical pathway requires the presence of antibodies, which are products of adaptive immune responses, while the alternative pathway and the lectin pathway are initiated during inflammatory responses upon contact with, for example, bacterial cell surfaces.

The functions of complement are to:

- kill target cells
- regulate inflammatory responses by enhancing phagocytosis and increasing leukocyte recruitment from the circulation

The classical pathway

The first component of the classical pathway is the C1 complex, consisting of one molecule of C1q bound to two molecules of C1r and two molecules of C1s. The classical pathway is activated when C1q binds to IgM- or IgG-containing immune complexes (see *Figure 4.3*). This leads to a conformational change in the C1 complex, which activates the serine protease activity of the C1r molecules. The active C1r molecules cleave and activate the C1s molecules, which also have serine protease activity, yielding the active C1 complex. This active C1 complex cleaves C2 and C4, producing C2b and C4b (the cleavage products C2a and C4a are released), which bind together

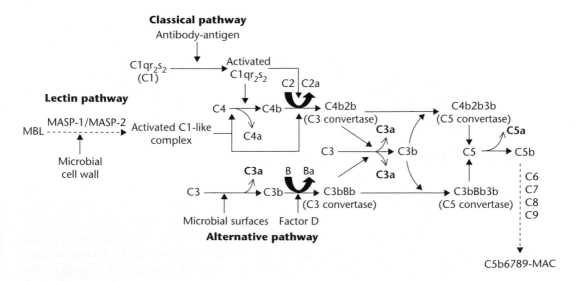

Figure 4.3
Overview of the classical, alternative and lectin pathways of complement activation. Activation of the classical pathway is initiated by antigen–antibody complexes, whereas the alternative and lectin pathways can be activated directly by microbial surfaces.

to form the classical pathway C3 convertase (C4b2b). C3 convertase cleaves C3 into C3a and C3b. C3 is the central component of all three pathways of complement activation. It is the most abundant of the complement proteins, reaching concentrations of up to 1 mg ml^{-1} of plasma during the acute phase of an immune response. Following cleavage of C3, C3a is released and C3b binds to the C3 convertase to form the C5 convertase (C4b2b3b).

The alternative pathway

The alternative pathway is initiated by spontaneous hydrolysis of the thioester bond in C3 to yield C3a and C3b. These cleavage products of C3 are unstable and are rapidly eliminated in the absence of infection. If there is a pathogen nearby, however, C3b can covalently bind to proteins or polysaccharides on the microbial surface. Surface-bound C3b will bind the plasma protein Factor B. The bound Factor B (B) is then cleaved by another plasma protein, Factor D, to give the alternative pathway C3 convertase (C3bBb) with the release of Ba. The surface-bound C3 convertase hydrolyses plasma C3, resulting in many more C3b and C3bBb molecules becoming bound to the microbial surface. This greatly amplifies the pathway. Deposition of C3b on microbial surfaces enhances the ability of phagocytes to engulf these pathogens. Some of the C3b generated by the C3 convertase will bind to the convertase to form the alternative pathway C5 convertase (C3bBb3b).

The lectin pathway

Activation of the lectin pathway is similar to classical pathway activation, with mannan-binding lectin (MBL), and sometimes ficolins, taking the place of C1q. MBL binds to mannose residues on the microbial surface. This leads to activation of the MBL-associated serine proteases, MASP-1 and MASP-2. Ficolins are homologous to MBL and activate MASP-1 and MASP-2 in a similar manner. Analogous to the active C1 complex in the classical pathway, MASP-1 and MASP-2 cleave C4 and C2. This leads to the formation of C4b2b, the same C3 convertase as in the classical pathway.

Late steps of complement activation

The late steps of complement activation are common to all three pathways. C5 convertase cleaves C5 into C5a and C5b. C5a is released and C5b recruits the complement proteins C6, C7, and C8, to the microbial surface. The C5b678 complex is anchored to the surface by the C7 and C8 components, which insert into the lipid membrane. Once C8 has bound it recruits the last member of the pathway, C9. C9 polymerizes and inserts itself through the plasma membrane, forming a cylindrical pore with a hydrophilic core through which water and ions can enter (see *Figure 4.4*). The C5b6789 complex is called the membrane attack complex (MAC). Insertion of the

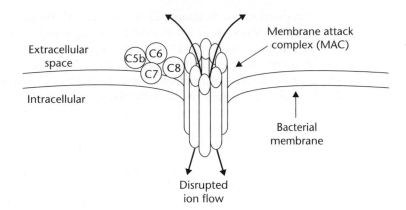

Figure 4.4
Insertion of polymerised C9 into the bacterial membrane leads to the formation of the membrane attack complex (MAC). The resulting disruption of membrane integrity leads to lysis of the bacterium.

MAC into the membrane of a target cell disrupts the normally continuous hydrophobic barrier. The passage of charged particles between the interior and the exterior of the cell cannot then be controlled. When several of these complexes are present on a single cell, the normal ionic gradients are disrupted and the cell dies. In this way, complement activation can directly curtail the spread of the pathogen. Some enveloped viruses are also susceptible to MAC-mediated lysis.

Regulation

Once complement activation gets underway it is essential that it is regulated so that excessive cell killing or inflammation is not promoted. Complement activation could cause damage to host tissues, therefore its activation is tightly regulated by complement control proteins. Some of these control proteins are present in high concentration in plasma. Other regulatory proteins are expressed on the membranes of host cells and prevent these cells from being lysed by complement. Several measures used to control complement activation are listed below.

■ The existence of complement inhibitors, especially C1 inhibitor (C1 INH), that restrict the extent of complement activation via the classical pathway by inhibiting the serine protease activity of C1r and C1s.
■ The anchoring of complement proteins to the target cell surface by attachment to antibodies (classical pathway), to focus the attack on the invading pathogen.
■ The expression of proteins on the surfaces of normal cells that interact with complement proteins to inactivate or degrade them. These factors are effective against both classical and alternative pathways of

complement activation. They are called regulators of complement activity (RCA) and they reduce the activation of C3 and C5. Decay accelerating factor (DAF or CD55) binds to the C3 convertases of both the classical pathway (C4b2b) and the alternative pathway (C3bBb) and enhances their decay. It also binds to C3b and prevents the assembly of the C5 convertase of the classical pathway (C4b2b3b) and the C5 convertase of the alternative pathway (C3bBb3b). Membrane cofactor of proteolysis (MCP or CD46) aids in the Factor I-mediated degradation of C3b to the inactive iC3b. Factor I further degrades iC3b to generate C3c and C3d. C3d remains covalently bound to the antigen and can modulate B cell responses against the antigen by binding to the B cell co-receptor (see *Section 7.7*).

■ Inhibition of the insertion of the MAC into lipid bilayer membranes. This is the function of molecules such as CD59 (inhibits C9 polymerisation) and vitronectin.

■ Proteolytic cleavage to degrade already formed active fragments. For example, C5a is rapidly inactivated by carboxypeptidase N.

Phagocytosis (see *Section 4.6*) is enhanced when complement proteins, in particular C3b, 'coat' or opsonize a foreign particle. Phagocytosis in its most basic form is a relatively non-specific phenomenon. This is because phagocytes have receptors on their surfaces, including PRRs, that allow them to bind to a wide variety of pathogens or non-self antigens. These receptors must be able to bind to a wide variety of pathogens; therefore they do not bind to all species of pathogens with high affinity. In other words, the receptors that a phagocyte uses to bind to pathogens are designed to suit a large number of pathogens but, as a consequence, these receptors do not suit any pathogen particularly well. 'Coating' the pathogen with complement greatly enhances phagocytosis because neutrophils and macrophages have a specific receptor on their surfaces called CR1. CR1 binds with high affinity to the C3b that is coating the pathogen. This greatly enhances the ability of the phagocyte to bind to and, subsequently, to ingest the foreign particle. Similarly, phagocytes have surface receptors that allow them to bind to the Fc portion of antibody molecules, allowing the phagocyte to efficiently ingest a particle that has bound antibody. Therefore the complement and antibody are acting as opsonins (see *Figure 4.5*). This function of complement is particularly important for elimination of immune complexes (antibody–antigen–complement complexes). Because of this, complement-deficient individuals do not efficiently clear immune complexes and are susceptible to immune complex diseases (see *Section 12.3*).

The recruitment of leukocytes from the circulation is enhanced by the small fragments cleaved from complement factors C3 and C5, called C3a and C5a, respectively. C5a binds to its high affinity surface receptor C5aR (CD88) on phagocytes such as neutrophils and is a potent chemoattractant for these cells. In addition, C3a and C5a cause mast cells to release the contents of their cytoplasmic granules. The enzyme carboxypeptidase B cleaves the C-terminal amino acid from C5a to form C5a des-Arg. Although C5a des-Arg is a potent neutrophil chemoattractant, unlike C5a it only

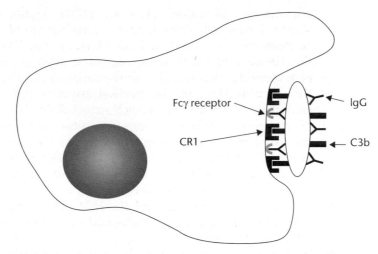

Figure 4.5
Opsonization, or coating, of microbes with IgG and C3b greatly enhances the ability of phagocytes to engulf the microbes via binding to CR1 and Fcγ receptors.

weakly stimulates mast cells to degranulate. Degranulation of mast cells plays an important role in acute inflammation.

4.4 DEGRANULATION OF MAST CELLS

With the activation of the complement cascade leading to formation of the MAC in susceptible pathogens, the immune system can curtail the spread of the invaders. The generation of C5a together with the production of chemokines and other chemoattractants at the site of the infection attracts immune cells to the infected tissue. The cells arrive via the circulation, but the infection is in the tissue. The cells must therefore get from the bloodstream into the tissue. This is where degranulation of mast cells plays an important role.

Mast cells have granules in their cytoplasm that contain a variety of biologically active mediators, including cytokines, chemokines, eicosanoids (see *Section 2.6*) and vasoactive amines. When mast cells become activated they degranulate, or empty their granules into the surrounding area. C3a and C5a, generated following activation of complement, stimulate mast cells and trigger mast cell degranulation. The vasoactive amine histamine, as well as prostaglandins (e.g. PGE_2) and leukotrienes (e.g. LTB_4) released by the activated mast cells, bind to arteriolar smooth muscle cells and cause them to relax. This causes the diameter of the arteriole to increase, a process known as vasodilation. Histamine also binds to endothelial cells lining the adjacent venules and causes them to contract. This causes an early, brief (15–30 minute) increase in vascular permeability. Spaces between the endothelial cells widen, allowing fluid to seep from the circulation into the tissues.

Mast cells also secrete the cytokines TNF-α and IL-1. Release of these cytokines by mast cells is induced not only by stimulation with C3a and C5a, but also by stimulation of TLRs on mast cells. IL-1 and TNF-α affect a variety of cells to induce many similar responses. These include fever, cytokine secretion, endothelial gene regulation, leukocyte adherence, phagocytosis, and fibroblast activation. Together they are responsible for the systemic effects of inflammation, such as loss of appetite and increased heart rate. They also induce the production of acute-phase proteins (see *Section 2.6*) such as complement components and α_1-antiproteinase inhibitor. A locally increasing concentration of IL-1 and TNF-α will cause heat, swelling, redness and pain.

IL-1 and TNF-α bind to receptors on vascular endothelial cells and induce cytoskeletal re-organization. This causes the junctions of the endothelial cells to retract. This effect takes approximately 4–6 hours and lasts in excess of 24 hours. The increase in vascular permeability allows more fluid to leave the venule and enter the tissue. This fluid is called the inflammatory exudate and its accumulation in the tissue leads to swelling. The exudate will contain more complement and will also contain bradykinin. Bradykinin is a nonameric peptide that is generated by the action of the enzyme kallikrein on high-molecular-weight kininogen. Bradykinin causes vasodilation and also acts on local nerve endings to cause pain. Like histamine, bradykinin will also cause an increase in vascular permeability.

The dilation of blood vessels by histamine, eicosanoids and other mediators (especially the plasma-derived bradykinin), increases the flow of blood to the affected tissue and leads to the redness associated with acute inflammation. Vasodilation must be strictly controlled since massive dilation of blood vessels can be harmful and can result in hypotension, which may lead to shock, loss of consciousness, or death.

It is important to note that stimulation with C3a and C5a are not the only mechanisms whereby mast cells can be activated. Mast cells express TLRs on their surface and can be stimulated directly by certain antigens. In addition, a class of antibody called IgE can bind to the surface of mast cells and cause the mast cells to degranulate if the IgE antibody binds to antigen. This is the major mechanism responsible for mast cell degranulation during allergies (see *Section 9.2*).

Activated mast cells also release chemokines such as IL-8. IL-8, C5a and LTB$_4$ all attract leukocytes to the infected site. As well as allowing immunologically active molecules to enter the tissue, an extremely important aspect of the increase in vascular permeability is that it allows activated leukocytes to squeeze between the cells lining the blood vessel and get to the site of infection. This process is called extravasation.

4.5   EXTRAVASATION OF LEUKOCYTES

The release of C5a, IL-8 and LTB$_4$ attracts leukocytes to the site of the infection. The leukocytes arriving via the circulation must stop and pass through the vascular endothelial cell layer and enter the tissue in order to attack the

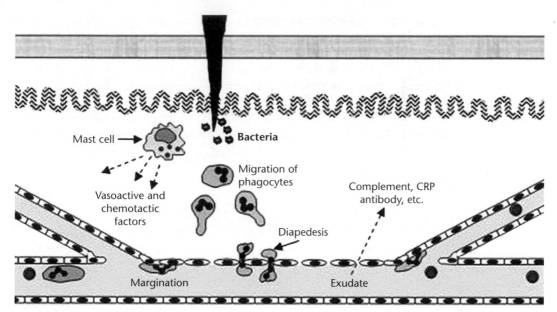

Figure 4.6
Neutrophils are attracted by chemotactic factors produced at sites of infection. On reaching the infected area, the neutrophils move to the wall of the blood vessel (margination) and roll along it until the adhesive contacts between the neutrophils and the vascular endothelial cells are sufficiently strong to bring the neutrophil to a halt (arrest). The neutrophils then pull themselves through gaps in the endothelial layer into the infected tissue (diapedesis).

pathogen (see *Figure 4.6*). This is facilitated by the action of IL-1 and TNF-α on vascular endothelial cells. When exposed to these cytokines the endothelial cells rapidly respond in the following ways.

- They alter shape, becoming more circular. This allows intercellular ('between cells') gaps to form.
- They release cytokines and chemokines (such as IL-8), which increase the rate and extent of the inflammatory response. In this way endothelial cells can amplify the inflammatory response.
- They produce the mediators PAF and nitric oxide (NO), both of which enhance vasodilation, bringing more leukocytes to the area.
- They express adhesion molecules, which make their luminal surfaces 'sticky'. This allows infiltrating leukocytes to bind tightly to the endothelial cells and 'pull' themselves through the gaps between them.

Adhesion molecules

There are four main families of adhesion molecules expressed on the surface of cells (see *Figure 4.7*). Integrins are largest of these groups and are found in the form of membrane glycoproteins that are made up of two subunits – α and β. Importantly, integrins can exist in two states – resting and active.

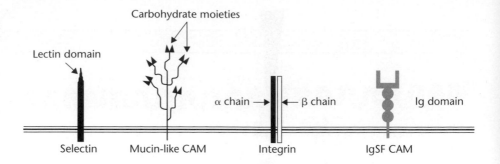

Figure 4.7
Four major families of cell adhesion molecules (CAMs) are selectins, mucin-like CAMs, integrins, and immunoglobulin gene superfamily (IgSF) CAMs.

When a cell becomes activated, an intracellular signalling pathway is initiated that ultimately increases the affinity of the integrins. This usually happens when a chemokine binds to a chemokine receptor on the cell that expresses the integrin. This 'activation step' allows the integrin to bind with high affinity to its counter-receptor. This step is crucial to allow the infiltrating cells to resist the shear force in the bloodstream and 'arrest' their movement on the vessel wall.

Immunoglobulin gene superfamily members contain, as a basic structural unit, regions of polypeptide sequence that resemble immunoglobulin domains. Members of this family include the cellular adhesion molecules (CAMs), e.g. intercellular adhesion molecule-1 (ICAM-1). All members of this group are expressed or induced on the surface of vascular endothelium. These molecules bind to integrins. Mucin-like cell adhesion molecules are a group of serine- and threonine-rich cell surface proteins, such as sialyl-Lewis^X (CD15), that are highly glycosylated. These molecules bind to selectins. Selectins have a membrane-distal lectin-like domain that allows them to bind to particular carbohydrate ligands on leukocytes and endothelial cells.

The process of extravasation of leukocytes into tissues is a four-step process. These steps are:

1. rolling – the leukocyte rolls along the wall of the blood vessel
2. tethering – the leukocyte makes firmer adhesive contacts with the endothelial cells; this leads to:
3. arrest – when the leukocyte stops due to activation of integrin molecules (see *Figure 4.8*); just prior to:
4. diapedesis – crossing the endothelial monolayer.

The steps outlined above allow inflammatory cells, predominantly neutrophils, to enter the infected tissue during an acute inflammatory response. Once in the tissue the neutrophil attempts to eliminate the

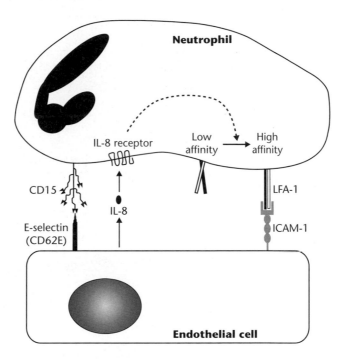

Figure 4.8
The initial, weak adhesive interactions between neutrophils and endothelial cells are due to binding of the mucin-like CAM CD15 on neutrophils to E-selectin (CD62E) on endothelial cells. Activated endothelial cells produce IL-8 which causes the integrin LFA-1 on neutrophils to adopt a conformation that binds to ICAM-1, an IgSF CAM expressed by activated endothelial cells, with high affinity. This high affinity interaction causes the neutrophils to arrest on the surface of vascular endothelial cells.

pathogen via phagocytosis, a process that is enhanced by IL-1, IL-8 and TNF-α.

4.6 PHAGOCYTOSIS

Phagocytosis is defined as the engulfment of solid particles by a cell (see *Box 4.3*). When a neutrophil encounters a pathogen, it sends out cytoplasmic processes called lamellipodia (or pseudopodia) to surround the pathogen and engulf it (see *Figure 4.9*). This process is made much more efficient if the pathogen is 'coated' or opsonized with complement or antibody. As explained above (see *Section 4.3*), this is because on its surface the neutrophil has receptors that bind to complement and receptors that bind to antibody. This enables the neutrophil to efficiently take up anything that has antibody or complement bound to it. This also helps to focus the phagocyte's activity on substances that have been recognized as being non-self.

After ingestion, the pathogen is enclosed within a vacuole, called a phagosome, inside the neutrophil. Neutrophils have two major mechanisms for

Box 4.3 Phagocytes

The phagocytic function was first described by Ilya Metchnikoff, who also coined the term phago-cyte. He shared the Nobel Prize for medicine with Paul Ehrlich in 1908.

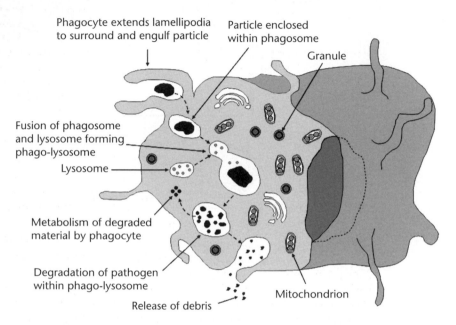

Phagocyte extends lamellipodia
to surround and engulf particle

Particle enclosed
within phagosome

Granule

Fusion of phagosome
and lysosome forming
phago-lysosome

Lysosome

Metabolism of degraded
material by phagocyte

Degradation of pathogen
within phago-lysosome

Release of debris

Mitochondrion

Figure 4.9
Phagocytosis and subsequent degradation of a particle by a neutrophil. The degraded material can cross the membrane of the phago-lysosome and be metabolized by the phagocyte. Non-utilizable material is released as debris.

killing ingested pathogens. The first mechanism involves activation of the respiratory burst. This requires the assembly of the multimolecular nicoti-namide adenine dinucleotide phosphate (NADPH – the reduced form) oxidase enzyme complex. This complex consists of two membrane-associ-ated proteins, gp91^{PHOX} and p22^{PHOX} (collectively termed cytochrome b$_{245}$) as well as several cytosolic components. NADPH oxidase catalyses the produc-tion of superoxide (O$_2^-$) from oxygen and NADPH (see *Figure 4.10*). This ultimately leads to destruction of the pathogen by oxidative attack with hydrogen peroxide (generated by superoxide dismutase) and hypochlorite ions (the active ingredient of household bleach) generated by the enzyme myeloperoxidase.

The second mechanism of pathogen destruction during phagocytosis is through digestion with lysosomal enzymes. These are delivered to the phagosome following fusion of this vacuole with lysosomes. Acidification of

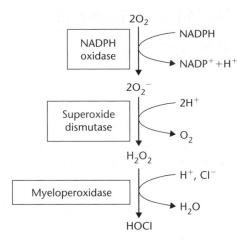

Figure 4.10
The superoxide generated by NADPH oxidase is converted into hydrogen peroxide by superoxide dismutase. The enzyme myeloperoxidase converts this hydrogen peroxide into hypochlorous acid.

the contents of the phago-lysosome, with the assistance of an H^+–ATPase pump, is an essential early step in non-oxygen dependent killing because lysosomal enzymes are active only in low pH environments (optimum pH 4.5–5.0). There are up to 50 different lysosomal enzymes that include lysozyme, nucleases, proteinases, cathepsins, glucuronidases, glycases, lipases, phosphatases, phospholipases and sulfatases. While bacterial cell walls are a major target of the enzymes, e.g. lysozyme degrades cell wall peptidoglycan, together they can catalyse the breakdown of all classes of biological macromolecules to small molecules. The small molecules can be transported across the phago-lysosomal membrane into the phagocyte's cytoplasm and contribute to its metabolism (see *Figure 4.9*). Cationic proteins from lysosomes also contribute to the bactericidal environment of the phago-lysosome.

4.7 RESOLUTION OF INFLAMMATION

Resolution of inflammation requires that the inflammatory cells be removed and that the tissue that hosted the inflammatory event returns to its pre-inflammatory state. Following phagocytic clearance of pathogens or other foreign material, the neutrophils undergo apoptotic cell death *in situ*. Dead neutrophils are a major constituent of pus. The dead, and dying, neutrophils are removed by infiltrating macrophages. Apoptotic cell death results in exposure of the phospholipid phosphatidylserine on the external surface of the neutrophil plasma membrane. This is recognized by specific receptors on infiltrating macrophages allowing the macrophages to engulf and digest the apoptotic neutrophils. These macrophages leave the tissue via the lymphatic drainage. The activity of released neutrophil proteases is counteracted by inhibitors, for example, the acute phase protein α_1-antiproteinase inhibits the activity of neutrophil elastase. Resolution of acute inflammation is further promoted by the dissipation of chemoattractant gradients and the induction of inhibitors of TLR activity.

Any tissue damage that led to, or resulted from, the inflammatory response must also be repaired to restore the tissue to its pre-inflammatory state. Wound healing consists of three phases:

- proliferation
- maturation
- remodelling

During the proliferation phase, there is growth of new blood vessels into the wound bed (angiogenesis) to supply oxygen to the healing tissue. Fibroblasts infiltrate the wound and deposit collagen (predominantly type III) and other extracellular matrix components. Granulation tissue, consisting of new blood vessels, endothelial cells and fibroblasts, fills the wound area and epithelial cells proliferate and migrate across this newly formed tissue. After about a week the wound begins to contract.

During the maturation and remodelling phases of wound healing, type III collagen is replaced by the stronger type I collagen and the collagen fibres are rearranged. The wound loses its red appearance due to the regression of unnecessary blood vessels.

Chronic inflammation

If the acute inflammatory response is not sufficient to eliminate the pathogen or harmful substance then the inflammatory reaction will mature into a chronic inflammatory response. Chronic inflammatory lesions are characterized by the accumulation of monocytes/macrophages and T cells. To allow this chronic inflammatory response to take place, antigenic material must be removed from the acutely inflamed site and taken to secondary lymphoid tissues. This is an important link between the innate and adaptive immune responses. This process will be examined in *Chapter 5*.

SUGGESTED FURTHER READING

Creagh, E.M. and O'Neill, L.A.J. (2006) TLRs, NLRs and RLRs: a trinity of pathogen sensors that co-operate in innate immunity. *Trends Immunol.* **27**: 352–357.

Kinet, J.-P. (2007) The essential role of mast cells in orchestrating inflammation. *Immunol. Rev.* **217**: 5–7.

Kono, H. and Rock, K.L. (2008) How dying cells alert the immune system to danger. *Nature Rev. Immunol.* **8**: 279–289.

Li, J., Chen, J. and Kirsner, R. (2007) Pathophysiology of acute wound healing. *Clinics Dermatol.* **25**: 9–18.

Nathan, C. (2006) Neutrophils and immunity: challenges and opportunities. *Nature Rev. Immunol.* **6**: 173–182.

Serhan, C.N., Brain, S.D., Buckley, C.D., *et al.* (2007) Resolution of inflammation: state of the art, definitions and terms. *FASEB J.* **21**: 325–332.

Stuart, L.M. and Ezekowitz, R.A.B. (2005) Phagocytosis: elegant complexity. *Immunity* **22**: 539–550.

Takeuchi, O. and Akira, S. (2007) Recognition of viruses by innate immunity. *Immunol. Rev.* **220**: 214–224.

SELF-ASSESSMENT QUESTIONS

1. What are the characteristic signs of acute inflammation?
2. What are the immunological processes which give rise to the observable characteristic signs of acute inflammation?
3. What is phagocytosis?
4. Describe the steps involved in the process of extravasation of leukocytes into tissues.
5. How does NK cell deficiency cause notable problems in an individual?
6. What is immunopathology?
7. What role does FMLP have in the immune response?
8. Name the three complement activation pathways.
9. What is the function of complement in the immune system?
10. Discuss the role of mast cell degranulation in acute inflammation.

Antigen acquisition and presentation

Learning objectives

After studying this chapter you should confidently be able to:

■ **Discuss how antigen is acquired in peripheral sites and taken to lymphoid tissues**

Antigen is acquired in peripheral sites by antigen-presenting cells (APCs). APCs transport the antigen and present it on major histocompatibility complex (MHC) molecules to lymphocytes in lymphoid tissue. Although monocytes/macrophages and B cells can function as APCs, dendritic cells (DCs) are the most efficient APCs and are particularly numerous at potential sites of entry of pathogens such as the skin and mucosae. There are a number of different subsets of DCs located throughout the body: epidermal Langerhans cells (skin); interdigitating DCs (paracortex of lymph nodes); marginal DCs (spleen); and thymic DCs. During a process known as immune surveillance, DCs migrate through peripheral tissues, constantly sampling their environment by pinocytosis and phagocytosis, in search of antigen to present to T cells.

■ **Describe the phenotypic and functional differences between mature and immature dendritic cells**

Immature DCs cannot activate naïve T cells; they require an encounter with antigen which results in changes in expression of many surface molecules. DCs prepare antigen by a process called antigen processing which involves digestion of antigen into small peptide fragments. The DC then presents the peptides, bound to MHC molecules, on its surface, where they can be recognized by T cells.

■ **Describe the structure and function of MHC molecules and understand the concept of MHC restriction**

MHC class I molecules consist of a polypeptide heavy chain (the α chain) and a small protein called β_2-microglobulin (β_2M). The heavy chain comprises three domains (α_1, α_2 and α_3). The α_1 and α_2 domains fold together to form a pocket where the antigenic peptide is bound. The α_3 domain has a binding site for CD8, explaining why CD8$^+$ T cells specifically recognize antigen presented on MHC class I molecules. MHC class II molecules have two peptide chains (α and β) each of which has two domains. The β_2 domain has a binding site for CD4, explaining why CD4$^+$ T cells specifically recognize antigen presented on MHC class II molecules. The α_1 and β_1 domains fold together to form a peptide-binding groove that is very similar to that found in MHC class I molecules. A T cell only recognizes antigen when it is presented by an APC that has a particular MHC molecule, a fundamental immunological concept that is termed MHC restriction. MHC restriction applies both to CD8$^+$ T cells recognizing MHC class I + antigen and to CD4$^+$ T cells recognizing MHC class II + antigen.

■ **Describe the pathways whereby antigen is processed and presented to T cells**

There are two major pathways by which antigens are processed and presented to T cells: the endogenous and exogenous pathways. The pathway that is used is determined by the source of the antigen. After the endogenous pathway of antigen processing, an MHC class I molecule with bound peptide is expressed on the surface of the APC cell and is recognized by the TCR of a CD8$^+$ T cell. Alternatively, the exogenous pathway results in presentation of peptide bound to an MHC class II molecule on an APC to the TCR of CD4$^+$ T cells. In addition to these major pathways of antigen presentation, a subset of dendritic cells can present peptides derived from endocytosed antigens on MHC class I molecules, via a process termed cross-presentation.

5.1 INTRODUCTION TO ANTIGEN ACQUISITION AND PRESENTATION

In the previous chapter the early, innate response against invading microbes was discussed. Although important in curtailing the spread of infections, innate responses usually cannot eliminate infectious organisms. Adaptive immune responses, mediated by T and B lymphocytes, are usually required to ensure this. Adaptive responses are initiated when antigen is presented to lymphocytes in organized lymphoid tissues by antigen-presenting cells (APCs). How antigen is acquired by APCs and presented to lymphocytes in peripheral lymphoid tissues will be discussed in this chapter.

5.2 ACQUISITION OF ANTIGEN

Activation of T cells, in particular of CD4$^+$ T cells, is crucial for generation of effective adaptive immune responses. T cells can only become activated when antigen is presented to them, on MHC molecules, by APCs. Therefore a critical step in the induction of an adaptive immune response is the acquisition of antigen.

Foreign antigen would usually enter the body via the skin, the respiratory tract or the gastrointestinal tract. Antigens injected directly into the bloodstream (e.g. arthropod-borne infections) are usually picked up by APCs in the spleen and presented to lymphocytes in that lymphoid organ. Otherwise, foreign antigens entering the tissues must be picked up and carried to peripheral lymphoid tissues where adaptive immune responses are initiated. The epithelia at the major portals of entry for antigen contain specialized APCs belonging to the dendritic cell (DC) lineage. Although monocytes/macrophages and B cells can also function as APCs, DCs are the most efficient APCs in the human body.

5.3 ANTIGEN UPTAKE BY DENDRITIC CELLS

DCs are a heterogeneous population of APCs found throughout the body. DCs are so named because they have extensive dendrite-like appendages that allow them to interact simultaneously with multiple lymphocytes. Generally, DCs are subdivided into myeloid DCs and plasmacytoid DCs (pDCs; also called lymphoid DCs), although there is considerable heterogeneity within these subclasses. DC subsets can be distinguished based on surface molecule expression, function, and anatomical localization. They include epidermal Langerhans cells (skin), interdigitating DCs (paracortex of lymph nodes), marginal DCs (spleen) and thymic DCs. Different DC subsets exhibit different functions, especially in the differentiation of T cells into different T cell subsets. DCs are particularly numerous at potential sites of entry of pathogens, such as the skin and mucosae.

DCs migrate into peripheral tissues, constantly sampling their environment by pinocytosis and phagocytosis, in search of antigen to present to T cells. This is known as immune surveillance. During an acute inflammatory response, DCs in the tissue will pick up antigen and carry it via lymphatic vessels to lymph nodes for presentation to T cells (see *Figure 5.1*). However, DCs are more than non-discriminating phagocytes. They express PPRs (see

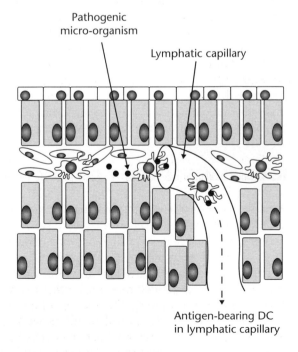

Figure 5.1
Dendritic cells pick up antigen in peripheral tissues and carry it via lymphatic vessels to draining lymph nodes.

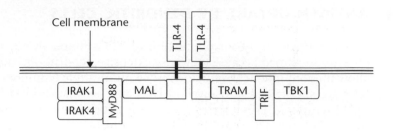

Figure 5.2
Most TLRs function as homodimers, although TLR-2 can form heterodimers with TLR-1 and TLR-6. Signalling through TLR-4 involves the adaptor molecules Mal and MyD88 (myeloid differentiation primary response gene 88) which recruit members of the interleukin-1 receptor-associated kinase (IRAK) family. TLR-4 can also use the adaptor molecules TRIF (TIR-domain-containing adapter-inducing interferon-β) and TRAM (TRIF-related adaptor molecule) to recruit the enzyme TBK-1 (TANK-binding kinase 1) to the receptor.

Section 4.2) that allow them to distinguish, at least at a gross level, between harmless substances and potentially harmful material. DCs express a variety of PRRs including the mannose receptor, DC-SIGN and 10 different TLRs. Since TLRs exist as dimers (see *Figure 5.2*) of either the same family member or of different family members, this allows macrophages and dendritic cells to interact with a wide variety of pathogens. Neutrophils, B cells and mast cells express a smaller number of TLRs.

Prior to their encounter with antigen, DCs remain in an immature state. In the absence of inflammatory signals, immature dendritic cells traffic through the blood, tissues and lymph. In this state they will actively engulf material, but with limited ability to present antigen to T cells, they are incapable of causing T cells to become activated. The following section discusses the requirements for activation of a naïve T cell.

5.4   REQUIREMENTS FOR T CELL ACTIVATION

A naïve T cell is a T cell that has not previously been activated. For a naïve T cell (either a $CD4^+$ T cell or a $CD8^+$ T cell) to become activated, it requires two signals (see *Figure 5.3*). The first signal (signal 1) comes via the TCR–CD3 complex when it interacts with MHC + peptide. The second signal (signal 2, also called co-stimulation) is transmitted via a molecule called CD28 on the T cell, when it binds to its counter-receptor on the APC. The counter-receptor for CD28 belongs to a family of molecules called the B7 family. The main B7 family members are B7.1 (CD80) and B7.2 (CD86), but other family members include B7-H (CD274), B7-H2 (CD275) and B7-H3 (CD276). This chapter will discuss mainly B7-1 and B7-2, referring to them collectively as B7. When CD28 on the T cell binds to B7 on the APC the T cell receives signal 2. Only when a naïve T cell receives both signal 1

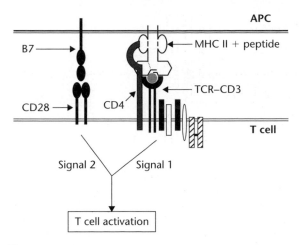

Figure 5.3
A naïve T cell requires two signals before it can become activated. Signal 1 is transmitted via the TCR–CD3 complex when it binds to an MHC–peptide complex on the surface of an antigen-presenting cell (APC). Signal 2 is transmitted via CD28 when it binds to its counter-receptor B7 on the APC.

and signal 2 will it become activated. However, a T cell that has previously been activated can be re-activated by signal 1 alone without the presence of signal 2.

If a naïve T cell receives signal 1 without signal 2, not only does it not respond, but also it is rendered incapable of responding to that antigen ever again. This state is called anergy and the T cell is said to be anergic. This is thought to play a key role in preventing reactions against self. As most cells in the body do not express B7, any naïve T cells recognizing antigen presented by most cells are rendered anergic. This is a major mechanism whereby potentially self-reactive T cells, not deleted in the thymus, are 'silenced' in the periphery. Silencing, or deletion, of T cells in the periphery is termed peripheral tolerance to distinguish it from central tolerance (see *Sections 3.6* and *10.2*).

5.5 DENDRITIC CELL MATURATION

As indicated above, immature DCs cannot activate naïve T cells. This is because:

- immature DCs have low levels of MHC on their surfaces and so provide little of signal 1
- immature DCs have little or no B7 on their surfaces and so cannot provide signal 2

The situation changes after a DC encounters antigen, or more correctly after it encounters potentially harmful antigen. After encounter with potentially

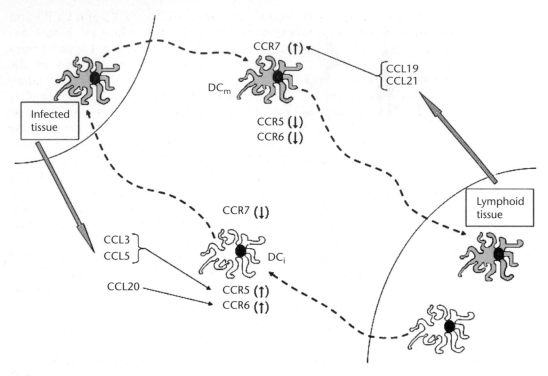

Figure 5.4
Immature DCs (DC$_i$) express high levels of CCR5 and CCR6 which allows them to respond to the inflammatory chemokines CCL3, CCL5 and CCL20 produced at sites of inflammation. Following maturation, mature DCs (DC$_m$) decrease surface expression of CCR5 and CCR6 and instead express high levels of CCR7. This allows them to migrate to lymphoid tissues in response to the chemokines CCL19 and CCL21.

harmful antigen the DC differentiates into a mature DC. A mature DC has high levels of MHC class II and B7 on its surface, as well as other adhesion molecules that will allow it to bind tightly to antigen-specific T cells. Unlike the immature DC, the mature DC is not actively phagocytic; it focuses its energy on processing and presenting the potentially harmful antigen it has taken up. Another important difference between immature and mature DCs is the responsiveness to particular chemokines. Major chemokines that are produced at sites of infection (termed inflammatory chemokines) include:

- CCL3
- CCL5
- CCL20

Immature DCs express receptors for these chemokines; the receptors CCR1 and CCR5 each bind the chemokines CCL3 and CCL5, whereas CCR6 binds the chemokine CCL20. Thus production of CCL3, CCL5, and CCL20 at sites of infection causes chemotaxis of immature DCs towards those sites (see *Figure 5.4*).

When DCs mature, they lose expression of CCR1, CCR5 and CCR6 and start to express the chemokine receptor CCR7. CCR7 binds to chemokines CCL19 and CCL21. CCL19 and CCL21 are frequently referred to as homeostatic chemokines, as they are constitutively produced by cells in the paracortex of lymph nodes (as well as the T cell areas of other secondary lymphoid tissues). Because of this, homeostatic chemokines regulate leukocyte migration through secondary lymphoid tissues. Since mature DCs lose expression of CCR1, CCR5, and CCR6 they are no longer attracted to the infected site, as they can no longer respond to the inflammatory chemokines produced there. Expression of CCR7 by mature DCs causes them to migrate towards the draining lymph node that is producing CCL19 and CCL21. Thus, the alteration in chemokine receptor expression that accompanies DC maturation directs DCs away from the inflammatory site and towards lymphoid tissue where they will present their antigenic cargo within their MHC molecule to antigen-specific receptors on lymphocytes.

One of the important signals involved in DC maturation is transmitted via the PRRs after they interact with PAMPs (see *Figure 5.5*). Stimulation of TLRs on DCs causes an increase in surface expression of B7 (in particular B7-1). Other important signals for DC maturation include:

- stimulation by IFN-α/β, which is made by cells after they become infected with a virus
- TNF-α and IL-1 which are both released by activated mast cells
- opsonized bacteria binding to complement receptors on immature DC

Thus, signals generated during acute inflammation can also induce DCs to mature after they have taken up antigen. In this manner the innate response is promoting the initiation of the adaptive response and possibly even the type of adaptive response that is generated.

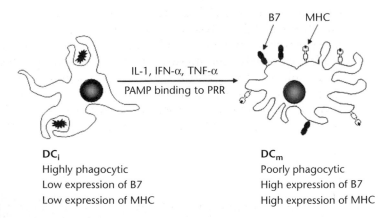

DC$_i$
Highly phagocytic
Low expression of B7
Low expression of MHC

DC$_m$
Poorly phagocytic
High expression of B7
High expression of MHC

Figure 5.5
DC maturation can be induced by inflammatory cytokines or by PRRs binding to PAMPs. Unlike immature DCs (DC$_i$), mature DCs (DC$_m$) are poorly phagocytic and express high surface levels of MHC and co-stimulatory molecules.

When immature DCs get signals to mature, they leave the tissue. In addition to the alteration in chemokine receptor expression discussed above, migration out of tissues is partially due to down-regulation of surface cell adhesion molecules that allow DCs to stay in the tissue. The DCs migrate via lymphatic vessels to the regional, or draining, lymph node. On the way to the lymph node, the DCs prepare the antigen that they have taken up so that it can be recognized by T cells. This process is called antigen processing and it involves the digestion of the antigen into small peptide fragments. The DC then presents these peptides, bound to MHC molecules, on its surface where they can be recognized by T cells.

5.6   THE MAJOR HISTOCOMPATIBILITY COMPLEX

The major histocompatibility complex (MHC) is located on the long arm of chromosome 6 in humans and spans approximately 4 Mb of DNA. As suggested by the name, MHC molecules constitute the major determinants of whether organ transplants are accepted or rejected (see *Box 5.1*). Organ rejection is a normal, albeit undesired, immune response directed against non-self MHC molecules (i.e. the MHC of the organ donor). In humans the MHC gene products are called human leukocyte antigens (HLA) as they were first identified on leukocytes. MHC genes are usually classified into three subgroups (see *Figure 5.6*).

Box 5.1 The MHC

In the 1940s George Snell generated strains of mice that were genetically identical except at the region we now call the MHC. Snell used these MHC-congenic mice to demonstrate that this region was the main genetic determinant of graft rejection.

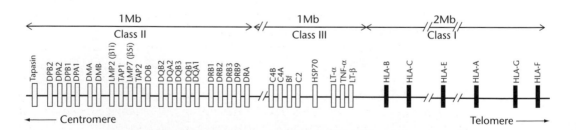

Figure 5.6
Organization of the human MHC on chromosome 6 showing the location of the MHC class I, class II and class III genes. In addition to MHC class II molecules, the MHC class II region encodes other proteins involved in antigen processing and presentation, including tapasin, TAP-1, TAP-2, HLA-DM and the immunoproteasome components β1i (LMP2) and β5i (LMP7). The MHC class III region encodes several proteins that are involved in immune responses such as the complement components C2 and C4 as well as factor B. Lymphotoxin (LT)-α, LT-β and TNF-α also are encoded in the MHC class III region.

MHC class I genes

These encode the MHC class I molecules that present antigens to CD8$^+$ T cells. There are three MHC class I loci in humans; HLA-A, HLA-B and HLA-C. The MHC class Ib molecule HLA-E is also encoded in this region.

MHC class II genes

This region encodes the MHC class II molecules that present antigens to CD4$^+$ T cells. In humans the MHC class II molecules are called:

- HLA-DP
- HLA-DQ
- HLA-DR

This region also encodes molecules that are involved in antigen processing and presentation to T cells, including HLA-DO, HLA-DM, TAP-1, TAP-2, tapasin, and components of a large cytosolic protease complex called the proteasome.

MHC class III genes

The MHC class III region is located between the MHC class I and MHC class II regions. It encodes several proteins involved in immunity, such as:

- TNF-α
- complement components C2, C4 and factor B

In addition, the MHC class III region encodes other proteins that have no clear known role in immunity. MHC class III genes are unrelated to MHC class I and II genes.

The function of MHC class I and II molecules is to present peptide epitopes to the TCR of reactive T cells. T cells are unable to recognize antigen unless it is processed and presented to them on MHC molecules. Thus MHC molecules determine what it is that T cells respond to, so MHC genes are sometimes called immune response genes.

The MHC is the most polymorphic locus in mammals, and so there are a great many alleles (slightly different versions of the same gene) of MHC class I and II within the population. For example, hundreds of alleles of HLA-B have been identified. The amino acid differences between these allelic forms are not dispersed equally throughout the primary sequence but are concentrated in the region of the molecule that is responsible for binding the peptide for presentation to T cells.

5.7 FUNCTION OF MHC MOLECULES

The function of MHC molecules is to present peptide antigen to T lympho-cytes. The research that led to this discovery was performed in the late 1960s by Peter Doherty and Rolf Zinkernagel (see *Box 5.2*). Their experiments showed that any given T cell only recognizes antigen when that antigen is presented by an APC that has a particular MHC molecule. Recognition by that T cell is said to be restricted by that particular MHC molecule. This fundamental immunological concept is termed MHC restriction, and is key to understanding adaptive immune responses. MHC restriction applies both to CD8$^+$ T cells recognizing MHC class I + antigen and to CD4$^+$ T cells recognizing MHC class II + antigen.

Box 5.2 MHC molecules present peptide antigen to T lymphocytes

A paper published in 1974 by Rolf Zinkernagel and Peter Doherty demonstrated that virus-specific cytotoxic T cells would only kill infected target cells if those target cells expressed the 'correct' MHC molecule. They shared the Nobel Prize for this work in 1996.

The experiments of Zinkernagel and Doherty demonstrated that virus-specific T cells would only respond against a virus if that virus was presented by an APC with the appropriate MHC molecule. A series of elegant experiments by Alain Townsend and colleagues provided the next leap forward in understanding this process (see *Box 5.3*). By using smaller and smaller pieces of a virus in his experiments, Townsend showed that the entire virus did not have to be presented by the APC in order for the T cell to respond against it. He went on to demonstrate that virus-specific T cells were able to respond against APCs (with the appropriate MHC) in the presence of short peptides derived from the virus. This suggested that MHC molecules presented small peptides from the virus to the TCR of the responding T cells. The ultimate confirmation of this result was obtained with the elucidation of the crystal structure of an MHC molecule with a bound peptide within it.

Box 5.3 MHC molecules present short peptides to the TCR of responding T cells

Alain Townsend was studying the recognition of target cells by cytotoxic T cells that were specific for influenza nucleoprotein (NP). He found that, by expressing shorter versions of NP in target cells, the entire protein was not necessary for cytotoxic T cells to be able to recognize the target cell. By using shorter and shorter fragments of NP he was able to demonstrate that the NP-specific T cells were actually recognizing a short peptide fragment of NP presented by the target cell.

5.8 STRUCTURE OF MHC CLASS I MOLECULES

MHC class I molecules are expressed on the surfaces of virtually all nucleated cells in the body with the notable exception of neurons. They consist of a heavy chain of 45 kDa (the α chain) that is non-covalently associated with a small 12 kDa protein called β_2-microglobulin (β_2M) (see *Figure 5.7*).

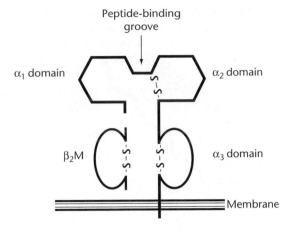

Peptide-binding groove

α_1 domain

α_2 domain

β_2M

α_3 domain

Membrane

Figure 5.7
The MHC class I molecule consists of a heavy chain that is non-covalently associated with β_2-microglobulin. The peptide binding groove is formed by the folding of the α_1 and α_2 domains of the molecule. The binding site for CD8 is located in the α_3 domain.

Unlike the MHC class I heavy chain, β_2M is not encoded within the MHC locus.

The class I heavy chain has a three domain structure. The α_1 and α_2 domains are distal from the cell membrane, whereas the α_3 domain is membrane-proximal. The α_3 domain is a classic immunoglobulin-like domain. This domain also has a binding site for CD8, explaining why CD8$^+$ T cells specifically recognize antigen presented on MHC class I molecules.

The structures of the α_1 and α_2 domains are quite different. They fold together to form a pocket where the antigenic peptide is bound. This pocket is often called the peptide-binding groove. The walls of the groove are formed by regions of α-helical protein structure, with the floor composed of β-pleated sheet. The peptide-binding groove is closed at both ends, limiting the size of peptides that can bind to MHC class I molecules (see *Figure 5.8*). Most of the differences between allelic variants of MHC class I (and between alleles of MHC class II) are concentrated in amino acid residues that line the peptide-binding groove. Consequently, the peptide-binding grooves of different MHC alleles are 'shaped' differently, therefore different MHC alleles will bind different peptide epitopes. Large numbers of molecules of a specific allele of MHC class I can be purified and treated with acid to remove the peptides from the peptide-binding grooves. Amino acid sequencing of the peptides demonstrates that:

■ the peptides are all approximately the same size (8–10 amino acids long)
■ at most positions the sequences of the peptides are very different from one another
■ at selected positions the sequences of the peptides are the same, or very similar

The sequences of the peptides are generally very different from one another at most positions because any MHC molecule has to be able to bind many different peptides. This is important because T cells can only respond against antigens that are presented by MHC molecules. Therefore, for T cells

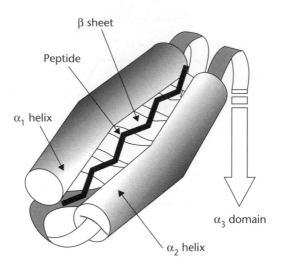

Figure 5.8
The peptide binding groove of class I molecules is restricted at both ends. This limits
the size of peptides that can bind to MHC class I molecules.

to be able to respond against a wide variety of pathogens, MHC molecules
must be able to present a wide variety of peptide antigens from those
pathogens.

Viewing the bound peptide in the groove of an MHC class I molecule
side-on reveals that some of the amino acid side chains in the bound peptide
point up towards the TCR. In the example shown (see *Figure 5.9*), that
would be amino acids 1, 3, 4, 6 and 8. It is a combination of these amino
acids and the surface of the MHC molecule that the TCR recognizes. Some
of the amino acids point down into the peptide-binding groove. In the
example shown they are residues 2 and 9. These are the amino acids that
allow the peptide to fit into the peptide-binding groove. For a peptide to be
able to bind to this class I molecule, that peptide must have certain amino
acid residues at positions 2 and 9. These residues 'anchor' the peptide in the
peptide-binding groove and are referred to as anchor residues. The arrange-
ment of the anchor residues is called the peptide-binding motif for that class
I molecule. There are usually only two or three anchor residues required for
binding to any given MHC molecule, and the anchor residues are different
for different MHC molecules. In the example given, if residue 2 of the
bound peptide is alanine and 9 is valine, then the peptide-binding motif for
this molecule is X–A–X–X–X–X–X–X–V, where X could be any amino acid.
All peptides binding to this molecule would have to conform to this motif.

Knowledge of the peptide-binding motifs for MHC molecules allows
computer-aided scanning of sequences of pathogens and prediction of
which epitopes from that pathogen are likely to be presented by those MHC

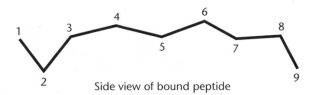

Side view of bound peptide

Figure 5.9
A side view of a peptide as it would be bound in the peptide binding groove of an MHC class I molecule. The amino acid residues at positions 1, 3, 4, 6 and 8 are pointing upwards and would be available to interact with a TCR. The amino acids at positions 2 and 9 point downwards and would serve to anchor this peptide in the peptide binding groove of the MHC class I molecule.

molecules. For several years there has been considerable interest in using this information to generate peptide-based vaccines to combat infectious diseases.

It is extremely important to have many different types of MHC molecules within the population. A pathogen would only have to mutate an amino acid residue at one of the anchor positions for a particular MHC class I molecule to be unable to present that peptide. Having multiple MHC class I molecules in the population (each with different binding motifs) ensures that some members of the population will be able to present an antigen from that pathogen, ensuring that the species does not all succumb to a particular infection. Fortunately, six class I MHC molecules are encoded in the human genome, three maternal and three paternal, so it is likely that one of our MHC alleles will be able to present an epitope from any given pathogen to our T cells.

5.9   STRUCTURE OF MHC CLASS II MOLECULES

MHC class II molecules consist of two transmembrane polypeptide chains, an α chain that is non-covalently associated with a β chain. Unlike MHC class I molecules, MHC class II molecules are expressed on the surfaces of a restricted set of cells in the body. MHC class II molecules are mainly found on the surfaces of professional APCs such as DCs, macrophages, and B cells. Expression of MHC class II molecules can be induced on the surfaces of certain other cells by the cytokine interferon-γ.

Each MHC class II chain has a two-domain structure (see *Figure 5.10*). The α_1 and β_1 domains are distal from the cell membrane, whereas the α_2 and β_2 domains are membrane-proximal. These membrane-proximal domains are classic immunoglobulin-like domains. The β_2 domain has a binding site for CD4, explaining why $CD4^+$ T cells specifically recognize antigen presented on MHC class II molecules.

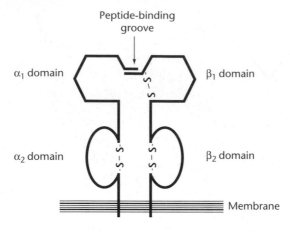

Figure 5.10
The MHC class II molecule consists of an α chain and a β chain. The peptide binding groove is formed by the folding of the α1 and β1 domains of the molecule. The binding site for CD4 is located in the β2 domain.

The α_1 and β_1 domains fold together to form a peptide-binding groove that is very similar to that found in MHC class I molecules. The major difference between the MHC class I and class II grooves is that the ends of the MHC class II groove are open (see *Figure 5.11*). Consequently, MHC class II molecules tend to present longer peptides than do MHC class I molecules. The average length of peptides bound to MHC class II molecules is 18–20 amino acids. Analogous to what was described above for MHC class I, most of the differences between allelic variants of MHC class II are in amino acid residues that line the MHC class II peptide-binding groove, explaining why different class II molecules bind different peptides. Peptide binding to MHC class II molecules follows the same rules as peptide binding to MHC class I molecules. This means that peptides must have particular anchor residues to allow them to bind to particular MHC class II molecules.

The phenomenon of MHC restriction described above for CD8$^+$ T cells applies equally to CD4$^+$ T cells. This means that a given CD4$^+$ T cell will recognize a particular epitope only when a given MHC class II molecule presents that epitope.

5.10 ANTIGEN PROCESSING AND PRESENTATION

There are two major pathways by which antigens are processed and presented to T cells; these are called the endogenous and exogenous pathways, respectively. The terms 'endogenous' and 'exogenous' refer to the source of the antigen. In the endogenous pathway, the antigen is made inside the presenting cell; in the exogenous pathway, the antigen is taken up from outside (i.e. exogenous to) the cell. All viral proteins have to be made inside host cells, therefore the endogenous pathway is used to present viral antigens to CD8$^+$ T cells. However, extracellular (exogenous) viral particles, or virions, can be taken up by an APC, so viral antigens can also be processed

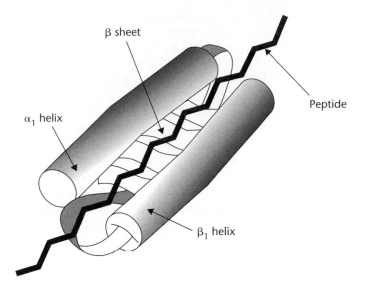

Figure 5.11
The peptide binding groove of class II molecules is open at both ends. As a consequence, longer peptides can bind to MHC class II molecules than can bind to MHC class I molecules.

via the exogenous pathway and presented to CD4$^+$ T cells. Virus-specific CD4$^+$ T cells will provide help to virus-specific B cells, enabling them to make antiviral antibody. Since most bacteria are capable of living outside host cells, these extracellular pathogens are usually processed and presented via the exogenous pathway.

The endogenous pathway

The endogenous pathway results in generation of peptide antigens that are presented, bound to MHC class I molecules, to CD8$^+$ T cells. This pathway is usually associated with presentation of viral antigens because viruses must make their proteins inside host cells, and the endogenous pathway is tailored towards presentation of antigens that are made inside the presenting cell. This means that the endogenous pathway also presents self antigens that are made inside the presenting cell. These self antigens can be tumour antigens, but the endogenous pathway also presents antigens from normal cells. In general, T cells that react against self antigens are killed during negative selection in the thymus (see *Section 3.6*) so, in most cases, there are no T cells in the periphery that will recognize the self antigens that are presented by the MHC molecules. The exception to this is the spectrum of diseases called autoimmune diseases (see *Chapter 10*).

The endogenous pathway of antigen presentation during a viral infection is given below as an example, although this will also apply to presentation of self antigens via this pathway. The first step in the pathway is the biosynthesis of antigen. In this case a virus infects a cell, transcribes its genes and uses host ribosomes to make viral proteins. Within the cytosol there is a large cylindrical multi-catalytic protease complex known as the proteasome. The cylindrical proteasome is made up of 14 different subunits, 7α subunits ($\alpha1$–7), and 7β subunits ($\beta1$–7) and its function is to degrade misfolded and spent proteins in the cell.

There is a subset of proteasomes in the cell called immunoproteasomes. These are responsible for the generation of the vast majority of peptides that are presented via the endogenous pathway. Immunoproteasomes differ from conventional proteasomes in that three of the normal β subunits are replaced by three other subunits. These new subunits are called $\beta1i$ (LMP2), $\beta2i$ and $\beta5i$ (LMP7), and their production is induced by the cytokines IFN-γ and TNF-α, cytokines that are produced during an immune response. These new β subunits alter the activity of the complex so that immunoproteasomes preferentially generate peptides that have hydrophobic or basic (positively charged) amino acids at their carboxy(C)-termini. This type of C-terminal amino acid is generally found in peptides that bind to MHC class I molecules. Most of the peptides generated by immunoproteasomes are too long to bind to MHC class I molecules, and these longer peptides are 'trimmed' to the correct length by aminopeptidases. Some aminopeptidases, such as an enzyme called leucine aminopeptidase, are present in the cytosol.

The peptides generated by the immunoproteasome bind to cytosolic 'carrier' proteins, such as particular heat shock proteins (HSPs). This protects the peptides from complete degradation by cytosolic peptidases. The carrier proteins also transport the peptides from the immunoprotea-

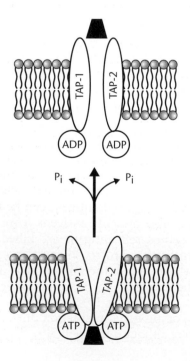

Figure 5.12
Binding of peptide (shown in black) to the cytosolic portion of the TAP heterodimer causes a conformational change leading to the translocation of the peptide into the lumen of the endoplasmic reticulum coupled to the hydrolysis of ATP.

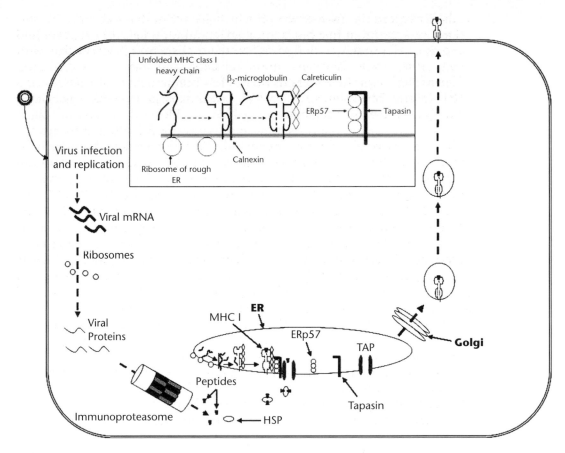

Figure 5.13
The endogenous pathway of antigen processing and presentation. Endogenously synthesized proteins
are degraded into peptides by the immunoproteasome. The peptides, coupled to carrier proteins, are
shuttled to the TAP complex and translocated into the lumen of the endoplasmic reticulum (ER). MHC
class I molecules are co-translationally translocated into the ER where they fold and associate with
calreticulin (inset). The MHC class I–calreticulin complex associates with a tapasin–ERp57 heterodimer
which in turn is associated with the TAP complex. The tapasin–ERp57 dimer assists in transfer of
peptide from TAP into the binding groove of the MHC class I molecule. Longer peptides may be
trimmed to size by the aminopeptidase ERAAP (not shown). Following peptide binding the class I
molecule is transported to the cell surface where is it available for recognition by CD8+ T cells.

some to the TAP (transporter of antigen presentation) complex, which spans
the membrane of the endoplasmic reticulum (ER). TAP is a heterodimer of
TAP-1 and TAP-2, and is an ATP-driven peptide pump. The peptides delivered by the carrier proteins are pumped from the cytosol into the lumen of
the ER by TAP (see *Figure 5.12*).

Like all membrane proteins, MHC class I molecules are made on the
ribosomes of the rough ER and, as they are made, the α and β chains are
translocated across the ER membrane. At this stage the proteins are
unfolded, until other proteins, called molecular chaperones (calnexin and

calreticulin), in the ER help the proteins fold. When the α chain is translocated into the ER, it first binds to calnexin. Calnexin helps the α chain fold and associate, weakly, with β$_2$M. When the α chain and β$_2$M associate with each other they dissociate from calnexin and bind to calreticulin. Calreticulin (with the associated MHC class I dimer) then associates with a heterodimer consisting of a protein called tapasin (for TAP <u>as</u>sociated prote<u>in</u>), which is disulphide-bonded to an ER-resident enzyme called ERp57. As the name suggests, tapasin associates with TAP. This brings the MHC class I molecule into close proximity with the peptides that have been translocated into the ER by TAP. The tapasin–ERp57 dimer assists in the transfer of these peptides from TAP into the peptide-binding groove of MHC I molecules. There is also an aminopeptidase in the ER called ERAAP (ER-<u>a</u>ssociated <u>a</u>mino<u>p</u>eptidase). Like the cytosolic aminopeptidases, ERAAP 'trims' peptides in the ER to the correct length (8–10 amino acids long) so that they can bind to MHC class I molecules. The multimeric complex consisting of MHC class I, calreticulin, tapasin, TAP, ERp57 and ERAAP, is referred to as the peptide-loading complex (PLC).

At this stage the peptide is bound to the class I molecule in the ER. The class I molecule then dissociates from the PLC and is exported to the cell surface via the Golgi complex along the conventional secretory pathway. The class I molecule with the bound peptide is expressed on the surface of the cell where it can be recognized by the TCR of a CD8$^+$ T cell (see *Figure 5.13*). If the class I molecule does not bind peptide, then it is degraded intracellularly by the proteasome.

An alternative TAP-independent pathway for presentation of endogenous antigens has also been described. Peptides presented via this pathway are mainly derived from signal peptides that are cleaved from precursors of secreted or transmembrane proteins by the enzyme signal peptidase. However, the majority of peptides presented by MHC class I molecules are processed via the conventional endogenous pathway described above.

The exogenous pathway

The exogenous pathway is so named because the antigens from which the presented peptides are derived are taken up by the cell from outside. As mentioned earlier, an example would be bacterial antigen, or extracellular virions. The first step in this pathway is very much like phagocytosis or pinocytosis. The antigen is taken up by the presenting cell, usually a professional APC, and isolated inside the cell in a vesicle called an endosome. The endosome is taken further inside the cell and the interior of the endosome is made progressively more acidic via the action of proton pumps in the endosomal membrane. The acidic pH activates enzymes called acidic proteases (proteases that are active at low pH) that are delivered to the endosome. The acidic proteases begin to act on the endocytosed antigen, degrading it into peptides.

MHC class II molecules are made just like MHC class I molecules and are translocated into the ER. As soon as the class II dimer folds in the ER it binds to another protein called the invariant chain. This complex is actually a nonameric complex consisting of three MHC class II dimers each bound to an invariant chain molecule. The invariant chain binds to class II in such a way that a portion of the invariant chain lies across and blocks the peptide-binding groove. This prevents class II from binding peptides in the ER. MHC class II molecules are used to present exogenously derived antigens, so it is important that they are prevented from binding peptides from the endogenous pathway (see above) in the ER. The portion of the invariant chain that blocks the MHC class II peptide-binding groove is called CLIP (for <u>cl</u>ass II-associated <u>i</u>nvariant chain <u>p</u>eptide). When the invariant chain binds to class II, this induces a conformational change that reveals a sequence in the cytosolic tail of the invariant chain. This sequence functions as an endosomal targeting signal and directs the class II-invariant chain complex to the endosomal pathway (see *Figure 5.14*).

Since the exogenous antigen is being brought into the cell via the endosomal pathway, the MHC class II molecules 'on the way out' meet up with the peptide antigen 'on the way in'. The vesicle carrying the MHC class II-invariant chain complex fuses with the endosome containing the antigenic peptides and an endosomal protease called Cathepsin S degrades the invariant chain. This leaves CLIP bound in the peptide-binding groove of the MHC class II molecule. Another protein, called HLA-DM catalyses the exchange of antigenic peptide for CLIP. The specialized endosomal compartment where this occurs is called the MHC class II loading compartment, or MIIC (see *Figure 5.15*).

When an MHC class II molecule binds peptide it moves to the surface of the cell. There, the class II peptide complex can be recognized by the TCR of CD4$^+$ T cells. The rest of the contents of the MIIC, including peptides that have not bound to class II, eventually fuse with lysosomes and are degraded.

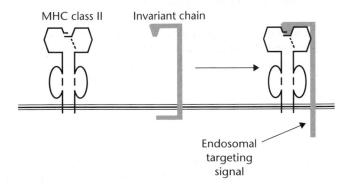

Figure 5.14
Binding of the invariant chain to an MHC class II molecule occludes the peptide binding groove. Following binding to class II, an endosomal targeting sequence is revealed in the cytosolic tail of the invariant chain.

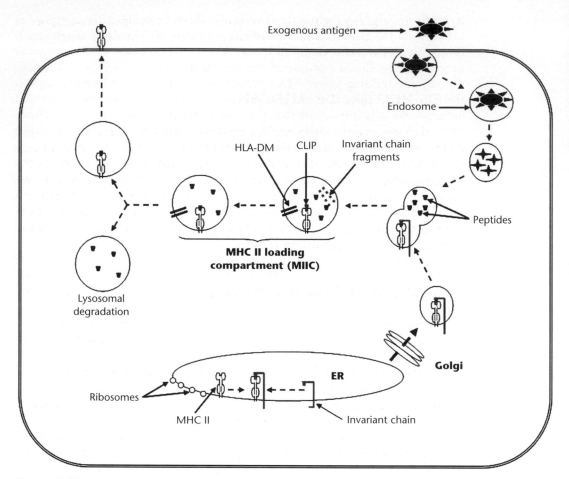

Figure 5.15
The exogenous pathway of antigen processing and presentation. Antigen is taken up by the cell into endosomes where it is degraded into peptides by acidic proteases. Vesicles carrying MHC class II-invariant chain complexes fuse with the endosomes to form the MHC class II loading compartment (MIIC). Cathepsin S digests the invariant chain but leaves a small portion, CLIP, in the peptide binding groove. HLA-DM catalyses the exchange of antigenic peptide for CLIP. Following peptide binding the class II molecule is transported to the cell surface where it is available for recognition by CD4+ T cells. Unbound peptides are degraded in lysosomes.

Cross-presentation

To enable effective immunological responses by cytotoxic T cells to virus or tumour cells, a phenomenon known as cross-presentation of antigens is essential. This allows exogenous antigen that is taken up by DCs to be introduced into the endogenous pathway of antigen processing. In this way, DCs can present peptides derived from exogenous antigens on MHC class I molecules. The precise mechanisms involved in cross-presentation remain to be elucidated. The main cell type involved in cross-presentation is thought to be plasmacytoid dendritic cells. These are a specialized subset of DCs central to the initiation of antiviral immunity, chiefly through secretion of type I interferon.

5.11 PRESENTATION OF ANTIGEN

Induction of adaptive immune responses requires antigen to be brought from infected sites to secondary lymphoid tissues. The DC acquires antigen in tissues and, in response to homeostatic chemokines, migrates to the draining lymph node. En route, the DC processes and presents its antigenic cargo and arrives in the paracortex of the lymph node bearing antigen in a form that can be recognized by T cells. In the next chapter we will examine the cellular and molecular interactions involved in generating an adaptive immune response against this antigen.

SUGGESTED FURTHER READING

Fritz, J.H., Ferrero, R.L., Philpott, D.J. and Girardin, S.E. (2006) Nod-like proteins in immunity, inflammation and disease. *Nature Immunol.* **7**: 1250–1257.

Jensen, P.E. (2007) Recent advances in antigen processing and presentation. *Nature Immunol.* **8**: 1041–1048.

Kumánovics, A., Takada, T. and Lindahl, K.-F. (2003) Genomic organization of the mammalian MHC. *Annu Rev. Immunol.* **21**: 629–657.

McGettrick, A.F. and O'Neill, L.A. (2007) Toll-like receptors: key activators of leucocytes and regulator of haematopoiesis. *Brit. J. Haematol.* **139**: 185–193.

McMichael, A.J. (2007) From influenza to HIV and back. *Nature Immunol.* **8**: 1149–1151.

Pulendran, B., Tang,H. and Denning, T.L. (2008) Division of labor, plasticity, and crosstalk between dendritic cell subsets. *Curr. Opin. Immunol.* **20**: 61–67.

Robinson, M.J., Sancho, D., Slack, E.C., LeibundGut-Landmann, S., and Reis e Sousa, C. (2006) Myeloid C-type lectins in innate immunity. *Nature Immunol.* **7**: 1258–1265.

SELF-ASSESSMENT QUESTIONS

1. What is the function of antigen-presenting cells (APCs)?
2. List three types of antigen-presenting cells.
3. What are the two signals that are required to activate naïve T cells?
4. What is anergy and how is it generated in T cells?
5. How are dendritic cells (DC) stimulated to mature and how do they differ from immature DC?
6. What are immune response genes?
7. Explain MHC restriction of T cells.

8. What is the benefit to a population of having many different MHC alleles expressed?

9. Name the two major pathways by which APCs can process antigen for presentation to T cells.

10. What are the functions of the invariant chain in antigen presentation?

Generation of adaptive immune responses

Learning objectives

After studying this chapter you should confidently be able to:

■ **Discuss how the structure of secondary lymphoid tissues enables antigen to be delivered to lymphocytes**
Secondary lymphoid tissues are highly organized structures designed to increase the probability that antigen-specific lymphocytes will encounter their cognate antigen. Lymph from tissues empties into the subcapsular sinus of lymph nodes where it is channelled via a series of conduits lined by antigen-presenting cells. The splenic circulation opens to the perifollicular zone adjacent to specialized antigen-trapping cells.

■ **Discuss the differentiation and functions of CD4$^+$ T cell subsets**
Naïve CD4$^+$ T cells can be induced to differentiate into one of five Th subsets depending on the cytokines that are produced by the antigen-presenting cell. Th1 cells develop under the influence of IL-12 and provide protection against intracellular infections. Th1 cells promote the expansion of CD8$^+$ cytotoxic T cells and secrete IFN-γ which activates macrophages to kill intracellular pathogens. Development of Th2 cells is promoted by IL-4. These cells produce high levels of IL-4, IL-5, IL-10 and IL-13. The cytokines produced by Th2 cells promote antibody production by B cells. In addition, IL-4 and IL-13 produced by Th2 cells trigger an alternative pathway of macrophage activation. Th2 cells are important in defence against parasitic infections and infections with certain extracellular bacteria. Th17 cells produce IL-17 and TNF-α and differentiate from Th0 cells under the influence of TGF-β and IL-6. Th17 cells play a role in defence against extracellular bacterial infections and have also been implicated in the pathogenesis of cell-mediated autoimmune diseases. Inducible regulatory (iT$_{REG}$) cells are important for controlling immune responses and are critical for maintenance of peripheral tolerance. They develop from Th0 cells under the influence of TGF-β. The final subset of Th cells is the follicular helper T (T$_{FH}$) cell. These cells are the main cell type involved in providing help for B cell responses. Their relationship, if any, to Th1 cells and Th2 cells remains to be elucidated.

■ **Describe the interaction between antigen-experienced CD4$^+$ T cells and naïve B cells**
Antigen-experienced CD4$^+$ T cells and B cells interact at the outer region of the paracortex of lymph nodes. The B cell internalizes antigen on its BCR and presents fragments of this antigen on MHC class II molecules to the T cell. Binding of the TCR to the MHC peptide complex activates the T cell and induces it to express CD154 which binds to CD40 on the B

cell. The signal generated by antigen binding to the BCR and the signal transmitted via CD40 result in B cell activation. The B cell then expresses surface receptors that allow it to respond to particular T cell-derived cytokines.

■ **Describe the germinal centre reaction**
Proliferating B cells re-enter a follicle and start to proliferate. They differentiate into centroblasts and lose surface BCR expression. The centroblasts mutate their rearranged V(D)J gene segments at a very high frequency. The centroblasts differentiate into centrocytes and express the mutated BCRs on their surfaces. They then compete with one another for binding to antigen deposits on follicular dendritic cells. Only those cells with high affinity BCRs will be able to bind to the antigen and receive a survival signal. Cells expressing low affinity BCRs die by apoptosis and are eliminated by tingible body macrophages.

■ **Discuss the generation of CD8⁺ T cell responses**
DCs acquire antigen, process it, and present it on MHC class I molecules to naïve CD8⁺ T cells. DCs deliver both signal 1 and signal 2 to the CD8⁺ T cell, priming it for activation. Proliferation and expression of cytotoxic mediators by CD8⁺ T cells require CD4⁺ T cell-derived IL-2. Following stimulation with IL-2, the CD8⁺ T cell is competent to kill infected cells, and it leaves the lymph node and migrates to sites of infection.

■ **Distinguish between primary and secondary immune responses**
Primary immune responses are those responses that are generated following the initial encounter with an antigen. Maximal responses are not generated until approximately 8–10 days following antigen exposure, with antibody responses frequently peaking much later. The level of antibody produced is modest and is generally of the IgM isotype. The generation and maintenance of memory cells following the primary response means that the immune system maximally responds much faster, generally within 3 days, following re-exposure to the same antigen. This rapid response upon re-exposure to antigen is called the secondary response. In general, the secondary response is also of greater magnitude than the primary response. The antibody produced during a secondary response is usually IgG, IgA or IgE and of higher affinity than that produced during the primary response.

6.1   INTRODUCTION TO ADAPTIVE IMMUNE RESPONSES

The innate immune response constitutes a relatively non-specific attack against invaders. Although innate responses may not eliminate the threat, they do serve two very important functions. First, they curtail the spread of infections until such time as an adaptive immune response can be generated. Secondly, they establish conditions conducive to elicitation of adaptive immune responses.

Early during the innate response, antigen is picked up by antigen-presenting cells (APCs). The milieu of pro-inflammatory cytokines that is generated during the innate response promotes the differentiation of these APCs into cells that are capable of activating lymphocytes, in particular CD4⁺ T cells. The activation of CD4⁺ T cells is a crucial step in the induction of adaptive responses. CD4⁺ T cells, by virtue of their secreted cytokines, regulate the adaptive response. They are critical for generation of most antibody responses and also provide help for generation of CD8$^+$ cytotoxic T cell responses.

Elicitation of adaptive immune responses requires antigen to be efficiently delivered to infrequent antigen-specific lymphocytes. The structure of secondary lymphoid tissues has evolved to promote this as well as to nurture the differentiation and expansion of the antigen-specific cells so that they can eliminate the antigenic threat.

After elimination of antigen, the immune response must stand down but maintain a state of vigilance. To enable this, memory cells are established during the initial encounter with an antigen. These memory cells persist after the antigen has been eliminated. They patrol the body and rapidly, and vigorously, respond to their specific antigen if they encounter it again.

6.2 THE FINE STRUCTURE OF SECONDARY LYMPHOID TISSUES

It has been estimated that the frequency of naïve lymphocytes that are reactive against any given epitope is between 1 in 10^5 and 1 in 10^6. Because of this, the chances of a random encounter between a naïve lymphocyte and its cognate antigen are slight. The task of ensuring that antigen is delivered to antigen-specific lymphocytes falls to secondary lymphoid tissues. Secondary lymphoid tissues are highly organized structures that facilitate the delivery of antigen to antigen-specific T cells and B cells, and provide an environment conducive to the proliferation and differentiation of these cells. We have encountered secondary lymphoid tissues already (see *Section 2.4*), but before we discuss the generation of adaptive immune responses, we need to examine the structure of the spleen and of lymph nodes in greater detail.

Fine structure of the spleen

Micro-organisms and their secreted products that are present in the bloodstream are filtered out, phagocytosed, and presented to lymphocytes in the spleen. Because of this, the spleen is important for protection against blood-borne pathogens and splenectomized patients usually require life-long prophylactic antibiotics. The spleen can be subdivided into two areas, the red pulp and the white pulp. The red pulp is primarily concerned with the removal of senescent erythrocytes from the blood and with recycling of iron. The white pulp is the lymphoid compartment of the spleen.

The splenic white pulp is organized into inner T cell areas and outer B cell follicles. The follicular areas are surrounded by the marginal zone. Unlike rodent splenic white pulp, human splenic white pulp does not contain a marginal sinus. Instead human splenic white pulp contains an additional outer area, the perifollicular zone, which is open to the general splenic circulation (see *Figure 6.1*).

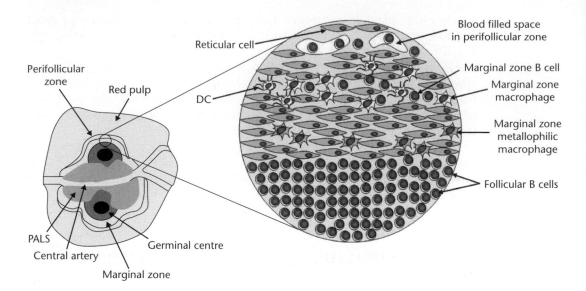

Figure 6.1
The splenic marginal zone overlies the B cell follicle and contains specialized antigen-trapping cells, such as marginal zone macrophages, marginal zone metallophilic macrophages, dendritic cells (DC) and marginal zone B cells, in addition to fibroblast-like reticular cells. Cells enter the white pulp via the perifollicular zone which contains blood-filled spaces that are open to the splenic circulation.

The marginal zone (MZ) contains B cells (primarily marginal zone B cells), macrophages, dendritic cells and reticular fibroblasts. MZ B cells express receptors for sphingosine-1-phosphate (S1P). S1P is a lysophospholipid chemoattractant for lymphocytes that is normally found bound to plasma proteins. Because of this, the concentration of S1P is approximately 100-fold higher in extracellular fluid than it is in tissues. Expression of S1P receptors by MZ B cells causes them to accumulate adjacent to the perifollicular zone, a site of high S1P concentration, where they are retained by interactions between LFA-1 and $\alpha_4\beta_1$ integrin on the MZ B cell and ICAM-1 and VCAM-1 on reticular cells, respectively. MZ B cells rapidly differentiate into IgM-secreting plasma cells after encounter with blood-borne antigens. They may also lose expression of S1P receptors after encounter with antigen and migrate into the T cell zone to present the antigen to specific T cells.

Two distinct populations of macrophages are found in the MZ. The first macrophage subset is called the MZ macrophage. MZ macrophages are found in the outer layer of the MZ. They express the C-type lectin DC-SIGN (see *Section 4.2*) and MARCO, a type I scavenger receptor, in addition to a range of TLRs. DC-SIGN binds to polysaccharide antigens on the surfaces of microbes such as *Mycobacterium tuberculosis* and *Streptococcus pneumoniae* (see *Section 8.3*) and are required for MZ macrophage-mediated phagocytosis of these organisms as well as for MZ macrophage-mediated clearance of certain viruses. MARCO also binds to surface antigens on a variety of pathogens such as *Staphylococcus aureus* and *Escherichia coli*. The second subset of macrophages found in the marginal zone is called the MZ metallophilic macrophage. These cells are located in the inner layer of the MZ close to the white pulp. MZ metallophilic macrophages express the adhesion molecule SIGLEC1 (sialic acid-binding immunoglobulin-like lectin) which can bind to surface antigens on micro-organisms such as *Neisseria meningitidis*.

The reticular fibroblasts secrete a network of type IV collagen fibres and extracellular matrix proteins that forms the splenic conduit system, a series of channels that allows the transport of blood-borne and locally produced molecules throughout the white pulp.

Cells, including lymphocytes and DCs, enter the spleen through the perifollicular zone (or through the marginal sinus in rodents). Entry of lymphocytes occurs via a similar process to the one leukocytes use to enter inflamed tissues (see *Section 4.5*). The nature of the initial weak interactions that mediate tethering between lymphocytes and endothelial-like fibroblasts in the perifollicular zone is unknown. It is possible that these weak interactions are unnecessary for entry of cells into the spleen because the rate of blood flow in this region is greatly reduced, resulting in a low shear stress. Arrest of lymphocytes is mediated by binding of LFA-1 and $\alpha_4\beta_1$ integrin on the lymphocytes to ICAM-1 and VCAM-1 on the endothelial-like fibroblasts. High affinity binding between these integrins and their receptors is dependent on chemokine-mediated activation of the integrins into their high affinity states (see *Figure 6.2*). This high affinity interaction allows the

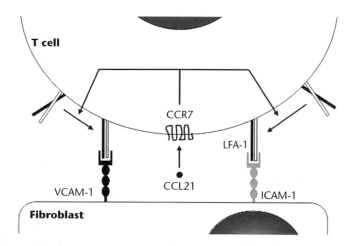

Figure 6.2
Lymphocyte entry into the spleen is facilitated by high affinity interactions between the integrin LFA-1 on the lymphocyte and its counter-receptors ICAM-1 and VCAM-1 on splenic fibroblastoid reticular cells. The high affinity interaction is dependent on a chemokine-induced alteration in the conformation of LFA-1. In the example shown, CCL21 binding to CCR7 induces a conformational change in LFA-1 on T cells.

lymphocytes to migrate from the leaky splenic microcirculation into the white pulp. Because T cells express the chemokine receptor CCR7, they migrate to the T cell area in response to the chemokines CCL19 and CCL21 that are produced by cells in the T cell zone. In contrast, B cells express the CXCR5 chemokine receptor and migrate into B cell follicles in response to CXCL13 that is produced by follicular stromal cells and follicular dendritic cells.

Fine structure of lymph nodes

Foreign material present in tissues is collected in lymph, the fluid that bathes the tissues. This material is then transported to lymph nodes where it is presented to antigen-specific lymphocytes. Because of this, lymph nodes are important for defence against infections in peripheral tissues.

The afferent lymphatic vessels drain into the subcapsular sinus of the lymph node. The subcapsular sinus gives rise to a three-dimensional network of channels called the lymph node conduit system. These conduits pervade the paracortex in particular (see *Figure 6.3*). The conduit system is produced by fibroblast-like reticular cells and, like the splenic conduit system, is composed of a central core of collagen fibres surrounded by extracellular matrix proteins. The lymph node conduit system ensures that material entering via the afferent lymphatic vessels is distributed throughout the T cell area. Interdigitating DCs are found along the conduits and constantly sample their contents for foreign antigen. Antigen-bearing DCs that enter the lymph node via the afferent lymphatic vessels localize to high endothelial venules (HEVs) in the paracortex, the site where lymphocytes enter the lymph node from the circulation.

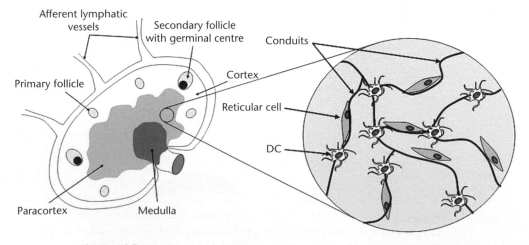

Figure 6.3
A network of channels called conduits ensures that antigen is distributed throughout the paracortex. DCs settle on the conduits and constantly sample the fluid for foreign antigen.

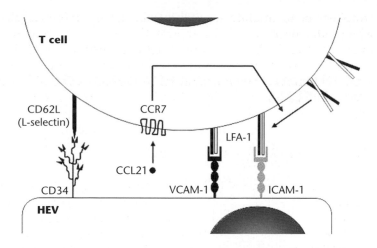

Figure 6.4
Lymphocytes enter lymph nodes at high endothelial venules (HEV). In the example shown, initial adhesive interactions between CD62L on a T cell and CD34 on the HEV cause the T cell to roll along the surface of the HEV. Migration across the HEV is facilitated by high affinity interactions between the integrin LFA-1 on the lymphocyte and its counter-receptors ICAM-1 and VCAM-1 on the HEV. CCL21 binding to CCR7 induces a conformational change in LFA-1 on T cells so that it binds with high affinity to ICAM-1 and VCAM-1.

Entry of lymphocytes into lymph nodes occurs via a four-step process similar to that used by leukocytes to enter inflamed tissues (see *Section 4.5*). The initial adhesive interaction is between CD62L on the lymphocyte and CD34 on the HEV (see *Figure 6.4*). This interaction is sufficient to tether the lymphocyte onto the surface of the HEV and prevent it from being flushed away by the high shear stress of the lymph node circulation. Arrest of lymphocytes on, and diapedesis through HEV is mediated by high affinity binding of LFA-1 and $\alpha_4\beta_1$ integrin on the lymphocytes to ICAM-1 and VCAM-1 on the HEV, respectively. This process is also dependent on chemokine-mediated activation of the integrins into their high affinity states.

As with the case of lymphocyte localization in the spleen, the CCR7[+] T cells settle in the T cell area and the CXCR5[+] B cells migrate to the follicles. This is due to the local production of T cell chemoattractants (CCL19 and CCL21) and B cell chemoattractant (CXCL13) at these sites, respectively.

The function of CD62L on lymphocytes and the expression of ICAM-1 on the HEV have been shown to be thermosensitive so that at 38–40°C, a temperature consistent with fever, lymphocyte migration into lymph nodes is increased. In addition, during inflammation lymph node arterioles can expand by as much as 50%. Collectively, these processes result in a greatly increased delivery of lymphocytes to lymph nodes in search of antigen. In the following sections the events that occur when lymphocytes encounter their specific antigen will be examined. The events that occur in lymph nodes will be focused on specifically, but similar responses take place in the splenic white pulp.

6.3   THE INTERACTION BETWEEN DENDRITIC CELLS AND CD4⁺ T CELLS

As outlined above, when antigen-bearing DCs enter lymph nodes they localize to sites adjacent to HEVs in the paracortex. Using their extensive dendrite-like appendages they scan the surfaces of naïve T cells that enter the node for TCRs that are capable of binding to the MHC class II-peptide complexes expressed on the DC cell surface. Because of their extensive appendages, DCs can interact with many T cells simultaneously. It has been estimated that DCs can scan the surfaces of as many as 5000 T cells per hour in search of antigen-specific T cells that are present in lymphoid tissues at very low frequency. Similarly, interdigitating DCs that acquire antigen from lymph node conduits process the antigen and present it on MHC class II molecules and use it to scan the surfaces of T cells for antigen-specific TCRs.

When a DC encounters a T cell that is specific for the antigen that the DC is presenting, it forms a stable interaction with the T cell. This leads to reorganization of the T cell cytoskeleton, resulting in the formation of an immunological synapse. Formation of the immunological synapse is made possible by the segregation of molecules that are important for T cell activation into cholesterol-rich microdomains, called lipid rafts (see *Box 6.1*), in the cell membranes. These molecules are recruited to the point of interaction between the T cell and the DC. The immunological synapse is not specific to T cell–DC interactions but is also generated at the points of contact between T cells and other APCs such as B cells.

Box 6.1 Lipid rafts

Lipid rafts are specialized membrane domains that are enriched in certain lipids, cholesterol and proteins. Lipid raft-associated proteins include glycosylphosphatidylinositol-anchored proteins and acylated Src family tyrosine kinases. Association of the TCR and BCR with lipid rafts is required for lymphocyte activation.

The immunological synapse has two main areas: a central supramolecular activation cluster (cSMAC) and a peripheral SMAC (pSMAC) surrounded by a ring of the cytoskeletal protein talin (see *Figure 6.5*). Molecules that have large extracellular domains, such as CD45, are excluded from the immunological synapse, whereas molecules that have smaller extracellular domains, that do not sterically hinder the interaction between the TCR and the MHC-peptide complex, are not excluded. During the first 15 minutes of interaction between a T cell and a DC, adhesion molecules on the T cell, such as LFA-1 and CD2, are localized to the cSMAC. By 30 minutes, however, as the synapse matures and the interaction between the two cells is stabilized, the adhesion molecules are redistributed to the

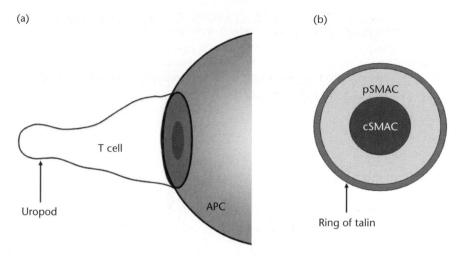

Figure 6.5
(a) Interaction between a T cell and APC results in formation of an immunological synapse at the site of interaction. (b) Face view of immunological synapse showing the central cSMAC surrounded by the pSMAC.

pSMAC and are replaced in the cSMAC by TCR complexes and associated signalling molecules, including the co-stimulatory molecule CD28 as well as protein kinase C-theta (PK-Cθ).

Formation of the immunological synapse allows T cell activation to occur. T cell activation is the result of the integration of signals derived from several different signal transduction pathways, including that initiated by the TCR binding to MHC–peptide complexes and that initiated by CD28 binding to B7 molecules (see *Figure 6.6*). The signalling pathways involve multiple kinases and adaptor molecules (see *Box 6.2*). The initial events involve phosphorylation of immunoreceptor tyrosine-based activation motifs (ITAMs; see *Box 6.3*) in the cytoplasmic tails of components of the CD3 complex by the tyrosine kinase Lck. Phosphorylation of the CD3-associated ζ (zeta) chain results in recruitment of the zeta-associated protein kinase ZAP-70 to the TCR. This ultimately leads to phosphorylation and activation of the enzyme phospholipase C-γ (PLC-γ). PLC-γ cleaves membrane phospholipids to generate inositol-1,4,5-trisphosphate (IP₃) and diacylglycerol (DAG). IP₃ causes an increase in intracellular Ca^{2+} leading to activation of Ca^{2+}-dependent enzymes and cellular processes, whereas DAG leads to activation of PK-C and Ras-exchange factors and activation of the mitogen-activated protein (MAP) kinase signalling pathway.

Box 6.2 Adaptor proteins

Adaptor proteins mediate protein–protein interactions during signal transduction cascades. They are usually devoid of any intrinsic enzymatic activity but recruit other proteins into short-lived active complexes.

Box 6.3 Immunoreceptor tyrosine-based activation motifs

An ITAM is a sequence of four amino acids that is repeated twice in the cytoplasmic tails of certain membrane proteins. An ITAM consists of a tyrosine separated from a leucine by any two other amino acids. ITAMs are important for signal transduction in cells of the immune system.

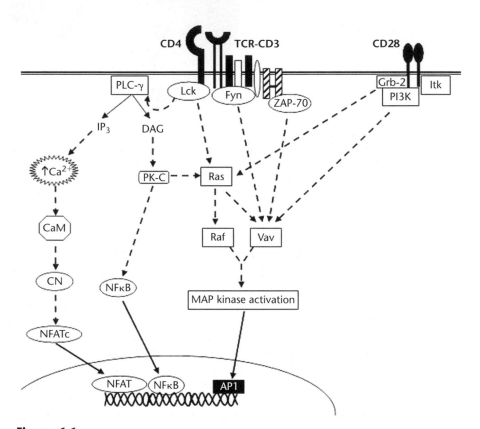

Figure 6.6
Stimulation of the TCR results in recruitment of the src family kinases Lck and Fyn to the TCR and CD4 co-receptor, where they phosphorylate components of the CD3 complex and the CD3-associated ζ (zeta) chain homodimer. This leads to recruitment and activation of the ZAP-70 kinase. The recruited kinases phosphorylate downstream targets that activate MAP kinase pathways leading to translocation of the AP1 transcription factor to the nucleus. Lck also activates phospholipase C-γ (PLC-γ) to release diacylglycerol (DAG) and inositol-1,4,5-trisphosphate (IP$_3$) from membrane phospholipids. DAG activates protein kinase C (PK-C) which relieves inhibition of the NFκB transcription factor allowing it to translocate to the nucleus and activate gene transcription. IP$_3$ causes an increase in intracellular Ca^{2+} which activates a range of Ca^{2+}-calmodulin (CaM) processes in the cell including activation of the phosphatase calcineurin (CN). CN activates the NFAT transcription factor allowing it to translocate to the nucleus and activate gene expression. Signals generated by the CD28 co-stimulatory molecule augment activation of the MAP kinase pathways.

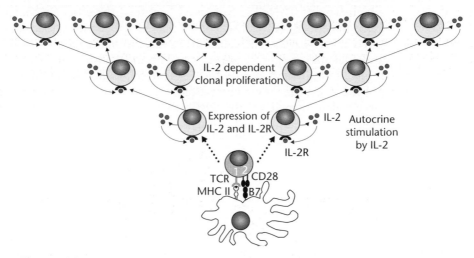

Figure 6.7
Interaction between an antigen-specific CD4⁺ T cell and an antigen-bearing DC results in delivery of signal 1 and signal 2 to the T cell. This leads to expression of the high affinity IL-2 receptor (IL-2R) by the T cell as well as to production of IL-2. Binding of IL-2 to the IL-2R results in T cell proliferation. For clarity, the CD4 co-receptor is not shown.

The signalling pathways initiated by the TCR and by CD28 result in transmission of signal 1 and signal 2, respectively, into the T cell (see *Section 5.4*). When the T cell receives signal 1 and signal 2, it enters the G1 phase of the cell cycle. The T cell will also express a molecule called CD154 (CD40L) on its cell surface. Expression of CD154 is transient but this molecule can be re-expressed if the T cell is stimulated again. Binding of CD154 to CD40 on APCs stimulates the APCs to secrete cytokines which promote T cell differentiation (see *Section 6.4*). The T cell also responds to signal 1 and signal 2 by making IL-2 and by expressing on its surface a high affinity IL-2 receptor. IL-2 is the major growth factor for T cells. Binding of IL-2 to its receptor allows the T cell to complete the cell cycle, i.e. to undergo cell division. These activated T cells can then divide approximately three times a day for several days. In this way the interaction between an antigen-bearing DC and an antigen-specific T cell can result in the generation of thousands of antigen-specific progeny T cells during this time period (see *Figure 6.7*). During this time the naïve CD4⁺ T cell will also differentiate into one of several different CD4⁺ T cell subsets.

6.4 DIFFERENTIATION OF CD4⁺ T CELL SUBSETS

Prior to its encounter with antigen, a naïve CD4⁺ T cell is called a Th0 cell. Following interaction with antigen, a Th0 cell can differentiate into one of several different helper T cell (Th) subsets (see *Box 6.4*). These different Th subsets promote different types of immune responses, and the choice of which type of Th cell is generated is crucial for efficient control of pathogenic infections. Five subsets of Th cells have been described (see *Figure 6.8*). These are Th1 cells, Th2 cells, Th17 cells, inducible regulatory T (iT$_{REG}$) cells, and follicular helper T cells (T$_{FH}$). The most important factors that determine the pathway along which a Th0 cell will differentiate are cytokines produced by the APC. The pattern of cytokines that an APC produces is largely determined by the PRRs that have been stimulated on the APC following encounter with antigen. In this way the nature of the antigen determines the type of T cell response that is generated.

Box 6.4 Th1 and Th2 cells

In the 1980s, Timothy Mosmann and Robert Coffman discovered that naïve murine CD4$^+$ T cells can develop into two distinct subsets following stimulation with antigen. They found that these two subsets could be distinguished from each other by virtue of the cytokines they secreted as well as by their effector function. They called these two subsets of CD4$^+$ cells Th1 cells and Th2 cells.

Differentiation of Th0 cells into Th1 cells is promoted by IL-12 which is secreted predominantly by DCs and macrophages. IL-12 is a heterodimeric cytokine consisting of a p40 subunit and a p35 subunit. Th1 cells express

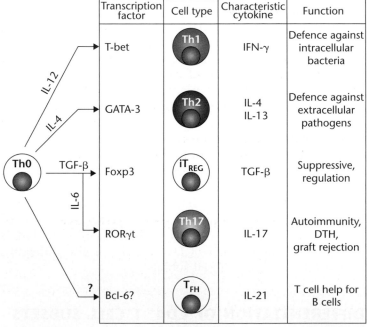

Transcription factor	Cell type	Characteristic cytokine	Function
T-bet	Th1	IFN-γ	Defence against intracellular bacteria
GATA-3	Th2	IL-4 IL-13	Defence against extracellular pathogens
Foxp3	iT$_{REG}$	TGF-β	Suppressive, regulation
RORγt	Th17	IL-17	Autoimmunity, DTH, graft rejection
Bcl-6?	T$_{FH}$	IL-21	T cell help for B cells

Figure 6.8
Differentiation of Th0 cells is determined by specific cytokines and the expression of subset-specific transcription factors. Factors controlling the differentiation of T$_{FH}$ cells are not known, but expression of Bcl-6 is thought to play a role in development of this subset of CD4$^+$ T cells.

the transcription factor T-bet which is required for expression of IFN-γ, the characteristic cytokine secreted by these cells. IFN-γ inhibits the differentiation of Th0 cells into Th2 and Th17 cells. Cross-regulation of Th subset development is a common feature of Th differentiation and it allows the establishment of polarized antigen-specific T cell responses. Th1 cells secrete IL-2 which drives the autocrine proliferation of these cells.

Differentiation of Th0 cells into Th2 cells is promoted by IL-4. The source of IL-4 during priming of Th2 responses is unclear; however, recent data suggest that production of IL-4 by basophils may be important for induction of Th2 responses. Expression of the transcription factor GATA-3 is required for commitment to the Th2 lineage. Characteristic cytokines produced by Th2 cells include IL-4, IL-5, IL-10 and IL-13. IL-4 inhibits the differentiation of Th0 cells into Th1 and Th17 cells. Another factor that is important for Th2 differentiation is the type of co-stimulatory molecule expressed by the APC. Co-stimulatory molecules are induced on APCs following interaction between PRRs on APCs and antigens. One of these co-stimulatory molecules, B7-H2 binds to a molecule called ICOS (CD278) that is expressed by T cells following activation. Binding of B7-H2 on the APC to ICOS on the T cell promotes production of Th2 cytokines by the T cell. Low concentrations of antigen may also favour the development of Th2 cells over Th1 cells. IL-4 produced by Th2 cells is the key cytokine responsible for driving the clonal proliferation of this Th subset.

Development of iT$_{REG}$ cells from Th0 cells requires TGF-β. iT$_{REG}$ cells also secrete TGF-β and this cytokine inhibits the generation of Th1, Th2 and Th17 cells. Commitment to the iT$_{REG}$ lineage requires expression of the Foxp3 transcription factor. In the presence of TGF-β and IL-6, expression of Foxp3 is inhibited and instead the transcription factor RORγt is expressed. This transcription factor is required for commitment to the Th17 lineage of Th cells. Expansion of Th17 cells is promoted by IL-23, a heterodimeric cytokine consisting of the p40 subunit of IL-12 together with a p19 subunit. The characteristic cytokine produced by Th17 cells is IL-17.

The final subset of Th cells is the T$_{FH}$ cell. It is currently unclear whether T$_{FH}$ cells develop as a separate lineage from Th1 and Th2 cells. T$_{FH}$ cells secrete a variety of cytokines including IL-4, IL-10 and IL-21.

6.5 FUNCTIONS OF CD4⁺ T CELL SUBSETS

Efficient elimination of potentially harmful material from our bodies requires the elicitation of appropriate Th responses. The different Th subsets promote disparate downstream effector responses by virtue of the specific cytokines that they release (see *Figure 6.8*).

Th1 cells

Th1 cells promote cell-mediated immune responses and are important for defence against intracellular bacterial infections, such as *Mycobacterium tuberculosis* (see *Section 9.10*), and viruses. This is primarily a function of IFN-γ, the characteristic cytokine produced by Th1 cells. IFN-γ activates macrophages and induces them to produce nitric oxide, and stimulates their microbicidal activity. IFN-γ also promotes NK cell activity. Th1 cells also are important in stimulating the proliferation of virus-specific CD8$^+$ T cells, the main cytotoxic cells active against viral infections. Unlike the situation in mice where Th1 responses are associated with the production of IgG2a, the antibody isotypes, if any, associated with Th1 responses in humans have not been completely elucidated.

Th2 cells

Th2 cells secrete IL-4, IL-5, IL-10 and IL-13, cytokines that are important for production of antibodies. IL-4 in particular stimulates B cell proliferation, Th2 cell proliferation, and isotype switch to IgE. Consequently, Th2 cells promote humoral immune responses. In particular, Th2 responses are associated with production of IgG1, IgG4 and IgE. Because of this, Th2 responses are important for control of infections with extracellular bacteria and parasitic worms. Opsonization of microbes by antibody enhances their elimination by phagocytosis, and antibody binding to Fc receptors can lead to pathogen destruction by ADCC (see *Figure 2.9*). Antibody can also prevent infection of cells by viruses and can promote clearance of extracellular virions. Th2 cell-derived IL-4 and IL-13 stimulate the alternative pathway of macrophage activation. Alternatively activated macrophages express the enzyme arginase and are important for control of parasitic infections such as schistosomiasis (see *Section 8.6*) and for tissue repair during wound healing (see *Section 4.7*). Exuberant Th2 responses are also associated with the development of Type I hypersensitivity responses (see *Section 9.2*).

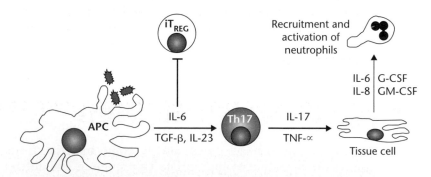

Figure 6.9
Th17 cells develop from Th0 cells in the presence of IL-6 (which inhibits the generation of suppressor iT$_{REG}$ cells) and TGF-β. IL-23 stabilizes the Th17 phenotype and induces Th17 cell proliferation. Production of IL-17 and TNF-α accounts for the pro-inflammatory effects of Th17 cells. IL-17 induces parenchymal cells to produce GM-CSF and G-CSF, which cause increased production of neutrophils, as well as IL-8, which leads to neutrophil recruitment.

Th17 cells

Th17 cells promote cell-mediated defence against extracellular bacterial infections especially via the expansion and recruitment of neutrophils. Th17 cells secrete IL-17 which acts on parenchymal cells to stimulate the production of IL-8 (see *Figure 6.9*), a potent neutrophil chemoattractant. IL-17 also causes bone marrow stromal cells to secrete GM-CSF and G-CSF, factors that cause an increase in neutrophil production (see *Figure 2.2*). Th17 cells also secrete the pro-inflammatory cytokine TNF-α. Recent data have implicated Th17 cells in the pathogenesis of cell-mediated autoimmune diseases (see *Section 10.7*).

iT$_{REG}$ cells

iT$_{REG}$ cells play an important role in suppressing immune responses and in maintenance of peripheral tolerance (see *Section 10.2*). The mechanisms of action of iT$_{REG}$ cells will be discussed later (see *Section 7.6*).

T$_{FH}$ cells

Following stimulation with antigen, a percentage of CD4⁺ T cells acquire expression of the chemokine receptor CXCR5 and, therefore, become sensitive to the chemokine CXCL13 which is produced by stromal cells in B cell follicles. The CD4⁺CXCR5⁺ T cells migrate to the follicles where they interact with antigen-specific B cells and promote antibody production. It is currently unclear whether these T$_{FH}$ cells arise from polarized Th1 and Th2 cells or whether they constitute a separate Th lineage. Although these three Th subsets have several features in common, they also differ in many respects (see *Table 6.1*). T$_{FH}$ cells are now considered to be the primary cells involved in providing T cell help for antibody production in lymph node follicles. Central to this function is their production of the cytokine IL-21 which binds to its receptor on B cells and promotes their differentiation into antibody producing cells.

6.6 GENERATION OF EFFECTOR AND MEMORY CD4⁺ T CELLS

Following activation by antigen, CD4⁺ T cells differentiate into short-lived effector cells or long-lived memory cells. Effector cells provide immediate defence against the antigen whereas memory cells confer protection upon re-exposure to the antigen. Effector and memory cells differ from each other in their expression of surface molecules (see *Table 6.2*). It is thought that effector and memory cell populations are established early following activation due to asymmetric cell division of antigen-specific T cells. This is made possible by selective recruitment of surface molecules into the immunological synapse during T cell–APC interaction (see *Figure 6.10*). Following cell

Table 6.1 Characteristics of Th1, Th2 and T$_{FH}$ cells^a

Cell	Function	Cytokines produced	Chemoattractant receptors
Th1	Defence against intracellular pathogens	IFN-γ, TNF-α, LT	CXCR3, CCR5
Th2	Defence against extracellular pathogens/parasites	IL-4. IL-5, IL-10. IL-13,	CCR3, CRTH2
T$_{FH}$	Provision of B cell help	IL-10, IL-21	CXCR5

^{a}**Abbreviations**: CCR, CC chemokine receptor; CXCR, CXC chemokine receptor; CRTH2, chemoattractant receptor homologous molecule expressed by Th2 cells; IFN, interferon; IL, interleukin; LT, lymphotoxin; TNF, tumour necrosis factor.

Table 6.2 Characteristics of naïve, effector and memory T cells

Molecule	Naïve	Effector	Memory
CCR7	+++	+/–	Subset
CD25	–	++	–
CD44	+	+++	+++
CD45RA	+++	+	+++
CD45RO	+	+++	+++
CD62L	+++	–	Subset
CD69	–	+++	–

division, one daughter cell will become an effector cell and one daughter cell will become a memory cell.

The effector T cells can leave the lymph node and migrate to the site of infection. Differential migration of T cells is controlled by changes in cell surface expression of chemokine receptors. Naïve CD4$^+$ T cells express the chemokine receptor CCR7 on their surfaces. This allows the T cell to traffic through lymphoid tissue in response to the chemokines CCL19 and CCL21. Following activation, T cells lose expression of CCR7 and acquire surface expression of the chemoattractant receptors CCR5 and CXCR3 (Th1 cells) or CRTH2 (chemoattractant receptor-homologous molecule expressed by Th2 cells) and CCR3 (Th2 cells). Thus Th1 cells will migrate to infected tissues in response to the inflammatory chemokines CXCL10 (which binds to CXCR3) and CCL3 and CCL5 (which both bind to CCR5). Effector Th2 cells will migrate to sites of production of CCL11 (which binds to CCR3) and PGD$_2$ (which binds to CRTH2). Egress of T cells from lymphoid tissue

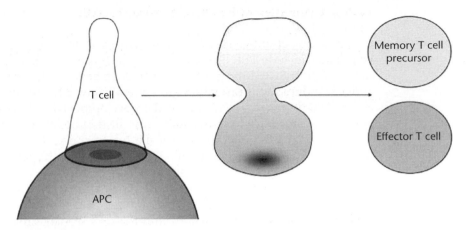

Figure 6.10
Formation of the immunological synapse leads to polarization of the T cell. As a result, subsequent cell division is asymmetric and results in daughter cells that are enriched for different effector molecules. Data from experiments using CD8$^+$ T cells suggest that the daughter cell proximal to the APC becomes an effector cell whereas the distal daughter cell becomes a memory cell.

is also dependent on S1P (see *Section 6.2*) binding to its receptor on the activated T cells.

Memory cells can be further sub-divided into central memory (C_M) and effector memory (E_M) cells. C_M T cells express CD62L and CCR7 but do not express either IFN-γ or IL-4. These memory T cells can reside for extended periods in secondary lymphoid tissues. E_M T cells are CD62L$^-$CCR7$^-$ cells which do produce effector cytokines and leave the lymph node and migrate through peripheral non-lymphoid tissues in search of antigen. Memory cells persist for many years after the initiating antigen has been eliminated from the body. Maintenance of CD4$^+$ memory T cells is dependent on the cytokine IL-7.

Following antigen stimulation, a subset of the antigen-specific T cells acquires expression of CXCR5 and differentiates into T_{FH} cells. Although these cells do not exhibit the polarized pattern of cytokine secretion characteristic of Th1 or Th2 cells, it is not yet known whether they constitute a separate CD4$^+$ T cell lineage, or whether they develop from Th1 and/or Th2 cells and subsequently acquire the ability to produce multiple cytokines. Following expression of CXCR5 T_{FH} cells migrate towards B cell follicles, in response to CXCL13, to interact with antigen-specific B cells.

6.7 ACQUISITION OF ANTIGEN BY B CELLS

Naïve B cells enter the lymph node via the HEVs in the paracortex and migrate to follicles in response to CXCL13. The B cells spend approximately 24 hours in the follicles, unless they encounter specific antigen, before exiting via the efferent lymph. If a naïve B cell does not encounter antigen within 8–10 days it will die.

A minority of antigens can directly activate B cells independent of T cell help. These include TLR ligands and microbial capsular polysaccharides that can cross-link BCRs on the B cell surface. In general, these T-independent antigens induce rapid production of generally low affinity antibody, usually of the IgM isotype, and stimulate the development of short-lived plasma cells. These short-lived plasma cells settle in the medullary cords of lymph nodes or in the bridging channels of the spleen and secrete antigen into the circulation. The generation of T-independent antibody responses is independent of B cell follicles. However, most antibody responses require help from T cells and are called T-dependent responses. Generation of T-dependent responses requires that the antigen be delivered to B cell follicles.

Antigen from the tissues drains into the subcapsular sinus of the lymph node which overlies the follicles. The subcapsular sinus contains macrophages that extend their cellular processes into the underlying follicles. These macrophages rapidly capture antigen from the lymph, in particular antigen that has complement bound to it, and transfer the antigen, bound on the surfaces of their long appendages, to the follicles. The antigen is retrieved from the subcapsular sinus macrophages by binding to the complement receptors CR1 and CR2 on the surfaces of follicular B cells. The follicular B cells carry the antigen through the follicle to follicular dendritic cells (FDC) and deposit the antigen on the surface of the FDCs. In the spleen, marginal zone B cells are thought to acquire antigen from the circulation and, following expression of CXCR5, transport the captured antigen to FDCs in B cell follicles.

Any B cells in the follicles that are specific for the antigen also can bind to the antigen via their BCR. Following binding, the antigen–BCR complex is internalized and the antigen is processed and presented on the B cell surface bound to MHC class II molecules. The antigen processing pathway used by B cells (see *Figure 6.11*) is just a modification of the conventional exogenous pathway. Importantly, this modification ensures that the epitope that the B cell presents on MHC class II molecules is a fragment of the antigen that was bound to the BCR. This ensures that B cells can only present antigen to, and receive help from, T cells that are specific for the same antigen (or antigenic complex). In other words, this is how B cells recruit antigen-specific T cell help. Note that because of the different ways that B cells and T cells recognize antigen (see *Figure 2.13*), the BCR and TCR generally will not recognize the same epitope, but different epitopes on the same antigen. The requirement for T cell help for antibody production guards against the generation of antibody responses against harmless antigens. To prevent such undesirable responses, an antigen-specific B cell must receive help from a T cell that is specific for the same antigen, and that has been activated by a DC that has sensed 'danger' (i.e. that has been induced to mature by inflammatory stimuli).

Like T cells, B cells also need two signals in order to become activated. Signal 1 for B cell activation is delivered through the BCR complex after it has bound antigen (see *Figure 6.12*). This pathway shares many general

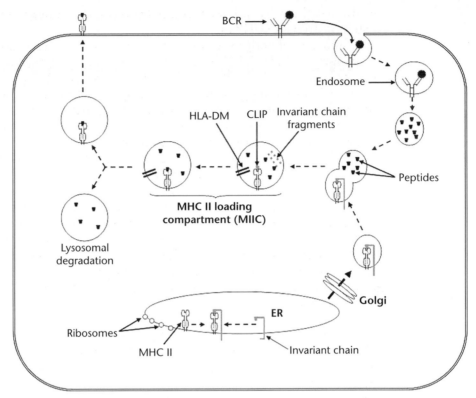

Figure 6.11
The exogenous antigen presentation pathway of B cells is a modified version of the conventional exogenous pathway of antigen presentation. Specific antigen is captured by binding to the BCR and is subsequently taken up into the B cell by receptor-mediated endocytosis. Processing and presentation of the antigen occurs as described for the conventional exogenous pathway of antigen presentation (see *Section 5.10*).

features with the signal transduction pathway initiated by the TCR–CD3 complex, including the activation of PL-C, PK-C and Ras-exchange factors. Signal 2 for activation of B cells is delivered following interaction with antigen-specific T cells.

6.8 B CELL–T CELL INTERACTION

Following binding of antigen to the BCR, follicular B cells increase their expression of CCR7. This allows them to leave the follicle and migrate to the boundary of the paracortex in response to CCL19 and CCL21. There they encounter T_{FH} cells that have localized to the edge of the follicle due to their expression of CXCR5. The B cell presents peptide fragments of its specific antigen on MHC class II molecules to the T cell. This results in the formation of an immunological synapse between the two cells. Since the T cell has previously been activated, it only requires signal 1 (via TCR–CD3)

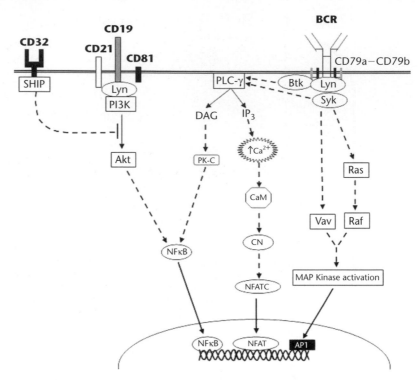

Figure 6.12
Stimulation of the BCR results in recruitment of the Src family kinase Lyn to the BCR complex where it phosphorylates residues in the cytoplasmic tails of CD79a and CD79b. This leads to recruitment and activation of the Syk protein kinase which phosphorylates downstream targets that activate MAP kinase pathways, resulting in translocation of the AP1 transcription factor to the nucleus. Bruton's tyrosine kinase (Btk) is also recruited to the BCR. Btk, in addition to Syk, activates phospholipase C-γ (PLC-γ) to release diacylglycerol (DAG) and inositol-1,4,5-trisphosphate (IP$_3$) from membrane phospholipids. DAG activates protein kinase C (PK-C) which relieves inhibition of the NFκB transcription factor, allowing it to translocate to the nucleus and activate gene transcription. IP$_3$ causes an increase in intracellular Ca^{2+} which activates the phosphatase calcineurin (CN). CN activates the NFAT transcription factor allowing it to translocate to the nucleus and activate gene expression. Signals generated by the CD19/CD21/CD81 co-receptor complex augment activation of the NFκB pathway. This is inhibited by signals generated by the inhibitory molecule CD32.

to become fully activated once more. The activated T cell expresses CD154 on its surface. This binds to CD40 on the surface of the B cell. The binding of CD154 to CD40 transmits signal 2 for activation to the B cell (see *Figure 6.13*). The B cell can now become fully activated.

The B cell next begins to express receptors for cytokines that are being produced by the activated T$_{FH}$ cell, especially the receptor for IL-4 which is a major growth factor for B cells. The T cell-derived cytokines cause the B cell to proliferate. Up to this point the B cells can secrete low levels of gener-

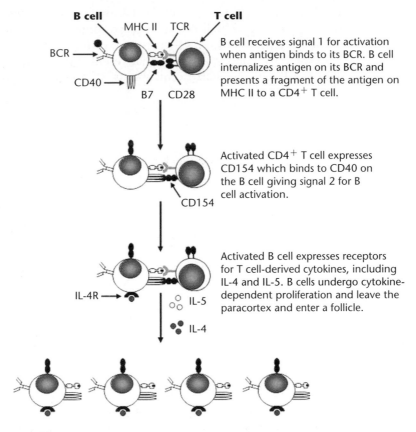

B cell

BCR

MHC II   TCR

CD40

B7   CD28

T cell

B cell receives signal 1 for activation when antigen binds to its BCR. B cell internalizes antigen on its BCR and presents a fragment of the antigen on MHC II to a CD4$^+$ T cell.

CD154

Activated CD4$^+$ T cell expresses CD154 which binds to CD40 on the B cell giving signal 2 for B cell activation.

IL-4R

IL-5

IL-4

Activated B cell expresses receptors for T cell-derived cytokines, including IL-4 and IL-5. B cells undergo cytokine-dependent proliferation and leave the paracortex and enter a follicle.

Figure 6.13
The interaction between an antigen-specific T cell and B cell in the paracortex of a lymph node.

ally low affinity IgM. At this stage some of the B cells differentiate into short-lived plasma cells and settle in medullary cords (lymph nodes) or in bridging channels (spleen) and secrete antigen into the circulation. A small number of antigen-specific B cells will re-enter the follicle, together with T_{FH} cells. Here the B cells will mutate their immunoglobulin genes and select those that encode BCRs that bind with highest affinity to the antigen. Collectively these processes result in production of high affinity antibody, a process that is frequently called affinity maturation of the antibody response. The cellular and molecular events that lead to affinity maturation are called the germinal centre reaction.

6.9   THE GERMINAL CENTRE REACTION

B cells that re-enter the follicle undergo several rounds of proliferation over the course of a few days. As the cells proliferate, the primary follicle expands and becomes a secondary follicle. Ultimately the intense cell proliferation gives rise to a germinal centre. The germinal centre consists of two main regions, a dark zone and a light zone (see *Figure 6.14*).

In the dark zone, the B cells that re-enter the follicle proliferate. At this stage the B cells are called centroblasts. Centroblasts no longer express the

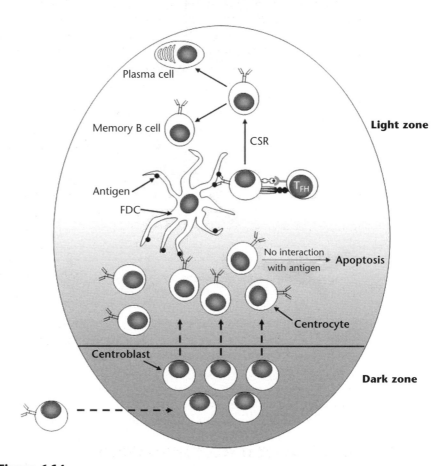

Figure 6.14
An activated B cell enters the follicle and proliferates, giving rise to many daughter cells and leading to the formation of a germinal centre. The proliferating B cells lose surface expression of their BCRs and become centroblasts. In the dark zone of the germinal centre the centroblasts undergo somatic hypermutation in which the rearranged V(D)J regions of their immunoglobulin genes are selectively mutated. The cells then express these mutated BCRs on their cell surfaces and become centrocytes. In the light zone of the germinal centre, the centrocytes compete with each other for binding to antigen deposits on the surface of follicular dendritic cells (FDCs). Only those cells whose BCRs can bind to the antigen get a survival signal. Those cells whose BCR binds to the antigen with low affinity are out-competed by the high affinity BCR-expressing cells and die by apoptosis. Following interaction with T_{FH} cells, the B cell undergoes class switch recombination and differentiates into a plasma cell or a memory B cell.

BCR on their surface but begin to mutate their immunoglobulin genes at a very high frequency ($\sim 10^{-3}$ per base pair per generation). This process is called somatic hypermutation (SHM). The mutations are targeted at the V(D)J regions of the heavy chain and light chain and do not occur in the constant region gene segments. SHM requires the activity of an enzyme called activation-induced cytidine deaminase (AID). AID catalyses the deamination of deoxycytidine which changes a C:G base pair into a U:G base pair. This U:G mismatch can be repaired by excision of the uracil base by uracil-DNA glycosylase (UNG) and replacement of the deleted base by any nucleotide. DNA polymerase η (eta) can also repair the U:G mismatch, but has a tendency to introduce mutations at A:T base pairs. Other DNA repair factors and error-prone DNA polymerases also contribute to the introduction of mutations into the V(D)J region. After SHM of V(D)J sequences, the centroblasts differentiate into cells called centrocytes and move to the light zone of the germinal centre. The mutated BCRs are then expressed on the surface of the centrocytes and tested for their ability to bind antigen.

BCRs are tested for their ability to bind antigen using the antigen that has been deposited on the surfaces of FDCs (see *Section 6.7*). B cells that have mutated their BCRs compete with one another for binding to the trapped antigen on the FDCs. The cells whose BCRs bind antigen with high affinity, out-compete the lower affinity B cells for binding to the antigen on the FDCs. Only cells that bind antigen get a survival signal via their BCRs that have bound antigen, as well as via interaction with antigen-specific T_{FH} cells. The other B cells die and are phagocytosed by cells called tingible body macrophages. Thus, after several rounds of proliferation and hypermutation, only B cells with the highest affinity BCRs remain. The overall result is the selection of B cells that are able to bind antigen with high affinity.

After mutating the immunoglobulin V(D)J sequence to 'improve the fit' of the antibody for the antigen, the B cell then alters the isotype of the antibody produced to make it more effective at eliminating the antigen. The process whereby this occurs is called class switch recombination (CSR).

6.10 CLASS SWITCH RECOMBINATION

The high affinity B cells again interact with antigen-specific T cells and, under the influence of T cell-derived cytokines, undergo CSR (also called isotype switching). The isotype that is produced is highly dependent on the predominant cytokine made by the T cell. For example, TGF-β induces class switching to IgA, whereas IL-4 is the major cytokine that induces class switching to IgE. The precise source of the cytokines that direct CSR is not completely understood. The predominant helper T cell in germinal centres is the T_{FH} cell and, *in vitro*, these cells are the most effective CD4$^+$ T cell subset at inducing CSR. However, Th2 cells, and to a lesser extent Th1 cells, have also been shown to localize to follicles and several studies have shown that populations of Th2 cells produce IL-21, a cytokine which promotes differentiation of B cells into antibody-producing cells. It is possible that the

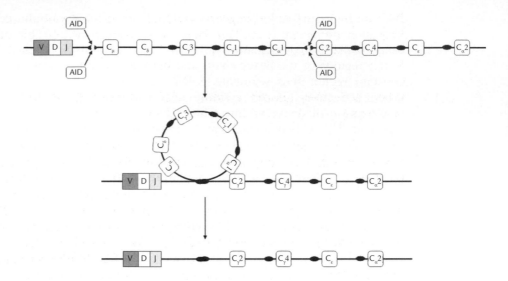

Figure 6.15
Class switch recombination is initiated by AID-mediated deamination of deoxycytidine bases on both strands of DNA in the switch sequence upstream of the selected constant region gene segments. The repair process results in the generation of double strand (ds) breaks. In the example shown, ds breaks are introduced in the switch regions flanking the C_μ and $C_\gamma 2$ gene segments. The intervening DNA is excised and ligation of the DNA strands results in a switch from IgM to IgG2.

production of Th1- and Th2-associated immunoglobulin isotypes requires the participation of Th1 cells and Th2 cells, but requires T_{FH} cells to promote high level B cell proliferation, antibody secretion and plasma cell differentiation in germinal centres. If T_{FH} cells develop from Th1 cells and Th2 cells, however, it is possible that they retain a degree of 'Th1-ness' or 'Th2-ness' that enables them to promote CSR to Th1- and Th2-associated immunoglobulin isotypes. An alternative explanation is that Th1- and Th2-driven CSR occurs outside of B cell follicles. This is consistent with the observations that extrafollicular CSR does occur and that CSR to IgE, a major Th2-associated isotype, is rarely observed within germinal centres.

The interaction between CD154 on the T cell and CD40 on the B cell is essential for initiation of CSR. Other important signals for induction of CSR are delivered by the T cell surface molecule ICOS binding to B7-H2 on the B cells, as well as by BAFF on the T cell binding to BAFF-R and TACI on the B cell (see *Section 3.3*).

CSR is initiated by induction of double strand breaks in regions of DNA called switch sequences (see *Figure 6.15*). These switch sequences are located upstream of each of the constant region gene segments. Like SHM, CSR requires the activity of AID. AID-mediated deamination of deoxycytidine residues in the switch sequences on both strands of DNA initiates a process that results in the generation of double strand breaks adjacent to the constant gene segments that are to be switched. The intervening DNA is deleted from the chromosome and the ends of the DNA strands are ligated. Transcription of the modified locus will produce mRNA encoding the switched immunoglobulin isotype.

6.11 GENERATION OF PLASMA CELLS AND MEMORY B CELLS

The events described in *Sections 6.7–6.10* allow a single antigen-specific B cell to proliferate and generate many thousands of antigen-specific daughter B cells. In particular, the germinal centre reaction results in the generation of high affinity, class switched antibody-producing B cells. These B cells develop into long-lived, high-level antibody-secreting plasma cells or into memory B cells. There is evidence that memory B cells may also be generated early during the germinal centre reaction. The factors that determine which pathway a B cell follows are as yet unclear. Unlike the short-lived plasma cells that are generated during extrafollicular responses, many long-lived plasma cells migrate to the bone marrow where they also secrete antibody into the circulation. The maintenance of memory B cells is thought to be dependent on homeostatic cytokines. Upon re-exposure to specific antigen, memory B cells rapidly differentiate into plasma cells that secrete high levels of high affinity antibody.

6.12 GENERATION OF CD8⁺ T CELL RESPONSES

The generation of CD8$^+$ cytotoxic T lymphocyte (CTL) responses is similar to that described earlier for CD4$^+$ T cell responses. DCs acquire virus, either in the tissues or after it has been carried in lymph to draining lymph nodes. The antigen is processed and presented, either via the endogenous pathway or via cross-presentation, on MHC class I molecules (see *Section 5.10*). Recent research indicates that the DC presents its antigenic cargo to CD8$^+$ T cells in the peripheral region of the lymph node, adjacent to the subcapsular sinus. Just like naïve CD4$^+$ T cells, naïve CD8$^+$ T cells require two signals before they can become activated; signal 1 delivered via the TCR after recognition of antigen–MHC class I molecules and signal 2 delivered via CD28 after it binds to B7 on the DC.

Just like proliferation of naïve CD4$^+$ cells, proliferation of CD8$^+$ T cells is dependent on IL-2. Although CD8$^+$ cells can themselves make some IL-2, most of the IL-2 required for generating CTLs comes from CD4$^+$ cells. One model of how this may happen is shown in *Figure 6.16*. In addition to presenting viral antigen on MHC class I to CD8$^+$ T cells, the antigen-bearing DC can simultaneously present its viral antigen on MHC class II molecules to CD4$^+$ cells, resulting in the generation of a Th1 response. These virus-specific CD4$^+$ cells provide the virus-specific CD8$^+$ cells with the IL-2 that they require for proliferation. Current research suggests that the interaction between DCs and virus-specific CD4$^+$ cells leads to the production of the chemokine CCL3. The released CCL3 causes chemotaxis of CD8$^+$ cells towards the site of production of this chemokine, i.e. the site of DC–CD4$^+$ cell interaction. This brings the CD4$^+$ and CD8$^+$ cells together so that the CD8$^+$ cell can receive 'help' (especially IL-2) from the CD4$^+$ T cell. Not only does IL-2 cause proliferation of CD8$^+$ cells, but it also causes them to make the major molecules that they use to kill infected cells. Following stimulation with IL-2, CD8$^+$ cells synthesize perforin and enzymes called granzymes, and store these molecules in granules in the cytosol of the cell. The CTL is now primed to kill and leave the lymph node and migrates to the site of infection.

Migration of CTL to infected tissue is promoted by alteration in cell surface chemokine receptor expression as described earlier for migration of activated CD4$^+$ T cells (see *Section 6.6*). Naïve CD8$^+$ T cells express the chemokine receptor CCR7 on their surfaces allowing them to traffic through lymphoid tissue in response to CCL19 and CCL21. Following activation, CD8$^+$ cells lose CCR7 expression and acquire surface expression of CCR5 and CXCR3. This alteration in surface chemokine receptor expression, as well as responsiveness to S1P, allows CTL to leave the lymph node and migrate to the site of infection where the ligands for CCR5 and CXCR3 are produced.

At the site of infection the CTL will recognize viral antigen presented on MHC class I of infected cells. The CTL will bind tightly to the infected cell and secrete the contents of its granules (degranulate) in the direction of the infected cell. The released perforin inserts into the membrane of the infected

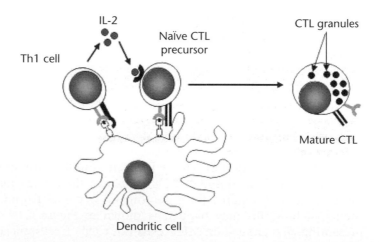

Figure 6.16
A DC can present antigen on MHC class I to CD8$^+$ T cells and on MHC class II to CD4$^+$ T cells. The CD4$^+$ T cell produces IL-2 which binds to its receptor on the CD8$^+$ T cell, inducing the cell to express perforin and granzymes. This causes the CD8$^+$ T cell to develop from a cytotoxic T lymphocyte (CTL) precursor cell into a mature CTL. For clarity, the co-stimulatory molecule CD28 has been omitted.

cell and forms polyperforin pores, very much like the membrane attack complex of complement (see *Figure 6.17*). These pores allow the granzymes to enter the infected cell where they initiate a cascade of events leading to apoptosis of the infected cell. CTL granules also contain granulysin, a lipid binding protein that can disrupt the membranes of many microbial pathogens.

Interaction between CD8+ cells and DCs results in the generation of an immunological synapse similar to that described for CD4+ T cell–DC interactions (see *Section 6.3*). In addition, it is thought that the differentiation of polarized effector and memory CD8+ T cells also results from asymmetric cell division. Memory CD8+ T cells also can be subdivided into CD62L+CCR7+ C_M cells that reside for extended periods in lymphoid tissues and CD62L−CCR7− E_M cells that migrate through peripheral non-lymphoid tissues in search of antigen. Analogous to memory CD4+ T cells, memory CD8+ T cells persist for many years after the stimulating antigen has been eliminated from the body. Maintenance of CD8+ memory T cells is dependent on the cytokines IL-7 and IL-15.

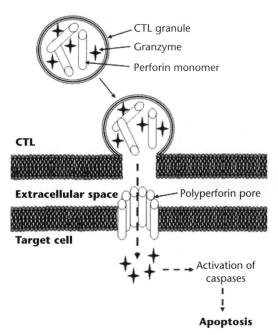

Figure 6.17
When the CTL recognizes a virus-infected cell it releases the contents of its granules, perforin and granzymes, towards that cell. The perforin polymerizes and inserts into the membrane of the infected cell forming a pore. The granzymes enter the infected cell through the polyperforin pore and activate caspases which causes the apoptotic death of the cell.

6.13 SECONDARY IMMUNE RESPONSES

The events described so far occur following the immune system's first exposure to a specific antigen. This response is called the primary response. The primary response against antigen is maximal at approximately 8–10 days following exposure. After elimination of antigen the majority (>90%) of the antigen-specific cells die (see *Section 7.5*). However, as described in the previous sections, memory B cells and memory T cells that are generated during the primary response are maintained. The persistence of these memory cells ensures that the immune system will respond more rapidly, and more vigorously, upon re-exposure to the antigen (see *Figure 6.18*). Unlike the primary response, this secondary response is usually maximal within 3–4 days of re-exposure to antigen. This anamnestic, or memory, response is a hallmark of adaptive immunity and promotes rapid elimination of antigen upon re-exposure. The secondary response also differs from the primary response in other respects. The antibody produced during the primary response is primarily of the IgM isotype and usually of low affinity. However, because of CSR and SHM, large amounts of high affinity antibody are produced during the secondary response and this antibody is usually of the IgG, IgA or IgE isotype.

Elimination of antigen, either during the primary or secondary response, results in down-regulation of the immune response. This is important to control immunopathology associated with uncontrolled immune cell activation. In the next section we will discuss mechanisms responsible for regulation of the adaptive immune response.

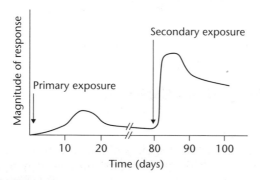

Figure 6.18
The secondary response differs from the primary response in that it occurs more rapidly following exposure to antigen. The magnitude of the secondary response also is much greater than that of the primary response.

SUGGESTED FURTHER READING

Bajénoff, M., Egen, J.G., Qi, H., Huang, A.Y.C., Castellino, F. and Germain, R.N. (2007) Highways, byways and breadcrumbs: directing lymphocyte traffic in the lymph node. *Trends Immunol.* **28**: 346–352.

Billadeau, D.D., Nolx, J.C. and Gomez, T.S. (2007) Regulation of T cell activation by the cytoskeleton. *Nature Rev. Immunol.* **7**: 131–143.

Chang, J.T., Palanivel, V.R., Kinjyo, I., *et al.* (2007) Asymmetric T lymphocyte division in the initiation of adaptive immune responses. *Science*, **315**: 1687–1691.

Crivellato, E., Vacca, A. and Ribatti, D. (2004) Setting the stage: an anatomist's view of the immune system. *Trends Immunol.* **25**: 210–217.

Dustin, M.L., Tseng, S.-Y., Varma, R. and Campi, G. (2006) T cell–dendritic cell immunological synapses. *Curr. Opin. Immunol.* **18**: 512–518.

Gordon, S. (2003) Alternative activation of macrophages. *Nature Rev. Immunol.* **3**: 23–35.

Klein, U. and Dalla-Favera, R. (2008) Germinal centres: role in B-cell physiology and malignancy. *Nature Rev. Immunol.* **8**: 22–33.

Mebius, R. and Kraal, G. (2005) Structure and function of the spleen. *Nature Rev. Immunol.* **5**: 606–616.

Pape, K.A., Catron, D.M., Itano, A.A. and Jenkins, M.K. (2007) The humoral immune response is initiated in lymph nodes by B cells that acquire soluble antigen directly in the follicles. *Immunity*, **26**: 491–502.

Reiner, S.L. (2007) Development in motion: Helper T cells at work. *Cell*, **129**: 33–36.

Sallusto, F., Geginat, J. and Lanzavecchia, A. (2004) Central memory and effector memory T cell subsets: function, generation, and maintenance. *Annu. Rev. Immunol.* **22**: 745–763.

Schwab, S.R. and Cyster, J.C. (2007) Finding a way out: lymphocyte egress from lymphoid organs. *Nature Immunol.* **8**: 1295–1301.

Shaw, A.S. (2008) How T cells 'find' the right dendritic cell. *Nature Immunol.* **9**: 229–230.

von Andrian, U.H. and Mempel, T.R. (2003) Homing and cellular traffic in lymph nodes. *Nature Rev. Immunol.* **3**: 867–878.

SELF-ASSESSMENT QUESTIONS

1. Name three functions of IL-4.
2. List three signals important for class switch recombination.
3. How do follicular dendritic cells acquire antigen in lymph nodes?
4. What causes follicular B cells to migrate to B cell follicles?
5. List three differences between primary and secondary immune responses.
6. What two processes in germinal centres are initiated by the enzyme activation-induced cytidine deaminase?
7. How do $CD8^+$ CTLs kill virus-infected cells?
8. What cytokines are required for the differentiation from Th0 cells into Th1 cells, Th2 cells, iT_{REG} cells and Th17 cells?
9. What is the lymph node conduit system?
10. What types of cells would you expect to find in the splenic marginal zone?

Regulation of the adaptive immune response

Learning objectives
After studying this chapter you should confidently be able to:

■ **Understand the requirement for immune regulation**
In order to mount an effective response to antigens, the immune system must rapidly generate sufficient numbers of antigen-specific T cells and B cells to counteract the threat. When the antigen has been eliminated the immune system must shut down the inflammatory response in order to avoid unnecessary damage to the host. It is also essential to eliminate the majority of the antigen-specific cells and restore the numbers of lymphocytes to normal levels.

■ **Discuss the role of antigen in shaping the immune response**
Antigen is the 'master switch' of the adaptive immune response. In a normal healthy immune system, without antigen, there is no response. The nature, dose and location of the antigen, all determine the type of immune response that is generated. When the antigen has been eliminated from the body the antigen-specific immune response diminishes as there is no longer sufficient antigen to stimulate T cells and B cells. Removal of antigen also results in decreased levels of cytokines that are required for maintaining the proliferation of antigen-specific lymphocytes. This cytokine deprivation leads to death of the cells.

■ **Describe the major mechanisms responsible for dampening the responses of antigen-specific lymphocytes**
A major mechanism of silencing antigen-specific immune responses is via induction of anergy. Binding of CTLA-4 on activated T cells to B7 on APCs transmits an inhibitory signal into the T cell. Other inhibitory co-receptors that can induce anergy include PD-1 and BTLA. Antigen-specific lymphocytes can also be silenced by induction of apoptosis. There are two major pathways by which this can occur. In activation-induced cell death (AICD), lymphocytes that have been stimulated through their antigen receptors are induced to undergo apoptosis following interaction between Fas, on the lymphocyte surface, and Fas ligand. Cytokine deprivation results in activated cell autonomous death (ACAD), an alternative apoptotic pathway that is independent of antigen receptor stimulation. B cell production of antibody may be modulated by feedback inhibition resulting from antibody binding to Fc receptors on the B cell surface. T cell responsiveness to cytokines can be inhibited by suppressor of cytokine signalling (SOCS) family members. T cell responses also may be inhibited by regulatory T cells.

■ **Discuss the modes of action of regulatory T cells**
There are at least three types of regulatory T cells; nT_{REG} cells, iT_{REG} cells and Tr1 cells. nT_{REG} cells develop in the thymus whereas iT_{REG} and Tr1 cells develop in the periphery from Th0 cells. nT_{REG} cells are thought to exert their immunosuppressive activity by cell–cell interaction via CTLA-4 or via membrane-associated TGF-β. In contrast, the immunosuppressive activities of iT_{REG} cells are believed to be mediated via release of the immunosuppressive cytokines TGF-β and IL-10. nT_{REG} and iT_{REG} cells also compete with effector T cells for binding of IL-2, leading to cytokine deprivation and death of the effector T cells. The suppressor activity of Tr1 cells is believed to be due to production of IL-10.

7.1   INTRODUCTION TO IMMUNOREGULATION

Cell-mediated and humoral immune responses must be tightly regulated following exposure to antigen. If this did not happen then the body would be overwhelmed by reactive lymphocytes and their secreted products, leading to substantial immunopathology. In essence, immunoregulation strives to attain a balance between immune activation and suppressor mechanisms to achieve an efficient immune response without damaging the host. Excessive activation of the immune system can lead to autoimmune disease whereas insufficient activation may lead to overwhelming infections.

Immunoregulation is complex, with regulatory mechanisms operative during the recognition, activation and effector phases of an immune response. Cytokines are important regulators of the immune system and can act at all these stages. Competition between lymphocytes for limiting amounts of cytokines is central to shaping the peripheral lymphocyte pool.

This chapter will focus on the down-regulation of adaptive immune responses by elimination of antigen-reactive cells and by inhibition of the function of these antigen-reactive cells. As the majority of B cell responses are T cell-dependent, inhibition of T cell function will also inhibit most humoral responses. However, there also are specific regulatory mechanisms that act directly on B cells.

A clearer understanding of the mechanisms that determine the balance between immune responses and tolerance could help in the design of novel therapies. For example, induction of tolerance could be used to treat autoimmune diseases (such as rheumatoid arthritis) or to prevent rejection of transplanted organs.

7.2   THE ROLE OF ANTIGEN

Adaptive immune responses are essentially antigen-driven responses. The nature, amount and site of entry of the antigen into the body determine the type of immune response that is generated, for example a Th1 or a Th2 response. This is predominantly determined by signals transmitted into the APC following the interaction between the antigen and a PRR (see *Section*

4.2). The amount of antigen also determines the magnitude and duration of the immune response. There is a threshold of antigen concentration that is required to induce T cell and B cell responses. Following an immune response, as the antigen is almost eliminated, lymphocyte responses wane. Elimination of antigen results in less antigen available to stimulate T cell and B cell responses. This in turn means that the levels of cytokines, in particular the levels of IL-2, IL-4, IL-9 and IL-21, secreted by activated T cells will also diminish. IL-2 and IL-4 are the main factors that drive the proliferation of Th1 cells and Th2 cells, respectively, and IL-9 and IL-21 also induce lymphocyte proliferation. Without these cytokines to sustain the clonal expansion of lymphocytes, a large proportion of the proliferating cells will die due to cytokine deprivation by a process that has been termed activated cell autonomous death (ACAD, see *Section 7.5*).

Additionally, persistent high levels of antigen also can down-regulate immune responses. For example, during chronic viral infection, high levels of persisting viral antigen can shut down virus-specific CD8$^+$ T cell function. The CD8$^+$ T cells may persist for some time but they are no longer responsive to stimulation by antigen. This phenomenon has variously been termed clonal paralysis or clonal exhaustion.

7.3   FEEDBACK INHIBITION

A key regulatory feature of many biological systems is feedback inhibition. A simple example of this is when the secreted products of a cell act on that same cell to inhibit synthesis of more of the same products. The classic example of feedback inhibition of immune function is mediated by antibody binding to CD32 on B cells. CD32 is a low affinity receptor for IgG (FcγRII) that is present on virtually all mature B cells. Binding of IgG-containing immune complexes to CD32 sends a signal into B cells that leads to down-regulation of antibody production. As CD32 is a low affinity receptor for IgG this negative signalling will normally only occur when the levels of IgG-containing immune complexes are high. Thus, antibody production is inhibited under conditions where antibody levels are high.

A similar mechanism of feedback inhibition controls IgE production. CD23 is a low-affinity IgE receptor (FcϵRII). Binding of IgE to CD23 on B cells leads to interaction between CD23 and CD21, a negative signalling molecule. This results in a signal being transmitted into B cells that leads to inhibition of IgE production. In this way IgE secretion can be inhibited when IgE levels are high.

Responsiveness of T cells to their secreted products, cytokines, also can be controlled by feedback inhibition. Many cytokines, including interleukins, interferons and colony stimulating factors, activate the Janus kinase (JAK) signal transducer and activator of transcription (Stat) pathway of signal transduction (see *Figure 7.1*). Suppressor of cytokine signalling (SOCS) proteins inhibit JAK-Stat signalling pathways. Eight members of the SOCS family have been identified so far; cytokine-inducible SH2-domain-containing protein (CIS) and SOCS-1–7. The expression of most SOCS

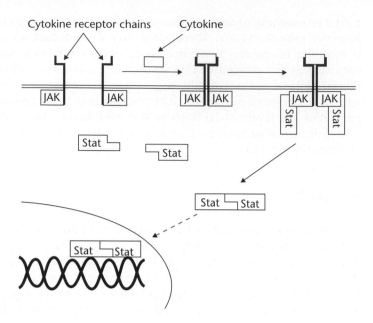

Figure 7.1
The chains of many cytokine receptors are associated with Janus kinases (JAKs). When cytokine binds to these receptors this brings the chains together so the JAKs can activate each other and then phosphorylate amino acid residues in the cytoplasmic tails of the receptors. Members of the Stat (signal transducers and activators of transcription) family of transcription factors bind to the phosphorylated cytokine receptors and are themselves phosphorylated by the JAKs. The phosphorylated Stat proteins dimerize and translocate to the nucleus where they activate gene transcription.

Table 7.1 Cytokines that induce or are inhibited by selected SOCS proteins[a]

SOCS	Induced by	Inhibits
CIS	IL-2, IL-3, IL-6, IL-9, IFN-α, TNF-α	IL-2, IL-3
SOCS-1	IL-2, IL-4, IL-6, IL-9, IL-13, IFN-α/β, IFN-γ, TNF-α	IL-2, IL-4, IL-6, IL-12, IL-15, IFN-α/β, IFN-γ, TNF-α
SOCS-2	IL-6, IFN-α, IFN-γ	IL-6
SOCS-3	IL-1, IL-2, IL-6, IL-9, IL-10, IL-13, IFN-α, IFN-γ	IL-2, IL-4, IL-6, IL-9, IL-11, IFN-α/β, IFN-γ
SOCS-5	IL-6 IL-4, IL-6	

[a] **Abbreviations**: CIS, cytokine-inducible SH2-domain-containing protein; IFN, interferon; IL, interleukin; SOCS, suppressor of cytokine signalling; TNF, tumour necrosis factor.

proteins is induced by cytokines and they therefore act in a classical feedback loop to inhibit cytokine-dependent signal transduction (see *Table 7.1*). SOCS proteins usually function by inducing the ubiquitin-dependent degradation of the cytokine receptor signalling complex, although some can directly inhibit JAK activation or recruitment of Stat proteins to the receptor. As a result of SOCS activity, the responding cell is rendered less susceptible to cytokine-mediated stimulation and this can lead to down-regulation of cell function or proliferation in a manner similar to that seen following cytokine deprivation.

7.4 ANERGY

An important mechanism of down-regulating adaptive immune responses is to render the antigen-specific cells non-responsive, or anergic, to antigen. Activation of lymphocytes is mediated by positive signals transmitted via their antigen receptors and co-stimulatory molecules. In contrast, anergy is frequently induced through the delivery of inhibitory signals via co-receptor molecules. Negative signalling co-receptors transmit signals into cells that attenuate their responses and, therefore, are also important in maintenance of self-tolerance (see *Section 10.2*). Three of these inhibitory receptors interact with members of the B7 family. These are:

- CTL-associated antigen-4, CTLA-4 (CD178)
- programmed death-1, PD-1 (CD279)
- B and T lymphocyte attenuator, BTLA (CD272)

CTLA-4 is not detectable on resting T cells but its expression is induced following several days of T cell stimulation. During T cell activation, B7 on the APC binds to CD28 on the T cell. With time, however, CTLA-4 expres-

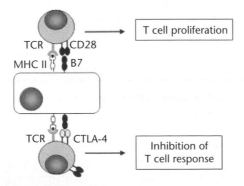

Figure 7.2
Signalling via CD28, when it binds to B7, is required for activation of naïve T cells and also augments T cell responses. By contrast, signalling via CTLA-4, when it binds to B7, inhibits T cell responses. Since the affinity with which CTLA-4 binds to B7 is 10–100 times greater than the affinity with which CD28 binds to B7, CTLA-4 will preferentially bind to B7 when both CD28 and CTLA-4 are expressed on a T cell.

sion is induced on the T cell. CTLA-4 has a greater affinity for B7 than does CD28 and it therefore successfully competes with CD28 binding to B7 (see *Figure 7.2*). The binding of CTLA-4 to B7 transmits an inhibitory signal into the T cell that inhibits T cell function. The T cells are rendered non-responsive to stimulation by antigen. The importance of this mechanism of immune regulation is evidenced by CTLA-4-deficient mice which exhibit uncontrolled T cell proliferation and die within 4 weeks of birth.

PD-1 is expressed on activated T cells, B cells and macrophages. There are two ligands for PD-1: B7H1 (CD274) and B7-DC (CD273). The cytoplasmic domain of PD-1 contains an immunoreceptor tyrosine-based inhibitory motif (ITIM; see *Box 7.1*) which is responsible for initiating transmission of a negative signal when PD-1 binds its ligand. The negative signal transmitted after ligation of PD-1 inhibits T cell function. Expression of B7H1 on tumours is believed to constitute a mechanism whereby they attempt to evade immune-mediated elimination. In addition, inactivation of HIV-specific CTLs is thought to occur via PD-1-dependent anergy.

Box 7.1 Immunoreceptor tyrosine-based inhibitory motifs

An ITIM is an amino acid sequence found in the cytoplasmic tails of many inhibitory receptors of the immune system. Phosphorylated ITIMs recruit protein phosphatases to the cell membrane where they deactivate signal transducing molecules.

BTLA is widely expressed on mononuclear leukocytes. Like PD-1, the cytoplasmic domain of BTLA contains an ITIM which is responsible for transmitting an inhibitory signal into the cell when BTLA binds to its receptor. The receptor for BTLA is CD270 which is expressed on T cells, monocytes and immature DCs. Ligation of BTLA by CD270 leads to inhibition of T cell function and may constitute a mechanism whereby immature DCs induce tolerance in naïve auto-reactive T cells.

7.5   APOPTOSIS

Exposure to antigen leads to expansion of antigen-reactive lymphocytes. In some viral infections the degree of expansion of the virus-specific $CD8^+$ T cell pool is quite remarkable, increasing from approximately 1 in 10^6 prior to infection, to greater than 1 in 10^2 at the peak of the adaptive immune response. After the virus has been eliminated, some of the virus-specific $CD8^+$ T cells persist as memory cells; however, most of the virus-specific $CD8^+$ T cells (>90%) must die to prevent serious immunopathology and to restore lymphocyte homeostasis (see *Figure 7.3*). This contraction of the antigen-specific immune response is largely due to apoptotic cell death.

Cell death is a daily occurrence in the immune system. The size of the peripheral lymphocyte pool remains relatively constant despite daily production of new B cells and T cells by the bone marrow and thymus,

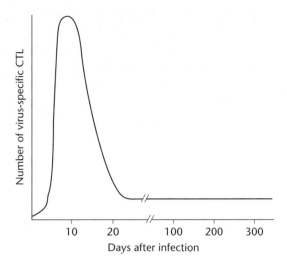

Figure 7.3
Viral infection results in a massive expansion of virus-specific CTLs. In general, peak numbers of virus-specific CTLs are detected 8–10 days following infection. Following elimination of the virus there is a precipitous decline in the numbers of virus-specific CTLs so that by 3 weeks following infection the numbers have declined by greater than 90%. The remaining CTLs consist of memory cells which may persist for many years after infection.

respectively. It has been estimated that approximately 10^{11} lymphocytes must die each day to maintain the constant size of the peripheral lymphocyte pool.

There are two main mechanisms whereby antigen-specific lymphocytes are eliminated, activation-induced cell death (AICD) and activated cell autonomous death (ACAD).

Activation-induced cell death

AICD refers to the induction of apoptosis in previously activated lymphocytes by restimulation of their antigen receptors. Early during the initiation of a T cell response, T cells are resistant to AICD but with time they become AICD-sensitive. Acquisition of AICD sensitivity in T cells is dependent on IL-2. A major pathway of AICD is initiated by binding of Fas (CD95) to its ligand FasL (CD178). Fas, a member of the TNF family, is expressed on the surfaces of activated B and T cells. FasL is expressed on activated T cells and certain epithelial cells. When FasL binds to Fas, a signal is transmitted through Fas that induces the apoptotic death of the Fas-expressing cell.

Binding of Fas to FasL induces the formation of a death-inducing signalling complex (DISC). The DISC contains trimerized Fas together with an adaptor molecule called Fas-associated death domain (FADD). The death domain on FADD binds to the death domain on Fas and recruits pro-caspase 8 and pro-caspase 10.

Freshly activated T cells express high levels of the anti-apoptotic B cell leukemia-2 (BCL-2) family member BCL-X_L which blocks Fas-induced apoptosis. During the expansion phase of the T cell response the levels of BCL-X_L drop. Under these conditions, ligation of Fas leading to activation of caspase 8 causes cleavage of another BCL-2 family member called Bid. Cleavage of Bid results in the generation of a truncated, pro-apoptotic form of the molecule, tBid. tBid is targeted to the mitochondria where it releases cytochrome c into the cytosol. The released cytochrome c binds to the cytosolic protein Apaf-1, ultimately leading to the formation of the multi-molecular apoptosome complex. The apoptosome recruits and activates pro-caspase 9. Caspase 9 ultimately activates caspase 3 and caspase 7 leading to death of the cell (see *Figure 7.4*).

Similarly, antigen-stimulated B cells are susceptible to Fas-mediated

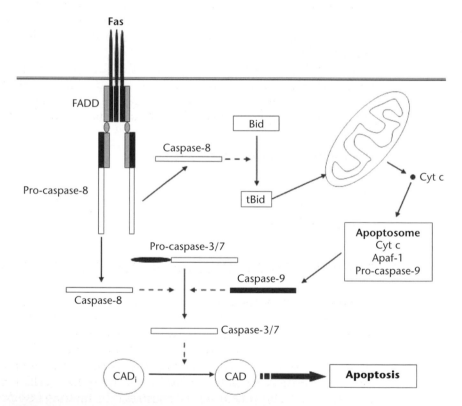

Figure 7.4
Binding to FasL induces trimerization of Fas which recruits the adaptor molecule FADD (Fas-associated death domain) to the cytoplasmic tails of the Fas trimer. This leads to the recruitment and cleavage of pro-caspase-8 to the Fas–FADD complex, forming the death-inducing signalling complex (DISC). Caspase-8 cleaves Bid, generating tBid, which releases cytochrome c (Cyt c) from mitochondria. Cyt c binds to Apaf-1 and pro-caspase-9 to form a complex called the apoptosome. This results in generation of caspase-9 which then activates caspases 3 and 7. Caspase-8 can also directly activate caspases 3 and 7. Caspases 3 and 7 then activate the caspase-activated DNase (CAD) leading to the apoptotic death of the cell.

AICD. This mechanism of apoptosis is important for purging the immune system of activated T cells and B cells. Mice that are deficient in either Fas or FasL are deficient in this form of AICD and exhibit profound lymphocytosis.

A Fas-independent pathway of AICD has been described for Th2 cells. In this pathway, AICD-sensitive Th2 cells synthesize granzyme B after stimulation of their TCRs. Granzyme B cleaves Bid leading to apoptosis of the cell as described above.

Activated cell autonomous death

This death pathway occurs in lymphocytes that are not restimulated by antigen when the concentration of antigen diminishes during an immune response. It is also sometimes called death by neglect or passive cell death. Because the cells are not restimulated they secrete lower levels of cytokines and/or express lower levels of cytokine receptors. This, ultimately, results in cytokine deprivation. Cytokine deprivation leads to an intracellular increase in the level of another pro-apoptotic BCL-2 family member called BIM (BCL-2 interacting mediator of cell death). BIM migrates to the mitochondria where it releases cytochrome c. This leads to the formation of the apoptosome complex and cell death as described above for AICD.

Perforin-mediated cell death

Studies using perforin-deficient mice have suggested a role for perforin in killing of antigen-specific CD8$^+$ T cells following elimination of antigen. The mechanism by which this occurs is unclear.

7.6 REGULATION BY CELL-MEDIATED SUPPRESSION

Recently it has become clear that cell-mediated suppression is a major mechanism for regulating immune responses. Several subsets of regulatory T cells exist, the best characterized ones being CD4$^+$ T$_{REG}$ cells. Even within the CD4$^+$ population of regulatory T cells there is considerable heterogeneity. A major subset of these cells that is important in maintaining immunological tolerance to self antigens, is the CD4$^+$CD25$^+$Foxp3$^+$ natural regulatory T (nT$_{REG}$) cell that develops in the thymus (see *Section 3.6*). In addition to thymically-derived nT$_{REG}$ cells, at least two other populations of CD4$^+$ regulatory/suppressor T cells exist. Unlike nT$_{REG}$ cells, the other regulatory T cells are thought to develop from naïve Th0 cells in secondary lymphoid tissues. One of these adaptive subsets is called Tr1. Tr1 cells develop from Th0 cells in the presence of IL-10. Unlike nT$_{REG}$ cells, Tr1 cells are Foxp3$^-$ T cells. The other subset of extra-thymically derived adaptive regulatory cells develops from Th0 cells in the presence of the cytokine TGF-β (see *Section 6.4*). Like nT$_{REG}$ cells, these inducible T$_{REG}$ (iT$_{REG}$) cells also are CD4$^+$CD25$^+$Foxp3$^+$.

Suppressor mechanisms of regulatory T cells

The suppressor mechanisms used by regulatory T cells is an area of intense research and several different mechanisms have been proposed (see *Figure 7.5*). The disparate mechanisms of action that have been described may be attributable to heterogeneous populations of regulatory T cells. Several experiments have demonstrated that the immunosuppressive activity of nT_{REG} cells is mediated by cell–cell contact. The precise molecular interactions are unclear, but may involve binding of CTLA-4 on the nT_{REG} cell to B7 on DCs. This interaction induces the expression of the enzyme indoleamine 2,3-dioxygenase (IDO) in DCs. IDO catalyses the conversion of the essential amino acid tryptophan into immunosuppressive catabolites such as kynurenine. CTLA-4-dependent signalling through B7 may also decrease the level of B7 on the DC surface, rendering it unable to provide

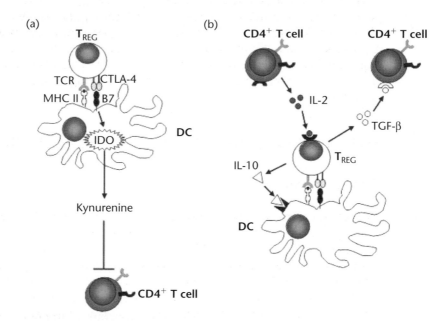

Figure 7.5
Mechanisms of T_{REG}-mediated inhibition. (a) Interaction between CTLA-4 on the T_{REG} and B7 on a DC induces expression of the enzyme indoleamine 2,3-dioxygenase (IDO) in the DC. IDO generates immunosuppressive metabolites, such as kynurenine, which are inhibitory to T cells. The interaction between CTLA-4 and B7 may also lead to down-regulation of B7 from the DC surface, rendering it unable to stimulate naïve T cells. (b) Cytokine-dependent inhibition by T_{REG} cells. T_{REG} cells may produce IL-10 which acts on DCs to render them tolerogenic. T_{REG} cells may also directly inhibit T cell function via the production of soluble or membrane-associated TGF-β, a potent immunosuppressive cytokine. Finally, T_{REG} cells express high levels of the IL-2 receptor and so can compete with other T cells for binding of this important T cell growth factor.

signal 2 to T cells leading to T cell anergy (see *Section 5.4*). Another model of nT_{REG} function proposes that membrane-associated TGF-β on the nT_{REG} binds to its receptor on effector T cells and inhibits proliferation of the effector T cell. Similarly, iT_{REG}-mediated suppression seems to be dependent on TGF-β; however, in this case the TGF-β is secreted by the iT_{REG}.

An alternative model for T_{REG}-mediated suppression has recently emerged. Both nT_{REG} cells and iT_{REG} cells express the IL-2 receptor, CD25. This allows them to compete successfully with effector T cells for binding of IL-2 produced by the effector T cells. This results in ACAD of the effector T cells due to cytokine deprivation (see *Section 7.5*). IL-2 stimulation also induces production of IL-10 by T_{REG} cells, a feature that is shared by Tr1 cells. Tr1 cells can down-regulate both Th1 and Th2 responses. These regulatory cells secrete IL-10 and this immunosuppressive cytokine is thought to be, at least in part, responsible for Tr1 cell-mediated suppression. IL-10 also may act on antigen-presenting DCs. IL-10-treated DCs induce tolerance in naïve T cells.

There is still much that we do not know about T_{REG} cells. There appears to be an ever increasing number of regulatory T cell subsets described in the scientific literature. The relationship, if any, between these subsets is unclear and the mechanism(s) of action of these cells remain to be convincingly elucidated. Furthermore, while some reports describe antigen-specific T_{REG} activity, others provide evidence for non-antigen-specific mechanisms of action.

7.7   OTHER MECHANISMS OF IMMUNOREGULATION

Complement

Complement has long been recognized as a regulator of B cell activity. C3d, a complement activation product (see *Section 4.3*), binds to CD21 which, together with CD19 and CD81, forms the B cell co-receptor. Binding of C3d-opsonized antigens to CD21 results in signalling through the associated CD19 molecule. This signal augments the signals transmitted through the BCR and and allows B cells to be activated by lower concentrations of antigen. This enhances antigen-specific B cell responses and antibody production. A more recent finding has been the realization that complement can also modulate T cell responses. T cells express CD46 which binds to the complement activation products C3b and C4b. Binding of C3b to CD46 on T cells during T cell activation has been shown to promote the development of Tr1 cells. As noted above, Tr1 cells regulate immune responses via the secretion of the immunosuppressive cytokine IL-10.

Neuroendocrine regulation of the immune response

There is accumulating evidence for neuroendocrine regulation of lymphocyte responses. Lymphoid tissues are innervated by autonomic and primary sensory neurons and lymphocytes express receptors for a variety of neuropeptides and hormones.

Neuroendocrine factors can augment or suppress immune responses. For example, stress-induced IL-1 stimulates glucocorticoid synthesis by the adrenal cortex. This causes down-regulation of cytokine synthesis and of antibody production by B cells. By contrast, prolactin binding to its receptor on macrophages and T cells enhances macrophage activation and IL-2 production, respectively, and β_2-adrenergic receptor stimulation results in an increase in IgE production by human B lymphocytes.

SUGGESTED FURTHER READING

Benner, D., Krammer, P.H. and Arnold, R. (2008) Concepts of activated T cell death. *Crit. Rev. Oncol/Hematol.* **66**: 52–64.

Miyara, M. and Sakaguchi, S. (2007) Natural regulatory T cells: mechanisms of suppression. *Trends Mol. Med.* **13**: 108–116.

Puccetti, P. and Grohmann, U. (2007) IDO and regulatory T cells: a role for reverse signalling and non-canonical NF-kB activation. *Nature Rev. Immunol.* **7**: 817–823.

Romagnani, S. (2006) Regulation of the T cell response. *Clin. Exp. Allergy,* **36**: 1357–1366.

Yoshimura, A., Naka, T. and Kubo, M. (2007) SOCS proteins, cytokine signaling and immune regulation. *Nature Rev. Immunol.* **7**: 454–465.

SELF-ASSESSMENT QUESTIONS

1. Why is regulation of the immune system required?
2. Does antigen have any role in regulating the immune response?
3. Describe how responses of antigen-specific lymphocytes are regulated.
4. Name three different types of regulatory T cells.
5. How do the different types of regulatory T cells differ?
6. Does immunoregulation occur during recognition, activation or effector phases of an immune response?
7. How does anergy occur?
8. What is feedback inhibition?
9. What happens if immunoregulation is too strong or does not occur?
10. Does complement have any role in immunoregulation?

Infection and immunity

Learning objectives

After studying this chapter you should confidently be able to:

■ **Discuss the strategies used by the immune system to combat pathogens**
Efficient control of most pathogenic infections requires the coordinated actions of innate and adaptive immune responses. Whereas innate responses can limit the spread of, and sometimes eliminate, the pathogen, protection against re-infection is conferred by adaptive immunity. The elements of adaptive immunity that are key in combating infections are largely determined by the life cycle of the pathogen. Extracellular pathogens are effectively targeted by antibody-dependent mechanisms such as neutralization, agglutination, phagocytosis, ADCC and complement-mediated lysis. Intracellular pathogens are inaccessible to antibody and are largely controlled by the cell-mediated arm of the adaptive immune response.

■ **Describe the mechanisms used by pathogens to evade the immune response**
Pathogens utilize a variety of strategies to evade their host's immune response. These range from establishing infection at sites that are relatively inaccessible to the immune system, to more complex strategies involving the production of molecules that specifically target essential components of the immune response. Certain viruses have evolved mechanisms which inhibit the endogenous pathway of antigen presentation, and also mechanisms which neutralize the activity of cytokines and chemokines that are crucial for effective cell-mediated immune responses. Bacterial strategies of immune evasion include neutralization of antibody, inhibition of neutrophil chemotaxis, inhibition of phagocytosis and, in common with certain fungal infections, inhibition of complement. Alteration in surface antigen composition is a strategy common to viruses, bacteria, fungi, and protozoan and metazoan parasites that enables them to evade detection by antibodies.

■ **Discuss current approaches to vaccine design**
Current vaccine strategies include the use of attenuated and inactive organisms as well as subunit vaccines that consist of immunodominant antigens of pathogenic organisms. Toxoids are inactivated toxins that promote the generation of a neutralizing antibody response against the native toxin, but that do not induce immunity against the pathogen that produces the toxin. Recombinant vaccines allow the incorporation of antigens from different pathogens into non-replicating vaccine vectors.

8.1   INTRODUCTION TO INFECTION AND IMMUNITY

The immune system has evolved under constant selective pressure imposed by the microbial world around us and within us. It functions to maintain the integrity of our bodies by repelling pathogenic invaders while at the same time minimizing damage to body tissues. The clinical presentation of an infectious disease is the end result of the dynamic interaction between the immune system and the invading micro-organism.

It is never advantageous to an infectious micro-organism to kill its host, because when the host is dead, the micro-organism no longer has a place to live and replicate. Some of the most successful pathogens are those that have evolved to be able to live together with the host over sustained periods of time. This is known as persistent infection. Some pathogens, however, are known to 'jump' species from their primary host to humans. This is most likely as a result of human encroachment into the habitat of the primary host. Such pathogens are termed 'emerging pathogens' as they have not co-evolved with humans and can cause devastating human diseases, for example, the ongoing AIDS pandemic associated with HIV infection or Severe Acute Respiratory Syndrome (SARS).

Microbes which can only establish infections within individuals with deficits in their physical defences, for example, wounds or compromised immune systems, are known as 'opportunistic pathogens'. *Pseudomonas aeruginosa* is a common cause of opportunistic bacterial infection in burns patients, while cytomegalovirus is a common cause of opportunistic viral infection in AIDS patients.

The primary immune mechanism(s) involved in control of any given pathogen will depend on the components of immunity that the pathogen is accessible to (see *Table 8.1*), in addition to a variety of other pathogen-specific and host-specific factors. Clinical symptoms of infectious diseases usually develop because of the inability of host immune responses to eliminate the infectious micro-organisms rapidly. The nature and magnitude of the immune response generated by an individual in response to infection is determined by several factors, including:

- the life cycle of the infecting micro-organism
- the site of infection
- the extent of infection – this is partly determined by the infectious dose
- host-specific factors that determine the efficacy of the host immune response against particular pathogens, for example, the MHC haplotype of the host – some MHC alleles present immunogenic peptides from a given pathogen more effectively than do other alleles
- other host factors, such as the presence of other infections that may cause immunosuppression (e.g. HIV co-infection), the use of immuno-suppressive drugs, or the presence of primary immunodeficiency disorders
- pathogen-specific factors such as immune evasion strategies

Effective protection against infectious diseases requires a combination of both innate and adaptive immune responses. Within this section, human

Table 8.1. General innate and adaptive immune strategies to control infectious diseases[a]

Strategy	Component	Mechanism
Prevention of infection	Phagocytes	Phagocytic elimination of infectious particles
	Type I IFN	Induction of antiviral state
	Antibody	Blocking of receptors on pathogen required for infection
Elimination of infected cell	CD8[+] T cells and NK cells	Lysis of cells infected with viruses and intracellular bacteria
	CD4[+] cells/macrophages	Intracellular killing of pathogen
Elimination of extracellular pathogens	Phagocytes	Phagocytic elimination of pathogens
	Antibody/complement	Opsonization of pathogens to enhance phagocytic clearance; ADCC
	CD8[+] T cells	Granulysin-dependent elimination of fungal pathogens
Toxin neutralization	Antibody	Blocking of site on toxin required for activity

[a]**Abbreviations**: ADCC, antibody-dependent cell-mediated cytotoxicity; IFN, interferon; NK, natural killer.

diseases caused by five major classes of pathogens: viruses, bacteria, protozoa, fungi and parasitic worms will be considered.

8.2 VIRAL INFECTIONS

Viruses are the smallest genome-containing infectious particles, and range in size from approximately 20 nm to 300 nm. They consist of a DNA or RNA genome together with proteins that either protect the genome or are required for infection of host cells. They are obligate intracellular parasites, meaning that they cannot survive without a host cell and upon infection they hijack the protein synthesis machinery of host cells to make viral proteins. The major sites of viral disease within the body include: the respiratory system, the gastrointestinal system, the genito-urinary tract, lymphoid tissues, the liver and other organs, and the central nervous system.

Viral infection induces potent innate defence responses from infected cells. Central to these responses is the virus-induced production of type I IFN (IFN-α and IFN-β) and pro-inflammatory cytokines (see *Section 4.2*), largely due to the interaction of viral molecules with host PRRs. The type I IFN induces an antiviral state in which adjacent cells are rendered resistant to infection. Early innate responses to certain viruses also involve NK cells and NK cell activity is critical for control of some herpes virus infections.

These and other early innate responses are essential to curtail virus dissemination.

The most significant anti-viral effectors of the adaptive immune response are CTLs (normally CD8$^+$ T cells). CTLs recognize peptides derived from endogenously synthesized viral proteins bound to MHC class I molecules on the surface of the infected cell (see *Section 5.10*). Following recognition of viral antigen, the CTL forms a tight conjugate with the infected cell. Granules in the cytosol of the CTL fuse with the plasma membrane and the contents of the granules are secreted towards the infected cell, resulting in lysis of the infected cell (see *Section 6.12*).

CD4$^+$ Th1 cells also contribute to anti-viral immune responses by releasing cytokines that promote CD8$^+$ T cell and macrophage activation, and by stimulating B cells to produce anti-viral antibodies that can promote viral clearance as well as neutralize the infectivity of viruses.

Viruses cause a wide range of human diseases (see *Table 8.2*). Despite the wide variation between different viruses in sites of infection and modes of transmission, all viruses can essentially be categorized as either cytopathic or as poorly or non-cytopathic. Cytopathic viruses kill host cells as part of the viral life cycle while non-cytopathic viruses do not. Non-cytopathic viruses, therefore, cannot be eliminated by antibody because antibody cannot gain access to intracellular virus. Unless they can be eliminated, cells infected with non-cytopathic viruses will persist as virus factories, releasing progeny viruses that can then infect other cells. The main mechanism for eliminating these cells is via CTL-mediated killing. In contrast, cytopathic viruses can be controlled by antibody. However, optimal control of cytopathic and non-cytopathic viral infections requires antibody, promoted by CD4$^+$ T cells, and CTLs. Many primary isolates of HIV-1 are non-cytopathic or poorly cytopathic *in vivo* and HIV-specific CTLs are crucial for reducing plasma titres of HIV-1 during clinical latency (see *Section 12.7*). Within this section the immune responses against the cytopathic virus influenza A and against the chronic viral infection caused by Epstein–Barr virus will be discussed.

Influenza A

Influenza viruses are orthomyxoviruses and consist of three types: A, B and C, of which influenza A and B are important for causing human disease. The largest known outbreak of human infectious disease was the influenza A pandemic of 1918–1919 which resulted in approximately 50 million deaths worldwide. Influenza pandemics occur when a viral strain emerges to which the global population has not previously been exposed and therefore has no immunity against it. As a consequence, the virus spreads rapidly within the population. The recent emergence of the highly pathogenic H5N1 strain of avian influenza A virus has heightened concerns about a future influenza A pandemic.

Influenza A is a respiratory pathogen and is spread from person to person by aerosol transmission via coughs and sneezes. The virus has a negative-

Table 8.2. Selected viral diseases of humans

Major target tissue/site	Representative virusesª	Representative diseases	Major mode of transmission
Skin	HSV-1	Herpetic cold sores	Oral/saliva
	Varicella zoster	Shingles/chickenpox	Aerosol
	Measles virus	Measles	Aerosol
	Papillomavirus	Warts	Direct contact
	HHV-8	Kaposi's sarcoma	Sexual
Brain	HSV-1	Encephalitis	Oral/saliva
	Mumps	Meningitis	Aerosol
Mouth	HSV-1	Stomatitis	Oral/saliva
	Coxsackie virus	Herpangina	Faecal–oral
Throat	EBV	Pharyngitis	Saliva
	Adenovirus	Pharyngitis	Aerosol, faecal–oral
Upper respiratory tract	Rhinovirus	Common cold	Aerosol
	Coronavirus	Common cold	Aerosol
Lower respiratory tract	Influenza virus	Influenza	Aerosol
	RSV	Pneumonia	Aerosol
Heart	Coxsackie virus	Myocarditis	Faecal–oral
Liver	HAV	Infectious hepatitis	Faecal–oral
	HBV	Serum hepatitis	Sexual, saliva, bodily fluids
Gastrointestinal tract	Rotavirus	Infant diarrhoea	Faecal–oral
Urogenital tract	Papillomavirus	Genital warts, cervical cancer	Direct contact, sexual
	HSV-2	Genital herpes	Sexual
Lymphoid	EBV	Mononucleosis	Saliva
	HIV-1	AIDS	Sexual, body fluids

ª **Abbreviations**: AIDS, acquired immune deficiency syndrome; EBV, Epstein–Barr virus; HAV, hepatitis A virus; HBV, hepatitis B virus; HHV, human herpes virus; HSV, herpes simplex virus; RSV, respiratory syncytial virus.

sense, segmented RNA genome which can code for up to 11 proteins. One of the proteins is the surface haemagglutinin (see *Figure 8.1*) which acts as a receptor and allows the virus to bind to host cells. The viral haemagglutinin binds to sialic acid residues on the surfaces of respiratory epithelial cells. Once infected, these cells produce large amounts of virus which can then spread to alveolar macrophages in the lungs.

Typically, influenza A causes an acute infection and within 48 hours of exposure to the virus, infected individuals experience:

- chills
- fever

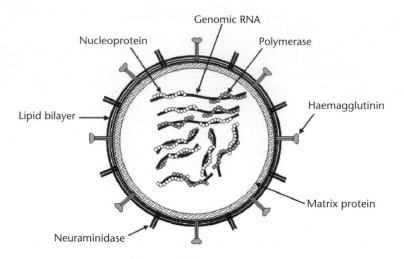

Figure 8.1
Influenza A virus is an enveloped, negative-sense, segmented RNA virus. The viral haemagglutinin binds to host cells and promotes fusion of the envelope with host cell membranes. The viral neuraminidase enhances the release of virions from infected cells.

- sore throat
- nasal congestion
- coughing and sneezing
- widespread aches and pains

Other symptoms include vomiting and diarrhoea and, less commonly, secondary bacterial pneumonia.

Influenza infection leads to the production of TNF-α and IL-1 as well as of the chemokines CCL2, CCL3, CCL5, CXCL10 and IL-8 by respiratory epithelial cells and alveolar macrophages. This leads to the infiltration of neutrophils and macrophages into the infected lung. Within the first 36 hours of infection, DCs carry viral antigen from the lungs to the draining lymph nodes, enabling the induction of an adaptive immune response against the virus. Subsequently virus-specific CD4$^+$ and CD8$^+$ T cells infiltrate the infected lung tissue. During infection with the highly lethal H5N1 strain of influenza A, these infiltrating leukocytes cause substantial immunopathology. In addition, influenza infection itself leads to death of epithelial cells and alveolar macrophages.

Efficient control of influenza virus requires the actions of virus-specific CD8$^+$ CTLs and antibody. Influenza-specific CD4$^+$ T cells are also essential but their role is primarily to promote optimal antibody and CTL responses. Influenza-specific antibody, in particular IgA and IgG, can protect against subsequent infections, although this may be thwarted by the propensity of influenza virus to alter the proteins that are recognized by antibody.

Influenza viruses alter their surface appearance via two main mecha-

---

Box 8.1 Antigenic drift and shift

The dynamic influenza virus continuously evolves through antigenic drift (all the time) or shift (occasionally). Antigenic drift refers to small, gradual changes that occur through point mutations in the two genes that contain the genetic material to produce the main surface proteins, haemagglutinin and neuraminidase, producing new virus strains that may not be recognized by antibodies to earlier influenza strains.

Antigenic shift refers to an abrupt major change and it occurs by direct animal (poultry) to human transmission or through mixing of human influenza A and animal influenza A virus genes through a process called genetic reassortment. Antigenic shift results in a new human influenza A subtype.

---

nisms: antigenic shift and antigenic drift (See *Box 8.1*). As the influenza genome is made up of RNA segments, mixing, or reassortment, of these segments between different strains of influenza viruses during infection can lead to acquisition of new RNA segments by viruses. Such reassortment events can lead to the alteration of the major antibody targets on the viral surface, the haemagglutinin and neuraminidase molecules. This is known as antigenic shift. Influenza viruses also undergo antigenic drift and can alter their surface haemagglutinin and neuraminidase molecules by mutating the genes encoding these molecules. As a consequence of antigenic shift and antigenic drift, influenza vaccines frequently have to be redesigned for successive 'flu seasons'.

Epstein–Barr virus

Epstein–Barr virus (EBV) is a gamma herpes virus (also known as human herpes virus 4 (HHV-4), that is widespread in the human population and which results in life-long infection. In the USA, more than 90% of the adult population is infected with EBV. Primary infection usually occurs during infancy, but in many Western countries exposure to the virus does not occur until adolescence or later. Acute infection with EBV results in infectious mononucleosis, which is also known as glandular fever or 'mono'. The symptoms of infectious mononucleosis include:

- fever
- malaise
- sore throat
- lymphadenopathy
- $CD8^+$ lymphocytosis

The receptor for EBV is CD21, the C3d receptor. This receptor is expressed on epithelial cells in the orthopharynx as well as on B cells (where it forms part of the B cell co-receptor). Following transmission, EBV initially infects orthopharyngeal epithelial cells. This is a lytic infection which results in the release of high levels of virus into the saliva, facilitating viral spread to other individuals, as well as establishing a viraemia that allows the virus to infect mucosal B cells and to spread to orthopharyngeal lymphoid tissue such as the tonsils. EBV stimulates B cell proliferation and during this acute stage of EBV infection as many as 10% of peripheral B cells may be infected. There is some evidence for a role of NK cells in early control of EBV infection; however, the primary cell responsible for controlling EBV is the CD8$^+$ CTL.

In response to infection with EBV there is a dramatic expansion of the CD8$^+$ T cell pool. In some individuals CD8$^+$ T cell numbers more than double during acute infection and these increased numbers largely consist of EBV-specific cells. There is a more modest expansion of EBV-specific CD4$^+$ T cells. The increase in CD8$^+$ T cell numbers (lymphocytosis) causes lymphadenopathy as well as splenomegaly. The profound antiviral T cell response and associated cytokine production causes fever and malaise. The EBV-specific CD8$^+$ CTLs kill infected B cells and drive the virus into latent infection of memory B cells. During latent infection the virus expresses only two genes, thus minimizing the number of target antigens that can be recognized by CD8$^+$ T cells. In addition, the product of one of these genes, Epstein–Barr nuclear antigen (EBNA)-1 inhibits antigen processing by the immunoproteasome.

EBV will periodically reactivate from latency and undergo lytic infection with the release of progeny viruses that infect new B cells. This lytic infection is rapidly controlled by the virus-specific CD8$^+$ T cells.

Early lytic infection of cells during acute infection results in the generation of antibodies against several EBV proteins, notably the early antigens. Although these antibodies play little part in control of infection, they are useful in distinguishing EBV infection from infections with other herpes viruses such as cytomegalovirus (CMV).

EBV-associated malignancies

EBV is a transforming virus and EBV infection has been linked to the development of various cancers. These most commonly occur in individuals who are immunosuppressed, for example, by malnutrition, by co-infection with HIV or other pathogens, or by immunosuppressive drugs.

The EBV-associated malignancy called Burkitt's lymphoma is a B cell lymphoma of the jaw and face (see *Box 8.2*). It occurs most frequently in equatorial Africa, where infection with the malaria parasite is a co-factor for the development of this malignancy. It is thought that malaria co-infection suppresses T cell-dependent control of EBV-infected cells, allowing the outgrowth of transformed B cells. Other B cell lymphomas can develop in immunocompromised patients. In contrast, nasopharyngeal carcinoma is an EBV-associated cancer of epithelial cells that is endemic in Asia.

See the Case study in *Box 8.3*.

Laboratory diagnosis of viral infections

Several approaches can be used in a diagnostic laboratory to confirm a clinical diagnosis of viral disease. The gold standard for proving the viral aetiology of a disease is the recovery, cultivation and identification of the viral

---

Box 8.2 Burkitt's lymphoma

A B cell lymphoma was discovered in 1956 in central Africa by Denis Burkitt, a Northern Irish surgeon. Burkitt described this unusual type of lymphoma, which was very common in children in Africa, and it is now known as Burkitt's lymphoma.

Box 8.3 Case study

George, a 16-year-old student, attends his doctor complaining of a sore throat and of swelling along his lower jaw. He tells his physician that he has had a fever, tiredness, and a general malaise that has persisted for several days. He also feels a slight soreness on the left side of his abdomen. On examination his doctor tells George that the swelling along his lower jaw is due to swollen cervical lymph nodes and that his abdominal discomfort appears to be due to enlargement of his spleen. A sample of George's blood was taken and, upon analysis, revealed elevated numbers of B cells and dramatically elevated numbers of CD8$^+$ T cells.

1. What virus is likely to be the cause of George's illness?
2. Why are George's lymph nodes and spleen enlarged?
3. George's baby sister has recently received a bone marrow transplant. Should this be a cause for concern?

Answers are given alongside the answers to the self-assessment questions for *Chapter 8* at the back of the book.

---

agent. Because many viruses are labile, samples for viral cultivation must be processed rapidly. Growth of some viruses results in dramatic changes in cell morphology, for example, cell fusion, vacuolation, and cell lysis. These are collectively termed virus-induced cytopathic effects (CPEs). CPEs can be detected by cytological examination of clinical specimens. If the level of virus is sufficiently high, for example, during high titre viraemia, then it may be possible to detect viral proteins by ELISA (see *Section 13.9*). A more sensitive technique to confirm the viral aetiology of a disease is to specifically amplify portions of the viral DNA or RNA genome from clinical specimens by polymerase chain reaction (PCR) or reverse transcriptase (RT)–PCR, respectively, and in some cases by real time PCR. Viral serology is also frequently used to confirm infection with a virus. This relies on the infected individual generating an antibody response against the virus. Although viral serology confirms exposure to the virus, the main drawback of this diagnostic technique is that it cannot distinguish between recent and previous infections, as antibody titres may remain elevated for many months after an acute viral infection.

8.3   BACTERIAL INFECTIONS

The body's physical and chemical barriers effectively prevent the entry of most bacteria. Those that do bypass these barriers are rapidly targeted by the innate immune response. Despite these efficient primary defences,

Table 8.3. The range of human bacterial diseases

Type of infection	Description	Example
Asymptomatic	No detectable symptoms	Asymptomatic bacterial vaginosis
Dormant	Generally asymptomatic carrier state	Dormant *Mycobacterium tuberculosis* infection
Opportunistic	Infection of immunocompromised patients with normal flora	*Pseudomonas aeruginosa* infection of burns patients
Primary	Clinically apparent infection	Pneumococcal meningitis
Secondary	Bacterial infection subsequent to initial infection	*Haemophilus influenzae* secondary to influenza virus
Acute	Rapid onset and brief duration	Salmonellosis
Chronic	Long-term infection	*M. tuberculosis* infection
Localized	Confined to a small area	Cutaneous staphylococcal abscess
Systemic	Widely disseminated	Septicaemia
Pyogenic	Pus-forming infections	Streptococcal infection
Fulminant	Sudden, intense infections	*Yersinia pestis* (bubonic plague)

pathogenic bacteria do cause a wide range of human infections, from asymptomatic to more severe fulminant infections (see *Table 8.3*). In addition, the inappropriate use of antibiotics has led to the emergence of antibiotic-resistant bacterial strains including multi-drug resistant *Staphylococcus aureus* (MRSA) and *Clostridium difficile* (see *Box 8.4*), which are major causes of serious nosocomial infections (infections associated with hospitalization and secondary to the original condition).

Box 8.4 *Clostridium difficile*

Clostridium difficile is so called as it was difficult to grow in the laboratory when it was first discovered. It is normally hospital-acquired, post antibiotic treatment, and causes diarrhoea. It usually causes a relatively mild illness, but occasionally in elderly patients it may result in serious illness and even death. It produces two toxins, responsible for the diarrhoea, which damage the cells lining the bowel.

Bacteria isolated from clinical specimens can be classified into three groups based on their capacity to cause human disease (pathogenicity).

These are:

- primary pathogens that are probable disease-causing agents, for example, *Enterococcus* spp. detected in a urine sample during urinary tract infection
- opportunistic pathogens isolated from immunosuppressed patients that may be disease-causing agents, for example, *Pseudomonas aeruginosa* detected in sputum of an immunocompromised individual
- non-pathogenic bacteria that never (or rarely) cause human disease, for example, *Bacillus subtilis*.

Pathogenic bacteria produce substances that aid in the infection of their host. Collectively these substances are termed virulence factors. Examples of virulence factors include:

- capsules – bacterial capsules confer a degree of protection from phagocytosis
- adherence factors – for example, projections called pili that many pathogenic bacteria use to colonize mucosae
- toxins – these include exotoxins that are synthesized and/or secreted from bacterial pathogens and the lipopolysaccharide (LPS) endotoxin of gram-negative bacteria
- superantigens – a special class of bacterial exotoxins; they bind simultaneously to MHC class II molecules and TCRs and stimulate activation of the T cells in an antigen-independent manner, and this can result in death of the T cells via AICD (see *Section 7.5*). Examples of bacterial superantigens include Staphylococcal enterotoxins A–E and toxic shock syndrome toxin-1 (TSST-1).

Septic shock is most commonly caused by endotoxins found as components of gram-negative bacterial cell walls; however, septic shock also may be induced by gram-positive bacteria. The most powerful stimulant of this syndrome is LPS, a component of certain bacterial cell walls. LPS is a potent stimulus for the production of pro-inflammatory cytokines by macrophages. LPS binds specifically to the CD14/TLR-4 complex on the surface of macrophages and causes them to produce high levels of the pro-inflammatory cytokines TNF-α, IL-1 and IL-6. Systemic release of these cytokines leads to profound vasodilation, increased vascular permeability, hypotension, and insufficient tissue perfusion. This can result in multisystem organ failure, mainly caused by hypoxia, and uncontrollable haemorrhaging. Management of the shock-specific symptoms is still one of the most challenging problems faced by clinicians.

The immune responses required to eliminate bacterial pathogens largely depend on whether the bacteria infect host cells or whether they replicate in the extracellular fluid. In general, intracellular bacteria are protected from antibodies and require cell-mediated immune responses for their elimination. One example of an intracellular bacterium is *Mycobacterium tuberculosis*, the causative agent of tuberculosis (see *Section 9.10*). Extracellular bacteria can be effectively targeted by phagocytes and antibodies. In addition, protection from the effects of bacterial toxins requires the generation of neutralizing anti-toxin antibodies which bind to the toxins and inhibit their activity.

Streptococcus pneumoniae

S. pneumoniae is the major cause of pneumonia in all age groups (approximately 500 000 cases annually in the USA), often as a sequela to a viral infection of the upper respiratory tract. *S. pneumoniae* is also a cause of otitis media (middle ear infections) and frequently disseminates leading to bacteraemia and, in more severe cases, pneumococcal meningitis. *S. pneumoniae* infection is associated with high rates of morbidity and mortality in children under 2 years of age and in adults over the age of 65.

Most people carry *S. pneumoniae* in their nose and throat and person-to-person spread occurs via inhalation of aerosolized bacteria expelled by coughing or sneezing. *S. pneumoniae* binds tightly to the nasopharyngeal epithelium. In some individuals it spreads from here to the lungs or via the eustachian canal to the middle ear. In the lungs, *S. pneumoniae* progresses to the alveoli. Invasion and growth is aided by the bacterial capsule which inhibits phagocytosis (see *Figure 8.2*). When the bacteria reach the lung, they trigger an inflammatory response characterized by the release of numerous cytokines and chemokines, such as IL-1, IL-6, TNF-α, CCL2, CCL3 and IL-8, and by a subsequent influx of neutrophils. Despite the anti-phagocytic properties of the capsule, exposed bacterial cell wall components activate complement via the alternative pathway (see *Section 4.3*), enabling phagocytes to engulf the opsonized bacteria. Normally this acute inflammatory response is sufficient to eliminate the bacteria; however, it can also cause substantial tissue damage, especially in conditions of high bacterial load.

S. pneumoniae infection also leads to production of antibodies against surface antigens. These antibodies protect against re-infection with the same serotype of bacteria. However, there are at least 90 different serotypes of *S. pneumoniae* and antibody responses against one serotype frequently do not protect against infections with other serotypes. The *S. pneumoniae* vaccine

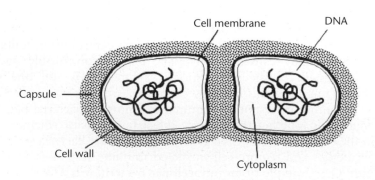

Figure 8.2
Cross-section through a *Streptococcus pneumoniae* diplococcus showing the protective outer capsule.

(pneumococcal vaccine) consists of extracts of 7–11 different serotypes and protects against 80% of life-threatening *S. pneumoniae* diseases.

Laboratory diagnosis of bacterial infections

Most laboratory diagnoses of bacterial infections rely on the cultivation of bacterial species from patient samples. The most common source for cultivation is peripheral blood, especially in cases of bacteraemia. However, other fluids such as cerebrospinal fluid and urine may be used if bacterial meningitis or urinary tract infections, respectively, are suspected, and bacteria that cause gastrointestinal infections can frequently be cultivated from faecal samples. Cultivated bacterial species may then be identified by morphological and cytological examination as well as by PCR-based molecular characterization. PCR can also be used to identify labile or non-cultivatable bacterial species in patient samples. Bacterial serology may be used to confirm exposure to specific bacterial pathogens, but, as with viral serology, it cannot distinguish between recent and previous infections.

8.4 PROTOZOAN INFECTIONS

Protozoan infections constitute major human health problems worldwide, and the incidence of many of these diseases has increased in recent years. Protozoa are single-celled, mostly free-living eukaryotes found worldwide in almost every possible habitat. Protozoan infections range from asymptomatic to life-threatening, depending on the parasite and the immune status of the host. Life-threatening protozoan infections are common in patients with AIDS, including infections with *Toxoplasma gondii* and *Pneumocystis jiroveci*, common protozoa that cause mild, if any, illness in immunocompetent individuals. Amoebiasis, or amoebic dysentery, is caused by ingestion of the cysts of *Entamoeba histolytica*, a protozoan parasite of the human intestine. Amoebiasis is one of the leading parasitic diseases worldwide. Infection of the large intestine with *E. histolytica* is frequently asymptomatic; however, invasion and ulceration of intestinal walls by this parasite can lead to diarrhoea, abdominal pain, and fever. In severe cases, the lungs, liver, spleen and brain may also be affected. Giardiasis is acquired by the ingestion of untreated water or consumption of fruits or vegetables contaminated with cysts of the intestinal parasite *Giardia lamblia*. Approximately 50% of *Giardia*-infected individuals are asymptomatic, while the remainder exhibit symptoms ranging from mild diarrhoea to severe weight loss due to nutrient malabsorption.

Certain protozoan parasites, for example, *Giardia* and *Trypanosoma* spp., live extracellularly and are therefore accessible to antibody-dependent elimination. The importance of antibody-mediated protection against extracellular protozoa is evidenced by the increased prevalence of *G. lamblia* infections in patients with primary immunoglobulin deficiency syndromes (see *Section 12.4*). Members of the *Trypanosoma* genus cause two strikingly different human diseases. *T. brucei gambiense and T. brucei rhodesiense* are the causative agents of African trypanosomiasis, or sleeping sickness, and are transmitted to man by bites of tsetse flies. By contrast, *T. cruzi* causes Chagas' disease, or American trypanosomiasis, and is transmitted to man by bites of reduviid bugs. *T. brucei* strains have evolved a highly effective strategy to avoid elimination by antibody. The surface glycoprotein of trypanosomes is called the variant surface glycoprotein (VSG). *T. brucei* VSG is highly variable and more than 1000 different VSG variants have been identified. Controlled expression of different VSG variants allows *T. brucei* to avoid antibody-dependent elimination.

Other protozoa, for example, *Plasmodium* and *Leishmania* spp., spend much of their life cycle inside human cells and are frequently referred to as intracellular protozoa. These parasites present a considerable challenge to the immune system as they are hidden from antibodies for much of their life cycle.

Malaria

Malaria is a major cause of human morbidity and mortality. The World Health Organization estimates that between 300 and 500 million clinical cases of malaria occur annually worldwide. Of these, approximately 2 million cases result in death, with the majority of deaths occurring in children. Approximately 90% of all cases of malaria are in sub-Saharan Africa, a region that also harbours 68% of all cases of HIV infection (see *Section 12.7*).

Malaria is caused by infection with members of the genus *Plasmodium*. There are four species of plasmodia that cause human disease. *Plasmodium ovale* and *P. malariae* cause relatively benign infections. Infection with *P. vivax* is a common cause of febrile illness, especially in Asia and South America, but is rarely fatal. The vast majority of malaria-related deaths are due to infection with *P. falciparum*. All these species of plasmodia are transmitted to humans via the bite of the female *Anopheles* mosquito, and they all have a common life cycle (see *Figure 8.3*). Following a bite from an infected mosquito, *Plasmodium* sporozoites are injected into the bloodstream. The sporozoites are carried in the circulation to the liver and infect hepatocytes where they replicate asexually for between 6 and 25 days. During this time the sporozoites differentiate into merozoites which are released into the bloodstream following lysis of the infected hepatocytes. In the bloodstream the merozoites infect red blood cells (RBCs) where they again reproduce asexually, each releasing up to 24 merozoites after lysis of the RBC. This period of infection and release from RBCs cycles every 48 hours and causes the classic periodic fevers associated with malaria.

P. falciparum encodes a protein called erythrocyte membrane protein 1 (EMP1) which is expressed on the surface of infected RBCs. EMP1 binds to intercellular adhesion molecule-1 (ICAM-1), vascular cell adhesion molecule-1 (VCAM-1), endothelial cell selectin (E-selectin) and several other cell adhesion molecules. Binding of EMP1 on infected RBCs to these

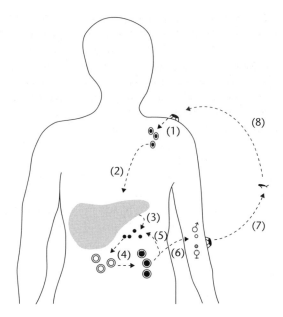

Figure 8.3
The life cycle of *Plasmodium falciparum*. (1) Plasmodium sporozoites are injected into the bloodstream from the bite of an infected *Anopheles* mosquito. (2) The sporozoites reach the liver and infect hepatocytes, and reproduce asexually for 6–25 days and differentiate into merozoites. (3) Merozoites are released from hepatocytes and (4) infect RBCs where they reproduce asexually and release merozoites into the bloodstream following lysis of the RBCs. (5) The released merozoites infect other RBCs. (6) Some of the merozoites within infected RBCs differentiate into male and female gametocytes which, when released, can be (7) picked up by an *Anopheles* mosquito when it feeds. (8) The parasite reproduces sexually in the mosquito, generating sporozoites which invade the mosquito's salivary gland, ready to be injected when the mosquito next feeds.

adhesion molecules leads to sequestration of infected RBCs in microvascular beds in tissues. As a consequence, the infected RBCs are not eliminated by the spleen.

Some of the merozoites differentiate into male and female gametocytes within RBCs. When released following RBC lysis, these gametocytes can be picked up by an *Anopheles* mosquito when it feeds on the infected individual. Sexual reproduction takes place in the gut of the mosquito, giving rise to oocysts which develop in the gut wall. Sporozoites develop in, and are released from, the oocysts. The sporozoites invade the mosquito's salivary gland and will be injected into a susceptible host when the mosquito feeds again.

Fever is the characteristic symptom of malaria, but other symptoms include headache, nausea, vomiting and chills. The classic periodic fever is not usually evident early in the course of infection, and therefore the absence of periodic fevers does not rule out a diagnosis of malaria. Life-threatening malarial infections are usually due to cerebral malaria, severe malarial anaemia (due to depletion of RBCs) or respiratory distress caused by metabolic acidosis. The apparently unchecked growth in the number of malaria cases worldwide has been attributed to the emergence of strains of *P. falciparum* that are resistant to the most effective antimalarials, particularly chloroquine, and to the emergence of insecticide resistance in *Anopheles* mosquitoes.

Plasmodium sporozoites infect hepatocytes within 30 minutes of injection into a human host. Because of this, the sporozoites are not usually targets of an immune response during natural infection. In addition, RBCs do not express MHC molecules so the erythrocytic stage of the plasmodium life cycle is inefficiently detected by the immune system. EMP1, which is exposed to the immune system, is antigenically quite variable, with each parasite being able to express at least 60 variants of this protein. Switching between EMP1 variants allows the parasite to evade EMP1-specific antibody responses. Consequently, the focus of the malaria-specific immune response is on the intrahepatocyte and merozoite stages of the plasmodium life cycle. There is evidence that protective immune responses do develop in malaria-infected individuals and cell-mediated and antibody-dependent immune responses are crucial for control of parasitaemia. Expression of the MHC class I molecule HLA-B53 is associated with a decreased risk of developing severe malaria. It is thought that this is due to efficient presentation of malarial antigens by HLA-B53-expressing hepatocytes to malaria-specific CTLs. In addition, high-level antibody responses against merozoite antigens are also associated with decreased risk of severe malaria. However, although these responses limit the clinical impact of the disease, they do not completely eliminate the parasite. In addition, maintenance of protective immune responses against *Plasmodium* spp. requires repeated infection and can be short-lived. The development of an effective vaccine against malaria is an area of intense biomedical research.

Laboratory diagnosis of protozoan infections

Diagnosis of protozoan infections is usually based on the microscopic identification of protozoan species in clinical specimens. Thorough clinical evaluation of the patient is essential to ensure that the correct samples are taken and processed for examination. For example, *Plasmodium* species can be detected in blood samples whereas faecal samples are required for the detection of *E. histolytica* and *Giardia* species.

8.5   FUNGAL INFECTIONS

Fungi are free-living saprotrophs (organisms that feed on non-living organic matter). *Candida albicans* and *Malassezia furfur* are the only fungal species that form part of our commensal flora. *C. albicans* colonizes the buccal cavity and gastrointestinal tract at birth and persists as a life-long commensal.

In general, fungal infections are accidental and fungal diseases are rare because immunocompetent individuals have a high level of innate resistance to fungi. Resistance to fungal infection relies primarily on intact physical barriers such as epithelial surfaces. When fungal diseases do occur they are usually a result of immunodeficiency or of other conditions that favour the invasion and growth of these organisms. Disease severity is determined by the immune status of the host together with other factors such as the size of the fungal inoculum and the ability of the fungus to replicate in tissue.

Most of the medically important fungi that can cause systemic illness initially enter via the respiratory tract where they encounter alveolar macrophages. Interactions between PRRs, in particular the mannose receptor, TLR-2 and TLR-4, on alveolar macrophages and fungal PAMPs lead to phagocytosis of the pathogen. This also leads to the production of the pro-inflammatory cytokines TNF-α, IL-1, IL-6 and IL-12, as well as the chemokines CCL3 and IL-8, which are important for generation of protective immune responses against fungal pathogens.

Unlike viral and bacterial pathogenesis, there is little information about mechanisms of fungal pathogenesis. Much more research is needed in this area because of the increasing incidence of opportunistic and iatrogenic fungal infections (see *Box 8.5*).

Box 8.5 Iatrogenic

The word 'iatrogenic' breaks down into: 'iatros' which is Greek for physician and 'genic', meaning induced by. Iatrogenic therefore translates to mean physician-induced and the term iatrogenic disease applies to any adverse effect associated with any medical advice or treatment.

Cryptococcosis

Cryptococcosis is caused by the fungi *Cryptococcus neoformans* and *C. gattii*. Infection occurs due to inhalation of the yeast form of the organism. The disease caused by *C. neoformans* is a characteristic infection of immuno-compromised individuals. There are three forms of the disease:

- cutaneous cryptococcosis
- pulmonary cryptococcosis
- cryptococcal meningitis

Cryptococcal meningitis results from dissemination of the fungus from the lungs via the circulation following pulmonary infection. Untreated cryptococcal meningitis is fatal.

In the lungs the inhaled yeast particle hydrates and acquires a thick polysaccharide capsule that confers a degree of protection from phagocytosis. This also results in decreased presentation of fungal antigens to T cells. In addition to interfering with phagocytosis, the capsule also blocks recognition by host PRRs. As a consequence, PRRs play a minor role in the immune response against *C. neoformans*. However, complement activation and opsonization of the encapsulated yeast cells enhance their uptake by APCs and promote the induction of T cell responses.

People with defective cell-mediated immunity, for example, individuals with AIDS (see *Section 12.7*), are especially susceptible to disseminated cryptococcosis. This is because the cell-mediated arm of the immune response is critical for control of infection. Studies in mice have shown that Th17 cells are critical for effective clearance of this fungus, most likely via the recruitment of neutrophils that will phagocytose the opsonized yeast particle. *C. neoformans* is also attacked and killed by NK cells and CD8$^+$ T cells. NK cell killing is perforin-dependent, but elimination of *C. neoformans* by CD8$^+$ T cells is dependent on granulysin. Granulysin is a member of the saposin-like family of lipid binding proteins, and is stored in the granules of CTLs and NK cells. It disrupts membranes and is toxic to a range of microbial pathogens.

Laboratory diagnosis of fungal infections

Diagnoses of fungal infections caused by primary fungal pathogens can frequently be made by microscopic examination of clinical specimens. In the case of opportunistic fungal pathogens, however, diagnoses are not so straightforward. Fungi that cause opportunistic infections are common in the environment and are frequent contaminants of diagnostic cultures. To confirm diagnoses of opportunistic fungal infections, the fungus must repeatedly be identified in lesional samples taken at different times.

8.6   HELMINTHIC INFECTIONS

More than two billion people worldwide are infected with parasitic helminthic worms. Although helminthic infections are usually not fatal, chronic infections with these parasites often cause anaemia and malnutrition. Most helminths are sufficiently large to be seen with the naked eye. The majority are extracellular parasites. There are three major classes of helminths.

Nematodes

Nematodes are segmented roundworms that live in animal or human intestines but must transmit through eggs or cysts to new hosts. The mode of transmission is primarily via the faecal–oral route. This class includes the most common worm infection in the world, *Ascaris lumbricoides*, which infects approximately 30% of the world's population. Pinworm, caused by the nematode *Enterobium vermicularis* is a common infection of small children in urban areas and trichinosis is caused by consumption of undercooked pork containing cysts of the nematode *Trichinella*. Lymphatic filariasis is caused by the nematodes *Wuchereria bancrofti*, *Brugia malayi*, and *B. timori*. Blockage of the lymphatic system by these parasites can lead to elephantiasis which is characterized by the dramatic swelling of the lower torso.

Cestodes

Cestodes, or tapeworms, are flat segmented worms. Clinically important cestodes are *Tenia saginata* (beef tapeworm) and *T. solium* (pork tapeworm). *T. saginata* can be up to 6 metres long and 1 cm wide. Infection occurs by ingestion of tapeworm larval cysts in poorly cooked, infected meat. The larvae escape the cysts and attach via suckers to the mucosa of the small intestine.

Trematodes

The most clinically important trematodes, or flukes, are the blood flukes, *Schistosoma mansoni* and *S. hematobium*. Human infection occurs following penetration of the skin by schistosomal cercaria in fresh water. The adult *S. mansoni* resides in mesenteric veins and releases millions of eggs into the intestine which are shed in faeces.

Schistosomiasis

Schistosomiasis, or snail fever, accounts for approximately 200 million infections in some 74 countries and ranks second only to malaria as a cause of parasite-associated morbidity worldwide. The disease is caused by worms of the genus *Schistosoma*. Schistosomes are parasites that live as adults in the blood vessels of mammalian and avian species. Unlike the majority of parasitic flatworms which are hermaphrodite, schistosomes live as an adult male and female pair in mesenteric veins. *S. mansoni* is the cause of the most widespread schistosomal infections and is endemic in South Africa, Saudi Arabia and Madagascar.

The life cycle of *S. mansoni* (see *Figure 8.4*) involves stages in humans and in freshwater snails. The free-living schistosomal larvae, cercaria, penetrate human skin and use proteolytic enzymes to digest a pathway to blood capillaries or to lymphatic vessels. En route, the cercaria develop into schistosomula. These migrate to the lungs and from there to the hepatic portal circulation where, if they meet a partner of the opposite sex, they develop into mature adult worms. Once they mature, the pair migrates to mesenteric veins where the female positions herself in a longitudinal groove, the gynacophoric canal, on the ventral surface of the male for copulation. The female produces approximately 300 eggs per day and these are deposited in the endothelial lining of the venous capillary walls. The developing miracidia larvae in the eggs secrete enzymes that allow the eggs to cross through tissue and penetrate the basement membrane and epithelium of the intestine where they are passed to the external environment in faeces. The eggs hatch in fresh water, releasing the motile miracidia which infect freshwater snails. There the miracidia form sporocysts which reproduce asexually giving rise to the free-living cercarial larvae which are released from the snails to again infect humans.

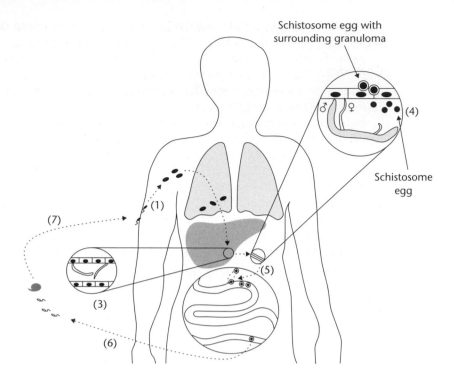

Figure 8.4
The life cycle of *Schistosoma mansoni*. (1) Free-living cercaria penetrate the skin,
develop into schistosomula and migrate to lymphatic vessels or blood capillaries. (2)
Schistosomula migrate via the lungs to (3) the hepatic portal circulation where they
mature into adult worms. (4) The mature male and female pair migrates to the
mesenteric veins where they mate. (5) The eggs cross though tissue to the intestinal
lumen where they are released. (6) The eggs hatch into miracidia which infect
freshwater snails and develop into sporocysts. (7) The sporocysts reproduce asexually
in snails and release cercaria which can infect humans.

Invasion of skin by cercarial larvae may give rise to localized, brief inflammation, and migrating schistosomula in the lungs en route to the liver may
cause bouts of coughing. Egg production and deposition leads to an inflammatory response that can cause fever, general malaise and abdominal pain.
Fatal schistosomiasis can result from liver damage caused by the inflammatory response. Chronic infection can lead to severe hepatomegaly and
splenomegaly and dissemination of eggs to the spinal cord can result in
neurological problems.

All stages of the *S. mansoni* life cycle in humans are too large for phagocytosis. Consequently, the main effector mechanism of innate immunity is
of no benefit during schistosomal infections. The infectious cercaria are
inefficiently targeted by the adaptive immune response during natural infection with *S. mansoni*. This may partly be due to the production of
prostaglandin D_2 by cercaria which inhibits migration of epidermal langerhans cells to draining lymph nodes. Adult schistosomes have an outer coat

called the tegument which absorbs host proteins, for example, MHC class I molecules, DAF and E-selectin. Expression of self-proteins on the schistosome surface fool the immune system into accepting the adult worm as 'self'. In addition, incorporation of DAF into the tegument prevents complement-mediated attack against the worm. E-selectin may play a role in adhesion of worms to vascular endothelium.

Schistosomal eggs induce a profound Th2 response and the production of high levels of IL-4, IL-5, IL-9 and IL-13 in particular. This Th2 response is beneficial to both the host and the worm. Fatal schistosomiasis can result from Th1-dependent inflammatory responses so the switch to a Th2 response is beneficial to the host. The Th2 response also leads to the formation of granulomata around schistosome eggs that seem to be important in allowing the eggs to pass from the mesenteric veins into the lumen of the intestine, and so is also of benefit to the parasite. Unlike the Th1-dependent granulomata seen during infection with *M. tuberculosis* (see *Section 9.10*), these Th2-dependent granulomata consist of the schistosome egg surrounded by eosinophils, Th2 cells and alternatively activated macrophages (macrophages activated by IL-4 and IL-13 as opposed to IFN-γ; see *Section 6.5*). Consistent with the biased Th2 response induced by

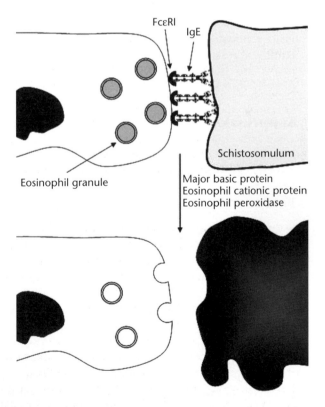

Figure 8.5
Schistosomula coated with IgE trigger FcεRI-dependent degranulation of eosinophils. The released granule contents cause the destruction of the schistosomula.

schistosomal infection, the major mechanism of immune-mediated protection is dependent on IgE. Binding of helminth-specific IgE to schistosomula targets these larvae for FcɛRI-dependent, eosinophil-mediated destruction (see *Figure 8.5*).

Laboratory diagnosis of helminthic infections

Helminthic infections are usually confirmed by detection of helminth eggs in stool samples. Quantification of egg output in faeces can be used to estimate the degree of infection and, therefore, to monitor the response of the patient to therapy.

8.7   IMMUNE EVASION STRATEGIES

The outcome of any given infection is the end result of a dynamic interaction between the invading pathogen and the host. In *Section 8.1* effector mechanisms used by the immune system to combat infections were alluded to; however, some pathogens have evolved mechanisms that allow them to evade the immune response and to persist in the host. Some of these immune evasion strategies are quite simple, for example, human papillomavirus replicates in cells in the basal layer of the epidermis, a site that is not readily accessible to immune surveillance. Other immune evasion mechanisms are more complex and involve pathogen-encoded molecules that directly interfere with the host's immune response.

Suppression of immune responses

Members of all the major groups of pathogens encode molecules that directly inhibit the immune response. Examples of these are given below.

Viruses

- EBV produces a cytokine-like molecule, termed viral IL-10 (vIL-10) that mimics the action of the immunosuppressive cytokine IL-10. This counteracts the cell-mediated immune response against the virus.
- Herpes simplex virus produces proteins that degrade complement factors.
- The US2 and US11 proteins expressed by human cytomegalovirus cause MHC class I and MHC class II molecules to be degraded inside host cells (see *Figure 8.6*).
- Poxviruses encode a variety of 'secreted cytokine receptors' that bind to and neutralize the activities of pro-inflammatory cytokines (e.g. IL-1, TNF-α) and therefore counteract antiviral immune responses.
- Herpes viruses and poxviruses encode a variety of secreted molecules that bind to and neutralize the activities of chemokines and therefore inhibit the recruitment of immune cells to the site of infection.

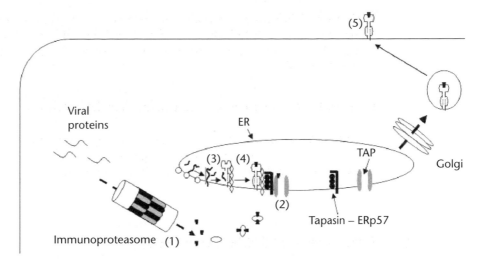

Figure 8.6

Examples of strategies used by viruses to inhibit the endogenous pathway of antigen processing and presentation (see *Section 5.10* and *Figure 5.13* for more details of the endogenous pathway). (1) The EBNA-1 protein of Epstein–Barr virus contains a Gly–Ala repeat that inhibits the activity of the proteasome. (2) The ICP47 gene product of herpes simplex virus inhibits peptide binding to the TAP complex and so prevents peptide translocation into the endoplasmic reticulum (ER). In addition, the US6 gene product of human cytomegalovirus binds to the ER luminal side of the TAP complex and blocks peptide transport. (3) The US2 and US11 gene products of human cytomegalovirus cause the MHC class I heavy chain to be removed from the ER and degraded by the proteasome. (4) The adenovirus E19K protein binds to MHC class I molecules and retains them in the ER. (5) The K3 and K5 proteins of human herpes virus-8 (HHV-8) and the Nef protein of human immunodeficiency virus (HIV)-1 cause MHC class I molecules to be internalized from the cell surface and degraded in lysosomes.

■ The K3 protein expressed by herpes viruses causes MHC class I molecules to be degraded inside host cells and the E19K protein expressed by adenoviruses binds to MHC class I molecules in the ER and prevents them from getting to the cell surface (see *Figure 8.6*). These strategies ensure that CD8$^+$ T cells cannot recognize the cells as being infected.

Bacteria

■ Gonococci and meningococci secrete proteases that degrade IgA and streptococcal proteases can degrade components of the complement system.

■ Streptolysin from streptococci is toxic for neutrophils.

- Mycobacteria prevent phagosome–lysosome fusion in macrophages and therefore prevent intracellular killing, and shigella can escape from phagosomes.
- Staphylococcal protein A and streptococcal protein G block the Fc ends of antibodies so that they cannot bind to Fc receptors. In addition, an *S. aureus*-encoded protein called SCIN inhibits the deposition of the opsonin C3b on the bacterial surface. These strategies inhibit phagocytosis of pathogens.
- An *S. aureus*-encoded protein called CHIPS binds to the FMLP receptor and to the C5a receptor on neutrophils and prevents ligand binding to these chemoattractant receptors. This inhibits neutrophil chemotaxis to the infected site.
- *S. pneumoniae* and meningococci surround themselves in an anti-phagocytic polysaccharide capsule and staphylococci form an outer coat of host fibrin that inactivates complement.
- *Leishmania* can produce a molecule similar to DAF that degrades complement.

Fungi

- The flavohaemoglobin enzyme of *C. neoformans* can neutralize the reactive oxygen species produced during the oxidative burst of phagocytes and can therefore inhibit intracellular killing of the fungus.

Parasites

- Toxoplasma inhibits phagosome–lysosome fusion and therefore inhibits intracellular killing.
- Roundworms secrete proteases that degrade antibodies, for example, *S. mansoni* secretes a protease that degrades IgE.

Replication inside host cells

Another common immune evasion strategy used by pathogens is to replicate inside host cells where they can hide from the immune response. All viruses must replicate inside host cells and the immune system has evolved a strategy to detect infected cells; it does so by displaying viral peptides on the surface of these cells bound to MHC class I molecules for recognition by CD8$^+$ CTL. Certain viruses, however, use cells of the immune system as their host cells, for example, HIV infects CD4$^+$ T cells and EBV infects B cells, in particular memory B cells. Destruction of these cells by the antiviral immune response can lead to immunosuppression. Certain intracellular bacteria, for example, *M. tuberculosis*, replicate in phagosomes of macrophages and *Bacillus anthracis* infects dendritic cells and alveolar macrophages. In addition, the fungus *C. neoformans* can persist inside macrophages and epithelioid cells. As previously discussed, *P. falciparum* replicates in RBCs where it can evade CTL-mediated elimination (see *Section 8.4*).

Antigenic variation

Many pathogens attempt to evade immune-mediated elimination by varying the structure of the antigens that the immune response is directed against, for example, HIV, influenza virus and rhinoviruses very frequently alter the structure of their surface antigens. Also, gonococci, streptococci and *Escherichia coli* vary the structure of their outer surface proteins so that they develop a large number of antigenically different bacterial strains. On each occasion that a person is infected with an organism it is treated as being a 'new' antigen and only primary responses can be mounted. This strategy circumvents the normally highly effective secondary antibody response. In addition, the complex life cycle of many parasites means that one organism can exist in several antigenically distinct stages and the surface antigens expressed at any one stage may vary within the species, for example, the highly variable VSG antigen in *T. brucei*. As previously discussed, *S. mansoni* can incorporate host molecules into its tegument so that it is not recognized by the immune system as being foreign (see *Section 8.6*).

Latency

Certain micro-organisms can infect host cells and remain dormant there, unseen by the immune system, for many years. This strategy is common to herpes viruses, for example, EBV, which latently infects B cells, and HSV, which latently infects nerve cells. HIV also latently infects $CD4^+$ T cells. In addition, intracellular bacteria such as *M. tuberculosis* may reside for many years within macrophages, only recommencing replication if the immune system is suppressed.

8.8 VACCINATION

Vaccination against infectious diseases is one of the major success stories of modern medicine. It is widely acknowledged that the modern era of vaccination began in May 1796 when the English physician Edward Jenner induced active immunity against the smallpox virus in a young boy by inoculating him with matter taken from a milkmaid's cowpox pustule. The boy's own immune system responded to the potential pathogen to bring about protective immunity. In 1980, the World Health Organization announced the worldwide eradication of smallpox. Other diseases such as polio, measles, mumps and chickenpox are also much less common than they were even a hundred years ago. Before 1985, when a widespread vaccination programme against *Haemophilus influenzae* was started, *H. influenzae* type b (Hib) was the most common cause of childhood meningitis in the USA, resulting in up to 20 000 cases and in excess of 500 deaths annually. As a consequence of vaccination, the prevalence of Hib meningitis has been reduced to a few hundred cases per year. The effectiveness of vaccination programmes relies on a phenomenon known as herd immunity.

This means that it is much more difficult for a disease to spread as long as the vast majority of the population is vaccinated.

A number of different types of vaccines have been developed to cope with a wide range of diseases. Most vaccine preparations contain an adjuvant. Adjuvants boost the immune responses against the antigen(s) in the vaccine. Alum is currently the only adjuvant licensed for use in human vaccines. The types of vaccine currently in use are described below.

Attenuated vaccines and inactivated vaccines

Attenuated (weakened) pathogens have been manipulated *in vitro* so that they can induce only a very mild infection. The risk attached is that a mutation may occur to restore virulence. A safeguard against this is either the removal of virulence genes or the inactivation (killing) of the organism so that it cannot replicate *in vivo*. Killed viruses usually generate only antibody-mediated immunity and, because the organisms in the vaccine cannot replicate, injections usually have to be repeated (booster injections) to maintain the required level of immunity. An example of an inactivated vaccine is the influenza A vaccine. Attenuated vaccines are more potent than inactivated vaccines as the immune response that is induced is more durable and resembles the natural response against the pathogen. The measles vaccine is an example of an attenuated vaccine.

Purified subunit vaccines

These vaccines comprise only some of the antigens expressed by the intact micro-organism. These normally represent the immunodominant antigens. In order to evoke a more powerful immune response, the purified subunit may be conjugated to a protein that will stimulate a strong CD4$^+$ T cell response and thus a powerful antibody-mediated response. These are known as conjugate vaccines. The Hib vaccine is an example of a conjugate vaccine.

Toxoids

A number of micro-organisms cause disease by producing toxins. Toxoids are inactivated toxins that induce immunity to a toxin, not to the micro-organism that produces the toxin. The tetanus vaccine is a toxoid vaccine.

Recombinant vaccines

Recombinant vaccines are generated by genetic engineering. Normally, the antigen of interest is expressed in a non-replicating vector that is then used for immunization. This technology potentially allows the incorporation of antigens from multiple pathogens into a single vaccine vector. The human papillomavirus vaccine is an example of such a recombinant vaccine.

Passive immunization

Passive immunization involves the administration of pre-formed antibodies (in antiserum) to a patient who has been exposed, or is at risk of exposure to an infectious pathogen. The antiserum must initially be made in another host, frequently in horses. Passive immunization does not allow the development of specific memory so antibodies that are given to a person are gradually removed from the circulation and so must be re-administered if needed in the future. Passive immunization is now carried out only in emergency situations. These include cases where:

- the patient has been exposed to something so toxic that they would die before an immune response was mounted, for example, tetanus toxin or snakebite venom
- the patient suffers from one of several immunoglobulin deficiency syndromes and must receive regular intravenous injections of pooled immunoglobulin (IVIG) to confer protection against common infections
- the patient is a pregnant woman and cannot be exposed to many of the current vaccines because of the risk to the fetus.

Vaccines against specific diseases

Measles vaccine

In 1988, the UK government introduced the combined measles, mumps and rubella (MMR) triple vaccine. The proportion of two-year-olds immunized increased to more than 90%. The vaccine contains live attenuated virus and is offered for babies, with a booster shot at about 4 years of age. This vaccine has been highly successful and has led to a dramatic reduction in the incidence of measles, once a common cause of blindness and brain damage. In recent years, the uptake of the MMR vaccine has been disappointingly low, and many health authorities are concerned about the possibility of measles outbreaks. This is a real concern as there have been several outbreaks of mumps in educational institutions over the past year. The low uptake of the MMR vaccine is related to highly publicized, though now discredited reports that the MMR vaccine was related to development of autism. This notion persists despite the lack of supporting scientific evidence and the MMR vaccine is often referred to as the 'controversial MMR vaccine'.

Human papillomavirus vaccine

The human papillomavirus vaccine (HPV) is a recombinant vaccine made up of the major capsid protein of HPV. When this protein is expressed in yeast cells it forms non-replicating virus-like particles (VLPs). The current HPV vaccine is a 'quadrivalent' vaccine made up of a mixture of the major capsid proteins of HPV-6, -11, -16 and -18, the main HPV types associated with cervical cancer. In clinical trials this vaccine was effective in preventing HPV infection with the HPV types from which the capsid proteins were derived.

Polio vaccine

The first polio vaccine to be developed was a formaldehyde-inactivated polio vaccine (IPV or Salk vaccine). This was developed by Jonas Salk and was used in the USA between 1955 and 1961. This was superceded by a live attenuated vaccine, also known as the Sabin or oral polio vaccine (OPV), developed by Albert Sabin. This became the preferred vaccine because it is easier to administer and because it promotes production of IgA, and therefore generates a protective mucosal immune response, in addition to stimulating the production of other antibodies. OPV contains live virus and reversion to virulence can cause a vaccinated child, the child's contacts, or immunosuppressed individuals, to develop vaccine-associated paralytic poliomyelitis (VAPP). VAPP cases due to OPV reversion to virulence occurs at a rate of about 8 to 10 cases annually. The polio eradication campaign has resulted in the restriction of endemic polio to parts of only four countries.

Hepatitis virus vaccines

The hepatitis A virus (HAV) vaccine consists of inactivated HAV. The vaccine has been shown to provide greater than 95% protection against HAV infection, and this protection persists for at least 10 years.

The hepatitis B virus (HBV) vaccine consists of recombinant HBV surface antigen (HBsAg) made in yeast cells. After an initial injection and two booster injections of the HBV vaccine, high levels of HBsAg-specific antibody are generated that protect against HBV infection.

Current problems in vaccinology

Not all vaccination programmes have been equally successful. In many cases the failure of particular vaccine strategies may be due to an incomplete understanding of the components of the immune response that are required to confer protective immunity against the pathogen. This is well illustrated by early attempts at developing a vaccine against HIV infection. The development of an effective HIV vaccine continues to frustrate the efforts of biomedical scientists and remains the focus of intense research. Similarly, malaria and schistosomiasis, the two other main infectious diseases worldwide, also lack effective vaccination programmes. Vaccination against these diseases 'in the field' also may present challenges. Due to the geographical distribution of these diseases, co-infections with various combinations of HIV, *P. falciparum*, and *S. mansoni* are relatively common and this may hamper attempts at vaccination. For example, infection with *S. mansoni* tends to bias immune responses against other antigens towards a Th2-type response. This sort of response would be of little benefit against HIV infection, so an individual with schistosomiasis may not respond appropriately to vaccination against HIV.

Many challenges remain in the field of vaccinology and effective vaccines against the current major infectious diseases are urgently needed. In addition, the acquisition of drug resistance by pathogenic organisms together with the global spread of current and emerging pathogens and the increased culture of worldwide travel ensures that vaccine development will be an active area of biomedical research for many years to come.

SUGGESTED FURTHER READING

Anthony, R.M., Rubitzky, L.I., Urban Jr, J.F., Stadecker, M.J. and Gause, W.C. (2007) Protective immune mechanisms in helminth infection. *Nature Rev. Immunol.* **7**: 975–987.

Doherty, P.C., Turner, S.J., Webby, R.J. and Thomas, P.G. (2006) Influenza and the challenge for immunology. *Nature Immunol.* **7**: 449–455.

Foster, T.J. (2005) Immune evasion by staphylococci. *Nature Rev. Microbiol.* **3**: 948–958.

Hislop, A.D., Taylor, G.S., Sauce, D. and Rickinson, A.R. (2007) Cellular responses to viral infection in humans: lessons from Epstein–Barr virus. *Annu. Rev. Immunol.* **25**: 587–617.

Lambert, P.-H., Liu, M. and Siegrist, C.-A. (2005) Can successful vaccines teach us how to induce efficient protective immune responses? *Nature Med.* Suppl. **11**: S54–S62.

Mansfield, J. M. and Paulnock, D.M. (2005) Regulation of innate and acquired immunity in African trypanosomiasis. *Parasite Immunol.* **27**: 361–371.

Marsh, K. and Kinyanjui, S. (2006) Immune effector mechanisms in malaria. *Parasite Immunol.* **28**: 51–60.

Rappleye, C.A. and Goldman, W.E. (2007) Fungal stealth technology. *Trends Immunol.* **29**: 18–24.

Schofield, L. and Grau, G.E. (2005) Immunological processes in malaria pathogenesis. *Nature Rev. Immunol.* **5**: 722–735.

van Rossum, A.M.C., Lysenko, E.S. and Weiser, J.N. (2005) Host and bacterial factors contributing to the clearance of colonization by *Streptococcus pneumoniae* in a murine model. *Infect. Immun.* **71**: 7718–7726.

Vossen, M.T., Westerhout, E.M., Söderberg-Nauclér, C. and Wiertz, E.J. (2002) Viral immune evasion: a masterpiece of evolution. *Immunogenetics,* **54**: 527–542.

Wright, P.F. (2008) Vaccine preparedness – are we ready for the next influenza pandemic? *N. Engl. J. Med.* **358**: 2540–2543.

SELF-ASSESSMENT QUESTIONS

1. What components of immunity are active against intracellular infections?
2. How does the capsule of *Streptococcus pneumoniae* confer protection against immune elimination?
3. Explain the difference between an attenuated vaccine and an inactivated vaccine.
4. Describe three ways in which *Staphylococcus aureus* can evade the immune response.

5. How does the tegument of adult schistosomes confer protection against the immune response?
6. Why is it often necessary to alter the influenza vaccine for successive 'flu seasons'?
7. What is meant by the term 'opportunistic pathogen'?
8. What is the causative agent of Chagas' disease?
9. Why are *Plasmodium falciparum*-infected RBCs not eliminated by the spleen?
10. Why do AIDS patients frequently suffer from disseminated cryptococcal infections?

CHAPTER 9 Hypersensitivity

■ Immunotherapy – hyposensitization or allergy immunization, with subcutaneous injections of increasing concentrations of the allergen(s).
■ Vaccination – an example is an oral allergy vaccine using a genetically modified grass pollen allergen (Grazax™) for immunotherapy.
Type II
■ For example, to prevent HDN after delivery, RhD⁻ women are given an injection of pre-formed anti-RhD antibody.
Type III
■ For example, for farmer's lung NSAIDs such as aspirin or antihistamines can be used to counteract the inflammatory response. Systemic administration of immunosuppressive corticosteroids may be required in more serious cases of Type III hypersensitivity reactions.
Type IV
■ Avoidance is the best solution for Type IV hypersensitivity reactions such as contact reactions to nickel or rubber.

9.1 INTRODUCTION TO HYPERSENSITIVITY

A hypersensitivity reaction is an immune or inflammatory response that occurs in an exaggerated or inappropriate form, or in an inappropriate situation. In such circumstances normal immune effector mechanisms damage host tissues, causing symptoms that range in severity from mildly debilitating to potentially life-threatening.

Gell and Coombs originally classified hypersensitivity reactions into four types in the 1960s (see *Table 9.1*). Types I, II and III are antibody-mediated reactions, whereas T cells and macrophages mediate Type IV hypersensitivity. All hypersensitivity reactions require the affected individual to be sensitized (pre-exposed) to the antigen that triggers the hypersensitivity reaction. During this sensitization phase, the susceptible individual develops the type of immune response that will lead to a hypersensitivity reaction upon re-exposure to the antigen. Therefore hypersensitive reactions do not present following the first exposure to antigens, only following the second or subsequent exposures. Re-exposure to antigen triggers the cellular and molecular events that result in the hypersensitive reaction. This phase of the response is called the activation or elicitation phase. In addition, an antigen may trigger multiple responses, so a particular disease may involve more than one type of hypersensitivity reaction.

An alternative classification to that of Gell and Coombs has been proposed which categorizes certain Type II hypersensitivity reactions as Type V hypersensitivity responses (see *Section 9.8*). In addition, other researchers have proposed the classification of septic shock (see *Section 8.3*) as innate hypersensitivity. This chapter adheres to the original Gell and Coombs classification of hypersensitivity reactions.

Table 9.1 Gell and Coombs classification of hypersensitivities

Type	Alternative names	Examples	Mediators
I	Immediate hypersensitivity, allergy	Hay fever Food allergy Allergic asthma	IgE
II	Antibody-dependent cytotoxicity	Erythroblastosis fetalis Goodpasture's syndrome Hyperacute graft rejection	IgG, IgM, complement
III	Immune complex disease	Serum sickness Lupus nephritis	IgG Complement
IV	Delayed-type hypersensitivity	Contact hypersensitivity Tuberculin reaction Granulomatous reaction Acute graft rejection	T cells, macrophages

9.2 TYPE I HYPERSENSITIVITY

Type I hypersensitivity, also known as immediate hypersensitivity, due to the appearance of symptoms within minutes, is frequently termed allergy or atopy (see *Box 9.1*) and affected individuals are said to be allergic or atopic. This type of response is associated with the generation of an IgE response against the eliciting antigen. Allergic diseases are prevalent in the developed world; therefore the pathological role of IgE in allergies is better known than the protective function of IgE in immune responses (see *Box 9.2*). It is thought that these responses have been conserved evolutionarily because of their role in elimination of parasitic infections (see *Section 8.6*), a significant cause of morbidity in developing nations.

Antigens that elicit Type I hypersensitivity responses are called allergens. A wide variety of different allergens have been identified (see *Table 9.2*).

Box 9.1 The 'allergy' concept

This was formulated in 1906 by Clemens von Pirquet to describe the hypersensitive reaction of some of his patients to normally harmless substances such as dust or pollen. von Pirquet called this phenomenon 'allergy' from the Greek words allos (other) and ergon (work).

Box 9.2 Discovery of IgE

Kimishige Ishizaka and his wife Teruko have performed ground-breaking studies on the causes and mechanisms of allergic diseases. Their early studies focused on the antibodies involved in human allergic reactions, and led to the discovery of IgE.

Table 9.2 Allergens commonly associated with Type I hypersensitivity

Class of allergen	Examples
Plant pollen	Ragweed
	Rye grass
	Birch trees
Food allergens	Nuts
	Seafood
	Milk
	Eggs
Insect products	House dust mite allergen
	Bee venom
	Wasp venom
Drugs	Penicillin
	Sulphonamides
	Salicylates
Miscellaneous	Animal dander
	Mould spores
	Latex
	Vaccines

Some of the more common allergens include grass pollen, cat dander, food antigens and insect venom. Individuals who are allergic to one substance are also frequently sensitive to other allergens.

The basis of the Type I hypersensitivity response is related to the production of IgE instead of any of the other immunoglobulin isotypes. This is generally associated with an exuberant Th2 response against the allergen. Studies have shown that when T cells from non-allergic patients are stimulated *in vitro* by specific allergen, they primarily produce IFN-γ (characteristic of a Th1 response), whereas T cells from allergic patients produce allergen-induced IL-4 and IL-13 (characteristic of a Th2 response). IL-4 and IL-13 are the major cytokines responsible for directing B cells to switch from making immunoglobulin of the IgM isotype to making IgE (see *Section 6.10*). The production of allergen-specific IgE is the crucial step in the development of Type I hypersensitivity reactions.

Compared with other immunoglobulin isotypes, IgE is present at very low concentration in the circulation (1–10 ng ml^{-1}). IgE differs also from the other immunoglobulin isotypes in that it has an extra constant region domain, $C_\varepsilon 4$, which enables it to bind to the high affinity IgE receptor, FCεRI, expressed on mast cells and basophils. This high affinity interaction ($K_d \sim 10^{-10}$ M) allows long-term, stable binding of IgE to these cells so that, even in non-allergic individuals, mast cells always have IgE bound on their surfaces.

Following exposure to an allergen, a susceptible individual generates a Th2 response and produces high levels of allergen-specific IgE. The IgE binds to the FcεRI receptors on the surface of circulating basophils and

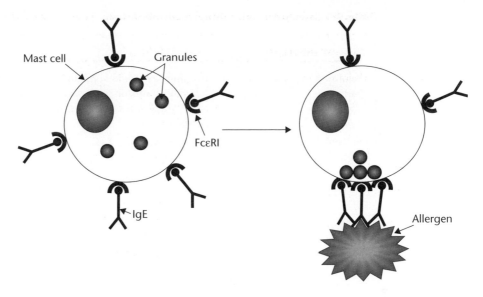

Figure 9.1
Following initial exposure to allergen, allergen-specific IgE binds to Fcε type I
receptors (FcεRI) on tissue mast cells and circulating basophils. Upon re-exposure to
the allergen, binding of allergen to FcεRI-bound IgE causes the IgE molecules to
aggregate, leading to degranulation of the mast cells.

tissue mast cells, for example, mast cells in the lungs or in the gastrointestinal tract. Consequently there are high levels of allergen-specific IgE
present in tissues of allergen-exposed individuals. This phase of the Type I
hypersensitivity response is called sensitization and the mast cells are
referred to as sensitized mast cells (see *Figure 9.1*).

On the second, and each subsequent, encounter with the same allergen,
this FcεRI-bound IgE binds antigen in such a way that adjacent IgE
molecules become cross-linked (see *Figure 9.1*). This causes the mast cells
to degranulate and release their preformed inflammatory mediators and also
to synthesize *de novo*, and release, lipid mediators and cytokines (see *Section
4.4*). This is the activation phase of Type I hypersensitivity and the mast cell-
derived mediators initiate the symptoms of this reaction (see *Table 9.3*). The
symptoms of an allergic response can be classified either as early phase or
late phase responses. The early phase responses occur within minutes of
exposure to allergen and are triggered by mast cell-derived mediators, such
as histamine, prostaglandins, leukotrienes and proteases.

Histamine binds to two major classes of receptors called H1 and H2
receptors. These receptors have different tissue distributions and mediate
different effects when stimulated by histamine. Binding of histamine to H1
receptors on vascular endothelial cells causes the cells to contract leading to
an increase in vascular permeability, whereas binding of histamine to H1
receptors on smooth muscle results in transient muscle contraction.

Table 9.3 Selected mast cell-derived mediators

Class of mediator	Examples[a]
Preformed mediators in granules	Histamine, heparin sulphates, neutral proteases (chymases and/or tryptases), major basic protein, acid hydrolases, cathepsins, carboxypeptidases, peroxidase
Lipid mediators	PGE_2, PGD_2, LTB_4, LTC_4, PAF
Cytokines	CCL2, CCL3, IFN-α, IFN-β, IFN-γ, IL-1α, IL-1β, IL-3, IL-4, IL-5, IL-6, IL-8, IL-10, IL-9, IL-11, IL-12, IL-13, IL-15, IL-16, IL-18, IL-25, TGF-β, TNF-α

[a]**Abbreviations**: CCL, CC chemokine ligand; IFN, interferon; IL, interleukin; LT, leukotriene; PAF, platelet activating factor; PG, prostaglandin; TGF-β, transforming growth factor-β; TNF-α, tumour necrosis factor-α.

Histamine binding to H2 receptors also increases vascular permeability and stimulates mucus secretion. Histamine also causes dilation of small blood vessels and stimulation of nerve endings. Mast cell-derived prostaglandins cause vasodilation while leukotrienes cause prolonged contraction of smooth muscle. The activity of mast cell-derived proteases (mast cell tryptases and chymase) can activate matrix metalloproteinases, leading to tissue damage. Collectively these mediators can cause the characteristic early phase responses, which include itching (pruritis), sneezing, increased mucus secretion (rhinorrhoea) and bronchospasm.

Mast cells themselves respond to and produce cytokines including IL-1, IL-4, IL-5, IL-13, TNF-α and CCL11 (formerly eotaxin-1, an eosinophil chemo-attractant). These cytokines, together with the degranulation products of mast cells, trigger the late phase responses of Type I hypersensitivity (see *Figure 9.2*). Late phase symptoms appear 2–24 hours after the

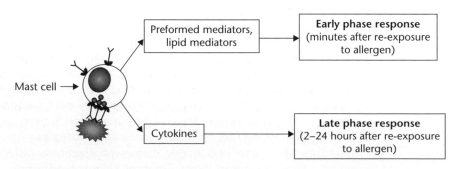

Figure 9.2
The two phases of an allergic reaction are caused by different mast cell-derived mediators. The immediate response is dependent on preformed mediators released from mast cell granules as well as on lipid mediators. The late phase response is largely dependent on mast cell-derived cytokines.

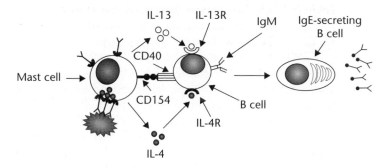

Figure 9.3
Cross-linking of FcεRI molecules on mast cells induces them to express CD154 on their surfaces. This can bind to CD40 on the B cell surface and, in concert with mast cell-derived IL-4 and IL-13, induce extrafollicular class switch recombination to IgE.

early phase reaction. Of all the mediators involved in promoting the late phase response, IL-4 and IL-13 may be particularly relevant. Cross-linking of surface IgE on mast cells causes them to express CD154 (CD40L) on their surfaces and this then can bind to CD40 on allergen-specific B cells. The IL-4 and IL-13 produced by the activated mast cells will induce isotype-switching to IgE (see *Figure 9.3*). IL-4 is also a growth factor for B cells, Th2 cells and mast cells. Thus IL-4 can promote the conditions necessary for a Type I hypersensitivity reaction. The interaction between mast cells and B cells can take place in mucosal-associated lymphoid tissues, the site of presentation of inhaled or ingested allergens. It may also occur in the inflamed tissue where B cells may accumulate in 'germinal centre-like' structures. Recent research indicates that basophils are essential for promoting IgE responses against allergens that have protease activity. IL-4 and IL-13 also induce production of CCL11 by epithelial cells. Although mast cells themselves can produce CCL11, the major source of this chemokine is epithelial cells. CCL11 production is important as this chemokine attracts eosinophils and Th2 cells to the site of exposure to the allergen.

Mast cell-derived IL-1 and TNF-α act on vascular endothelial cells to promote extravasation of leukocytes into the tissue (see *Section 4.5*). Unlike an acute inflammatory lesion where the predominant infiltrating cells are neutrophils, the major cells infiltrating the site of an allergic reaction are Th2 cells and eosinophils. Th2 cells infiltrate the tissue having been attracted to the site primarily by the mast cell-derived prostaglandin PGD_2, but also by CCL11. Th2 cells secrete the cytokines IL-3, IL-4, IL-5, IL-9, IL-13 and the chemokine CCL11. IL-3 is a major growth factor for mast cells and IL-4 promotes Th2 cell proliferation. IL-9 attracts additional mast cells to the tissue and promotes their differentiation. IL-4, IL-9 and IL-13 produced by the Th2 cells induce CCL11 production by tissue epithelial cells and, in the respiratory tract, promote differentiation of epithelial cells into goblet cells and enhance the secretion of mucus by goblet cells. This leads to obstruction of the airways causing difficulty in breathing. In this way, the recruitment of Th2 cells can exacerbate the hypersensitivity reaction. This is particularly true in allergic asthma where the increase in mast cell numbers in the lungs is thought to be due, at least in part, to Th2 cell-derived cytokines.

CCL11 is a potent eosinophil chemoattractant and leads to accumulation of eosinophils in the tissue. This is further promoted by IL-5, a growth and survival factor for eosinophils, produced by Th2 cells. Eosinophilia of lung tissue is a common feature of advanced allergic asthma, which can develop following allergen stimulation of mast cells in the bronchial submucosae. Like mast cells, the infiltrating eosinophils release leukotrienes, which induce bronchoconstriction, leading to difficulty in breathing. The sulphidopeptide leukotrienes LTC_4, LTD_4 and LTE_4, sometimes termed slow reacting substance of anaphylaxis (SRS-A), are particularly important in this regard. Activated eosinophils secrete major basic protein and eosinophil peroxidase, which are toxic for respiratory epithelial cells and induce tissue damage. Th2 cells are also attracted by the chemokines CCL17 and CCL22 that are produced by activated eosinophils, leading to further accumulation of Th2 cells in the tissue. Persistence of the allergen will lead to a chronic inflammatory response characterized by profound infiltration of Th2 cells and eosinophils as well as increased mast cell numbers. Recent studies suggest that pro-inflammatory Th17 cells (see *Section 6.5*) may also infiltrate the tissue during chronic disease and induce the accumulation of neutrophils, thus exacerbating the tissue damage.

The late phase of the Type I response leads to remodelling of respiratory tissue. The damage caused by the inflammatory cells and mast cells can cause extensive sub-epithelial fibrosis. Th2 cell-derived cytokines induce myocyte proliferation, resulting in an increase in airway smooth muscle mass. This is a major contributory factor to airway hyper-responsiveness. Permanent, allergen-independent, airway hyper-responsiveness to bronchoconstrictors such as histamine, is a hallmark of asthma. Asthma symptoms include coughing, wheezing, and shortness of breath due to a narrowing of the bronchial passages (airways) in the lungs and to excess mucus production. Asthma can be extremely debilitating and can sometimes be fatal. If wheezing and shortness of breath accompany allergy symptoms, it is a signal that the bronchial tubes have also become involved, indicating the need for medical attention.

Table 9.4 Symptoms of allergy

Site of exposure to allergen	Symptoms
Nose	Sneezing, itching, runny nose
Eyes	Redness, itching
Lungs	Sneezing, coughing, wheezing, shortness of breath
Skin	Eczema, hives
Gastrointestinal tract	Abdominal pain, vomiting, diarrhoea, bloating

A strong determinant of the seriousness of the allergy for the patient is the site in the body where mast cell degranulation occurred (see *Table 9.4*). In the case of a reaction to cutaneous exposure to an allergen, for example, the response may be little more than a painful or itchy swelling. But, if the allergen has been inhaled, the swelling could significantly affect breathing and progress to allergic asthma (as described above). Food allergies are believed to occur in approximately 7% of infants in the UK. These ingested allergens stimulate mast cells in the intestinal wall leading to increased fluid secretion and peristalsis, resulting in vomiting and diarrhoea. However, food allergy can also cause symptoms involving a number of different body systems. For some people, food allergies can be life threatening and others may have a mild reaction. Each individual's sensitivity will determine the degree to which the offending foods should be eliminated from the diet. The most common food allergens are nuts, fish, eggs, milk, wheat and soy. Of these groups, peanuts and shellfish are the most common foods that cause life-threatening allergies. Most restaurant menus and food packaging now provide warnings regarding potential allergen content.

9.3   THE NATURE OF ALLERGENS

Most allergens are low molecular weight soluble molecules borne on large particles such as pollen grains. Following inhalation or ingestion, these allergens are readily eluted into the mucosa where they can be acquired by DCs for presentation to T cells. It is thought that most allergens are presented to the immune system at very low doses, a condition that favours the induction of Th2 responses over Th1 responses (see *Section 6.4*).

Many allergens are enzymes. Der p 1, an allergen associated with the house dust mite, *Dermatophagoides pteronyssinus*, and Amb a, an allergen of ragweed pollen, are proteinases that break down tight junctions between epithelial cells. This induces production of thymic stromal lymphopoietin (TSLP) by the epithelial cells. TSLP binds to receptors on sub-epithelial DCs and activates them to induce the differentiation of CD4$^+$ T cells into Th2 cells, the T cell subset that is associated with development of allergy (see *Figure 9.4*). Basophils are also recruited to the paracortex of draining lymph nodes after allergen exposure. Exposure of basophils to allergens with protease activity stimulates them to secrete IL-2, IL-4, IL-13, and TSLP, cytokines that promote a Th2 response and IgE production.

The effects of airborne pollutants on the immune system have been widely studied in the respiratory tract. An airborne pollutant may enter the respiratory tract as a volatile gas (e.g. ozone, benzene), as liquid droplets (e.g. sulphuric acid, nitrogen dioxide), or as particulate matter (e.g. components of diesel exhaust fumes). These pollutants may cause local and systemic hypersensitivities. Most airborne pollutants function as haptens (see *Section 2.7*), and are small molecular weight chemicals that must be coupled with other substances (e.g. proteins or conjugates) before they can be recognized by the immune system and cause an effect. Occupational asthma can occur following exposure to toluene diisocyanate, a compound

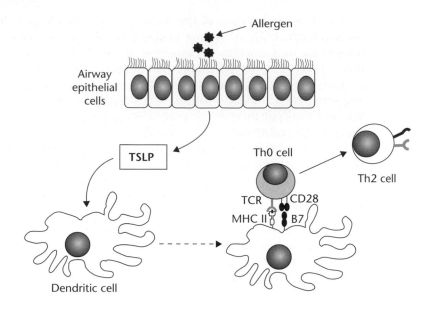

Figure 9.4
Certain allergens induce airway epithelial cells to produce thymic stromal
lymphopoietin (TSLP) which stimulates DCs to promote Th2 cell differentiation.

that is frequently used in the petrochemical industry, and exposure to certain other volatile chemicals. In contrast, immunosuppression can be demonstrated following exposure to the polycyclic aromatic hydrocarbon 2,3,7,8-tetrachlorodibenzo-*p*-dioxin, possibly via induction of the suppressor of cytokine signalling gene *Socs2* (see *Section 7.3*). Recent research has found that stimulation of the aryl hydrocarbon receptor (AHR), a receptor for a wide variety of environmental pollutants and drugs, can influence T cell differentiation following exposure to antigen. Further research in this area is likely to increase our understanding of the effects of airborne pollutants on local mucosal immune responses in the gastrointestinal and respiratory tracts.

9.4   SYSTEMIC ANAPHYLAXIS

Systemic anaphylaxis, also called anaphylactic shock, is a dramatic allergic reaction that can result in collapse of the affected person and sometimes death. The onset is rapid and symptoms can develop within 5–30 minutes of exposure to the allergen. Death may occur within a further 15 minutes. The symptoms of systemic anaphylaxis result from systemic release of allergic mediators from mast cells.

Anaphylaxis can occur after any route of administration of allergen, but episodes are more frequent and often more severe when antigen is injected rather than ingested. Urticaria (hives), angioedema and flushing are the most common initial signs of anaphylaxis. Frequently, the absence of such symptoms mitigates the diagnosis of anaphylaxis, although cardiovascular collapse with shock can occur immediately and without any cutaneous or respiratory symptoms in rare instances. Other common symptoms of anaphylactic shock are hoarseness, difficulty in breathing (angioedema of the airways can be fatal), feelings of great anxiety, abdominal pain, vomiting and dizziness, and ultimately collapse.

Two events participate in the production of shock symptoms. The first is profound vasodilation and the second is increased vascular permeability due to widespread release of mast cell-derived mediators. This increase in vascular permeability produces a shift of fluid from the intravascular to extravascular space and can result in rapid and profound loss of intravascular volume, leading to a serious drop in blood pressure (hypotension). Up to 50% of intravascular volume can be lost within 10 minutes. The biggest threat to life during anaphylactic shock is constricted airways, which can cause death within minutes.

The best possible treatment for allergy is avoidance of the known allergen. Unfortunately, this is not always possible. All persons with a known life-threatening allergy or a history of very severe allergy symptoms are advised to carry with them an allergy kit or auto-injectable adrenaline (epinephrine in the USA) kit. When the early symptoms are experienced the patient takes the pre-measured dose of adrenaline and this raises the blood pressure back to normal and reduces swelling (especially of the airways). It is the quickest and most effective way to stop the anaphylactic reaction.

9.5   DIAGNOSING ALLERGIES

When clinical evaluation indicates that particular symptoms are consistent with an allergy, a number of confirmatory tests can be carried out.

Skin prick test

A diluted extract of potential allergens (e.g. dust, pollen, etc.) is injected under the patient's skin or applied to a small puncture wound made on the arm or back. A positive reaction consists of a small, raised, pale area with a surrounding flush and is known as a wheal and flare reaction. The wheal is due to fluid build-up in the papillary body in the dermis and is an important clue in the diagnosis of an allergy. The flare is redness of the skin due to dilation of blood vessels. This wheal and flare response should be maximal within 30 minutes and will then diminish. Skin testing is not advisable in some people, such as those with widespread skin conditions like eczema, or if the individual has taken medications that interfere with skin testing. Due to the life-threatening nature of severe allergic responses, skin testing must be performed with caution, and with access to injectable adrenaline.

Blood test

Other tests can be done using a blood sample from the patient to detect levels of IgE antibody to a particular allergen. One such blood test is called the RAST (radioallergosorbent test). Unfortunately the RAST is expensive to perform, takes several days to yield results, and is somewhat less sensitive than skin testing. In many labs, the RAST test has been replaced by the more rapid ELISA (see *Section 13.9*). It is important to note that the RAST or ELISA only test if a person has generated an IgE response against a particular allergen. Although highly suggestive, this does not mean that the individual is certain to develop an allergic reaction to that allergen. The only test currently available to elucidate this is the skin prick test.

9.6   TREATING ALLERGIC DISEASES

Although no cure for allergies has yet been found, there are several strategies that, alone or in combination, can provide varying degrees of relief from allergy symptoms. The general approaches to the treatment of allergies are outlined below.

Avoidance of the allergen

Complete avoidance of allergenic substances, although an extreme solution, may offer only temporary relief, since a person who is sensitive to a substance may subsequently develop allergies to new allergens after repeated exposure. For example, people allergic to ragweed may leave that area and move to areas where ragweed does not grow, only to develop allergies to other weeds or even to grasses or trees in their new surroundings. This is particularly true if the individual is genetically predisposed to developing strong Th2 responses against antigens.

Medication to relieve symptoms

If allergen avoidance is not feasible, allergy symptoms may be controlled pharmacologically. Effective medications that can be prescribed include antihistamines, bronchodilators, topical nasal steroids, sodium cromoglycate and vasoconstrictors. These drugs can be used alone or in combination.

Antihistamines, such as diphenhydramine (e.g. Benadryl®) are H1 receptor antagonists. These drugs block the actions of histamine on H1 receptors and are effective against the early phase symptoms of allergy. Antihistamines are most effective when administered prophylactically.

Inhaled bronchodilators such as albuterol (e.g. Ventolin®) are prescribed for the treatment of asthma. These drugs are β_2-adrenergic receptor agonists, which relax airway smooth muscle leading to dilation of the bronchial passages. Daily use of these drugs can reduce the frequency of asthma attacks. In cases of severe asthma, long-acting β_2-adrenergic receptor agonists, such as salmeterol (e.g. Advair®), may be prescribed.

Topical nasal steroids such as prednisone (e.g. Meticorten®) are anti-inflammatory drugs that are effective against the late phase response of the allergic reaction. In addition to other beneficial actions, they reduce the number of mast cells in the nose and reduce mucus secretion and nasal swelling.

The direct link between mast cell degranulation and development of allergy symptoms is apparent when mast cell membrane stabilizers are used as treatment. One such drug is sodium cromoglycate (Cromolyn), which inhibits the release of the mast cell-derived mediators. Sodium cromoglycate interferes with the release of the inflammatory mediators but does not directly counteract the effects of the mediators themselves. The drug is most effective when given prophylactically. It is not a bronchodilator and has few general pharmacological effects.

Vasoconstrictors such as adrenaline (e.g. EpiPen® containing adrenaline) are the drugs of choice to counteract the vasodilation and increased vascular permeability associated with systemic anaphylaxis. Adrenaline is an α_1-adrenergic receptor agonist that acts on vascular smooth muscle to cause vasoconstriction. Like albuterol, adrenaline can also bind to β_2-adrenergic receptors causing bronchodilation.

Immunotherapy

Desensitization, also called hyposensitization or allergy immunization, is the only available treatment that may reduce the patient's allergy symptoms in the long term. Patients receive subcutaneous injections of increasing concentrations of the allergen(s) to which they are sensitive into the back of the upper arm. Initially, very low doses of allergen are injected. The dose of allergen is gradually increased over a period of 6–12 months. The rationale is to try to generate a competing Th1 response or, alternatively, a suppressive T_{REG} response, against the allergen. A Th1 or T_{REG} response would inhibit the allergen-specific Th2 response. This, in turn, would reduce the amount of IgE produced and, in the case of a Th1 response, promote production of IgG. The allergen-specific IgG would bind to and neutralize the allergen before it could bind to sensitized mast cells. Desensitisation has been shown to be effective in certain individuals with allergic responses against insect venom; however, this approach has not been beneficial in the treatment of food allergies. Current approaches to desensitization utilize recombinant allergens that are genetically modified or conjugated to carrier proteins to modulate the allergen-induced immune response.

Vaccination

One of the most exciting developments in the field of allergy treatment is the recent development of an oral allergy vaccine using a genetically modified grass pollen allergen (Grazax®) for immunotherapy. This vaccine has proven to be effective in clinical trials of hay fever sufferers. Recombinant vaccines against Der p 1 and against a cat allergen, Fel d 1, are currently being developed.

Helminth infection

The reduction in the incidence of allergic diseases in individuals infected with helminthic parasites, e.g. *Schistosoma mansoni*, suggests that these organisms may be beneficial in treating allergies. Several researchers are attempting to identify molecules expressed by these parasites that may be useful in allergy therapy.

9.7 CAUSES OF ALLERGIES

It is unclear why some individuals develop allergies while others do not. Elevated IgE responses alone are not sufficient, as these are sometimes seen in non-allergic individuals. There has been much research into risk factors that predispose to development of allergies, and these are usually classified as genetic or environmental factors.

Genetic factors

Allergic diseases tend to run in families. Studies have demonstrated that identical twins suffer from the same allergy about 70% of the time, whereas fraternal twins have shared allergies about 40% of the time. Furthermore, allergic parents are more likely to have allergic children than are non-allergic parents. In addition, children of allergic parents are likely to develop more severe allergies than children of non-allergic parents. However, children of allergy sufferers frequently develop allergies to different allergens than their parents. Thus, it is the likelihood of developing allergy, rather than a specific allergy, that is inherited. Young children are at greatest risk of developing allergies, possibly because levels of IgE are highest in childhood and decrease rapidly between the ages of 10 and 30 years.

Several studies have investigated genetic susceptibility factors for development of allergies. Among the genes found to be associated with allergy are allelic variants of CCL11, IL-4, IL-13, TNF-α, as well as an allelic variant of a gene encoding the β chain of FCϵRI. It has been proposed that the functions of these allelic variants enhance Th2 responses and/or mast cell hyper-responsiveness in allergy. Recent studies indicate also that suppressor T_{REG} function may be deficient in allergic diseases.

Environmental factors

Allergies are more common in industrialized nations than in developing nations, and children from large families or from families living in overcrowded conditions have a reduced risk of developing allergies. To explain these observations, it has been proposed that exposure to microorganisms or parasites early during childhood protects against the subsequent development of allergic disease later in life, possibly by biasing the development of immune responses towards Th1 responses. This notion is referred to as the hygiene hypothesis. This hypothesis proposes that the widespread use of disinfectants and antibiotics in developed nations to reduce the risk of exposure to potential pathogens concomitantly increases the risk of developing allergies (see the Case study in *Box 9.3*).

Box 9.3 Case study

David is a 5-year-old boy who is brought to his doctor by his mother because he has difficulty sleeping. At night he suffers from a non-productive cough, itchy and watery eyes, and his mother can hear him wheezing as he sleeps. David's mother prides herself on how clean her house is and she changes the bed linen frequently. She tells the doctor that David sleeps better after his bed linen is changed but that his coughing and wheezing return on subsequent nights. David's first episode of wheezing occurred on his fourth birthday on a visit to his grandparents who had just bought a cat. Before that time, David would occasionally play with his neighbour's cat, but that neighbour moved house shortly after David's third birthday. When David plays with his grandparents' cat he will sneeze and wheeze and sometimes his face will swell. David seems to be particularly susceptible to colds and sometimes going outdoors on a cold winter's evening is sufficient to make him cough and wheeze. He tires easily at play with his school friends and succumbs to episodes of coughing and wheezing if he takes part in strenuous exercise. He cannot play outside if his neighbours have just cut their lawn because this makes his eyes itchy and watery and makes his nose run.

On laboratory testing, David's differential blood cell count was normal, except for elevated numbers of eosinophils.

1. Provide an explanation for David's symptoms.
2. What are the potential environmental triggers of David's condition? What tests could you perform to confirm this?
3. What are the immunological mechanisms responsible for this condition and how do they affect the airways?
4. How may David's condition be treated?

Answers are given alongside the answers to the self-assessment questions for *Chapter 9* at the back of the book.

9.8 TYPE II HYPERSENSITIVITY

Like Type I hypersensitivity, Type II hypersensitivity is an antibody-mediated phenomenon. However, the antibody involved in Type II hypersensitivity is usually IgG or IgM. Type II hypersensitivity responses occur due to antibody-dependent destruction of cells. The pathogenic antibody is produced in response to a cell surface antigen. When the antibody binds to the antigen, it can target the cell expressing that antigen for destruction by phagocytes or NK cells (effector cells) which express Fcγ receptors on their surfaces. The antibody therefore forms a bridge between the target cell and the effector cell and triggers the release of cytocidal molecules from the effector cell. This process is called antibody-dependent cell-mediated cytotoxicity (ADCC, see *Section 2.9*). Studies using CD16-deficient mice suggest this as the major mechanism responsible for tissue damage in models of Type II hypersensitivity. Cell surface-bound antibody may also activate complement via the classical pathway (see *Section 4.3*), leading to complement-mediated lysis of the cell followed by elimination by phagocytes. However, with the exception of erythrocytes, complement-mediated destruction of cells requires the deposition of multiple active complement complexes to overcome the inhibition of complement activation mediated by membrane-bound inhibitors of complement activation that are expressed by most cells.

Clearly, antibody-dependent cytotoxicity is beneficial in the appropriate situation, for example, in the elimination of infectious micro-organisms. However, it is not beneficial when targets are cells such as those entering the body in blood transfusions or tissue transplants. On occasion, Type II hypersensitivity reactions can occur as side-effects of treatment with certain drugs. Drugs such as penicillin, cephalosporin, quinidine, or methyldopa can be adsorbed on to surface proteins of red blood cells and platelets. In particular individuals, these drug–protein complexes can induce the generation of antibodies (sensitization phase), which can then bind to the adsorbed drug. This can lead to elimination of the cells that have adsorbed the drug by complement-mediated lysis or by phagocytosis by splenic macrophages, resulting in drug-induced haemolytic anaemia or thrombocytopaenia. The pathologies of certain autoantibody-mediated autoimmune diseases, e.g. Goodpasture's syndrome, are caused by mechanisms that are analogous to those involved in Type II hypersensitivity reactions (see *Section 10.8*).

Certain antibodies bind to cell surface receptors and, instead of targeting the cell for destruction, either block the ligand binding site of the receptor or mimic the action of the natural ligand and stimulate the receptor. Examples of such diseases are the autoimmune disorders myasthenia gravis and Graves' disease (see *Section 10.8*). Some immunologists term these disorders Type V hypersensitivity responses, or stimulatory hypersensitivity responses, to distinguish them from cytotoxic Type II hypersensitivity reactions.

Rhesus incompatibility

A model of Type II hypersensitivity is provided by the phenomenon of Rhesus incompatibility. This reaction once caused considerable morbidity and mortality in newborn babies. Present day screening for this incompatibility is simple and routine and precautionary immunotherapy measures (see *Section 14.4*) are highly effective.

Rhesus incompatibility occurs when a woman who is negative for the Rhesus D antigen (RhD⁻) becomes pregnant with the child of a Rhesus D positive (RhD⁺) father. The RhD antigen is expressed on erythrocytes and is inherited as a dominant gene, and so offspring of a RhD⁺ father will, themselves, often carry the D antigen. A RhD⁻ woman's first pregnancy with a Rh⁺ baby should proceed normally and it is not until birth that some of the baby's RBCs will enter the maternal circulation. The mother is stimulated to mount an acquired immune response to the baby's RBC RhD antigen, leading to the synthesis of anti-RhD antibodies. During any subsequent pregnancy with an RhD⁺ child, some of the maternal IgG anti-RhD antibodies will cross the placenta to the developing fetus. A Type II hypersensitivity response then occurs which destroys the baby's erythrocytes (see *Figure 9.5*). This condition is known as erythroblastosis fetalis, or haemolytic disease of the newborn (HDN). The affected baby may be stillborn, or if it is a live birth, immediate blood transfusion is the only effective treatment.

In order to avoid this situation, pregnant women are screened for their blood type, including Rhesus status. At the time of delivery, RhD⁻ women are given an injection of pre-formed anti-RhD antibody (e.g. RhoGAM®). This will target the baby's RhD⁺ RBCs for elimination or complement-mediated destruction when they enter the maternal circulation, before the mother's immune system can generate an antibody response against the RhD⁺ cells. Anti-RhD therapy must be repeated each time an affected mother gives birth. The passively administered antibodies pose no threat to the fetus during a subsequent pregnancy, as the amount given is small enough to ensure that the antibodies are rapidly eliminated from the circulation.

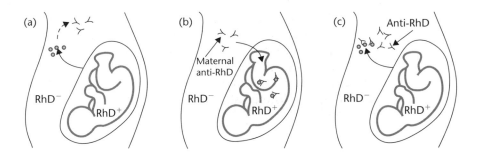

Figure 9.5
When a woman who is negative for the Rhesus D antigen (RhD⁻) becomes pregnant with the child of a RhD⁺ father, the child also may be RhD⁺. (a) At birth, exposure of the maternal immune system to the child's RhD⁺ red blood cells results in the generation of maternal antibodies against RhD. (b) If the mother subsequently bears another RhD⁺ child, the IgG anti-RhD will cross the placenta and target the fetal red blood cells for destruction. (c) Sensitization of the maternal immune system against RhD can be prevented by injecting the RhD⁻ mother with anti-RhD immediately post-partum.

Transfusion and transplant-associated reactions

A transfusion of blood, which is incompatible with the recipient's blood group, as defined by the ABO system (see *Section 11.4*), is destroyed by pre-existing antibodies in a Type II hypersensitivity response: this is known as hyperacute rejection and usually occurs within 24 hours of transplantation. In the case of a whole blood transfusion, an antibody response may also be generated against MHC class I or II antigens on the surfaces of leukocytes. In the case of chronic rejection of incompatible tissue transplants, which can occur months to years post-transplant, antibodies may be directed against MHC class I antigens on tissue cells and MHC class I and class II antigens on any leukocytes that may be included in the transplanted tissue. These cells are also attacked in a Type II hypersensitivity response.

Diagnosis and treatment

As indicated above, HDN is readily avoided by screening the patients in advance for their Rhesus D status. Transfusion and transplant-associated reactions can be minimized by blood or tissue typing (see *Section 11.3*). In autoimmune diseases that proceed via a Type II mechanism, laboratory tests together with clinical evaluation may be required to confirm the diagnosis. Patient serum may be tested by ELISA (see *Section 13.9*) or immunostaining (see *Section 13.8*) for the presence of antibodies against specific antigens. For example, Goodpasture's syndrome (see *Section 10.8*) is characterized by an autoantibody that binds to the glomerular basement membrane and this can be demonstrated using patient serum to stain sections of unaffected kidney tissue.

   For serious Type II reactions, such as drug-induced haemolytic anaemia, systemic administration of immunosuppressive corticosteroids, e.g. prednisolone, may be required together with cessation of drug treatment. In the most severe cases, transfusion to replace the erythrocytes, and possibly plasmapheresis to remove the pathological immunoglobulins from the circulation, may be required.

9.9   TYPE III HYPERSENSITIVITY

This class of hypersensitivity is frequently referred to as immune complex disease. It also involves antibodies, predominantly IgG and IgM and the sensitization phase of the Type III response involves the production of antibodies against particular soluble antigens. The antibodies involved in Type III responses usually bind to their specific antigens with low affinity. Consequently, the antibody–antigen complexes (immune complexes) formed tend to be small and, therefore, are not efficiently eliminated by phagocytes in the spleen and liver. The small immune complexes persist in the circulation and are ultimately deposited at susceptible sites in the body, including the renal glomeruli, choroid plexus, the skin, lungs, heart, small blood vessels and joints. Factors predisposing to immune complex deposition include high haemodynamic pressure (e.g. in glomeruli, capillary beds, choroid plexus), turbulence (e.g. at arteriolar junctions or bends in blood vessels) and tissue expression of Fc or complement receptors that can bind to the immune complex. Deposition of immune complexes in tissues is also promoted by the increase in vascular permeability triggered by complement activation *in situ*. Complement activation also leads to recruitment and activation of phagocytic cells. Binding of immune complexes to Fc receptors, in particular to the FcγRIII receptor, in tissues can trigger the release of inflammatory mediators that will enhance the inflammatory response (see *Figure 9.6*).

An early example of Type III hypersensitivity was observed with passive immunization for diphtheria when patients were given doses of preformed horse antisera against diphtheria toxin. When injected, the horse antibodies neutralized the diphtheria toxin; however, they themselves were foreign to the affected patients. The patients' immune systems generated antibody responses against the horse antibodies, which bound with low affinity to the horse antibodies, forming small immune complexes which were subsequently deposited systemically in susceptible sites. The deposited complexes attracted phagocytes, which attempted to phagocytose the tissue cells that had been 'opsonized'. Failing to complete phagocytosis, these cells released lysosomal enzymes and reactive oxygen species directly on to the tissue (see *Figure 9.6*). Thus many tissues sustained damage and their function was impaired. This condition is known as serum sickness and is characterized by fever, joint pain, lymphadenopathy and urticaria. Passive immunization

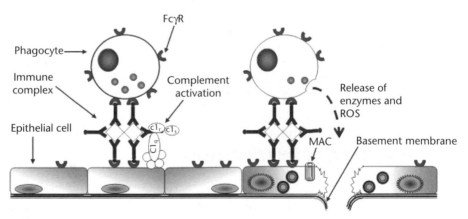

Figure 9.6
In Type III hypersensitivity, immune complexes deposit in susceptible sites (e.g. glomeruli, skin, joints). These complexes activate complement via the classical pathway and, therefore, attract phagocytes. The phagocytes attempt, but fail, to engulf the complexes deposited in the tissues ('frustrated phagocytosis'). Consequently, the lysosomal enzymes and reactive oxygen species (ROS) that are usually confined within the phagocytes are released on to tissues, causing damage. This is a major mechanism of joint damage in the autoimmune disease rheumatoid arthritis (see *Section 10.7*).

is now employed only in a very limited range of situations, e.g. where the patient is pregnant or immunosuppressed and cannot withstand exposure to an active immunogen and great care is taken to avoid the induction of serum sickness.

The conditions that predispose to Type III hypersensitivity are those where low affinity antibody is produced in low amounts over a period of time. Antigens which satisfy these criteria include some environmental antigens to which people may be exposed constantly over prolonged periods, e.g. in occupational environments. One of these is the thermophilic actinomycetes mould found in hay, which induces the condition known as farmer's lung or hypersensitivity pneumonitis. A second stimulus of low affinity antibody production is thought to be self antigen, leading to autoantibody-mediated autoimmune diseases. In cases where antibodies are generated against self antigens, the antigens cannot be eliminated so immune complex production does not stop. The ensuing chronic inflammation is characteristic of immune complex-mediated autoimmune diseases such as rheumatoid arthritis (see *Section 10.7*).

Because complement is important in uptake of immune complexes by phagocytes, individuals with specific complement deficiencies (see *Section 12.3*) are predisposed to development of Type III hypersensitivity diseases. In addition, immune complex disease is frequently seen in cases of persistent or chronic infection, e.g. leprosy and malaria. In these instances the rate of formation of immune complexes exceeds the rate at which they can be removed by the spleen and liver. The complexes therefore persist, ultimately depositing in susceptible sites leading to the inflammatory sequelae described above.

Diagnosis and treatment

Many cases of Type III hypersensitivity are benign and self-limiting following elimination of the antigen (e.g. serum sickness). In more serious cases laboratory tests may be required, together with clinical evaluation, to confirm the diagnosis. One such test is the measurement of serum levels of circulating immune complexes. In this test, immune complexes present in a serum sample are selectively precipitated by the addition of low concentrations of polyethylene glycol (PEG). The concentration of PEG used is selected so that only immune complexes are precipitated while uncomplexed immunoglobulins are not. The PEG-precipitated material is then tested for the presence of immunoglobulins by ELISA. To confirm a diagnosis of immune complex disease it may also be necessary to biopsy the affected tissue. The biopsy then is examined for the presence of immune complex deposition by immunostaining.

Different treatment regimens may be used depending on the severity of the reaction. In mild cases NSAIDs such as aspirin or antihistamines can be used to counteract the inflammatory response. Systemic administration of immunosuppressive corticosteroids may be required in more serious cases. In the most severe cases plasmapheresis may be considered. Successful resolution of pathogen-associated Type III responses may require treatment of the underlying infectious disease.

9.10   TYPE IV HYPERSENSITIVITY

Unlike the other types of hypersensitivity reactions, Type IV hypersensitivity does not involve antibody. Its defining characteristic is that it can be transferred between histocompatible individuals by transfer of T cells. Thus T cells are the central regulatory component. This type of response is also called delayed-type hypersensitivity (DTH) because the reaction takes 48–72 hours to develop. With Type IV responses the T cell is known as T_{DTH} (T cell of delayed-type hypersensitivity). The clinical features of this type of response will depend on the nature of the sensitizing antigen and the route of exposure. Variants of Type IV hypersensitivity reactions include contact hypersensitivity, tuberculin-type hypersensitivity and granulomatous hypersensitivity.

As in antibody-mediated hypersensitivities, prior exposure to antigen (sensitization) is required for development of a Type IV hypersensitivity response. The classical view of sensitization for this response is that DCs take up the antigen at the site of exposure and carry it to lymphoid tissue where they induce the differentiation and proliferation of antigen-specific Th1 cells. Following re-exposure to the antigen (the activation phase), the Th1 cells migrate to the site of exposure. Th1 cell-derived cytokines recruit macrophages to the site and the IFN-γ produced by the T cells activates the macrophages to release inflammatory mediators. This classical view of the generation of a Type IV hypersensitivity response has been challenged with the discovery of the pro-inflammatory Th17 subset (see *Section 6.5*). Studies in murine DTH models have revealed that Th17 cells are required for development of a Type IV hypersensitivity response. *In vivo*, the majority of IL-17-producing cells at inflammatory sites produce IFN-γ, in addition to IL-17, so these cells would also be capable of recruiting and activating macrophages during a DTH response (see *Figure 9.7*).

Most of the effector functions in a Type IV hypersensitivity response are mediated by activated macrophages. In the case of a Type IV response induced by a micro-organism, the macrophages ingest the organism. The macrophages are then activated by T cell-derived IFN-γ and attempt to destroy the ingested organism using lysosomal enzymes and reactive oxygen species.

Contact hypersensitivity

The characteristic feature of this response is the induction of localized eczema following contact with an antigen. The most common antigens to provoke contact hypersensitivity are nickel, chromate, rubber products and chemicals contained in poison ivy. These substances are all small molecules, termed haptens, that can penetrate the epidermis of intact skin and become

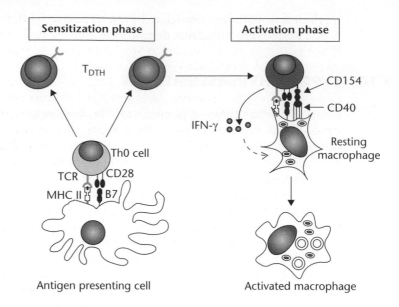

Figure 9.7
During the sensitization phase of a type IV hypersensitivity response, antigen presenting cells carry antigen from tissues to lymph nodes and present the antigen to T cells causing them to differentiate into T_{DTH} cells (Th1 or Th17 cells). Following re-exposure to antigen, during the activation phase of the response, the T_{DTH} cells activate macrophages, largely via the production of IFN-γ.

conjugated to normal body proteins. This conjugation has the effect of making the haptens more antigenic, because several haptens can bind to a single protein, thus increasing both the dose and the size of the antigen. The protein–hapten complex is taken up by epidermal Langerhans cells and presented to T cells, resulting in the generation of T_{DTH}. On subsequent contact with the allergen these T cells will migrate to the site of exposure and will be stimulated to mount a more rapid secondary response. An inflammatory response then ensues; however, the principal leukocyte type infiltrating the skin is not the neutrophil but mononuclear leukocytes. Keratinocytes also participate in this response by secreting cytokines including TNF-α and IL-1. They may also be involved in down-regulating the inflammatory response via the production of the immunosuppressive cytokines IL-10 and TGF-β.

Tuberculin reaction

This type of hypersensitivity is the basis of the widely used tuberculin skin test (TST), also called the Mantoux TST. This test involves the inoculation of an individual with a purified lipoprotein derived from *Mycobacterium tuberculosis,* called purified protein derivative (PPD), and it is the standard method for detecting infection by *M. tuberculosis*, the causative agent of tuberculosis (TB). The reaction is measured as millimetres of induration (hard swelling) of the skin after 48–72 hours. The basis of the tuberculin response is the reactivation of antigen-specific T_{DTH} cells within the dermal layer of the skin. Cytokines produced by these cells act on local vascular endothelial cells to promote the infiltration of leukocytes into the skin. By about 4 hours after exposure, the predominant infiltrating cells are neutrophils. By about 12 hours the predominant infiltrating cell types are T cells and monocytes, and their number reaches a peak at about 48 hours. By this time the infiltrate also involves the epidermis. The characteristic indurations are a result of the combination of a large number of cells with oedema. The signs of the reaction normally last for between 5 and 7 days, after which they resolve. This is in contrast to the situation where, if there is a constant source of antigen as a result of infection, the reaction progresses to become a granulomatous lesion.

Since TST is the only way to determine asymptomatic infection by *M. tuberculosis*, the false-negative rate cannot be calculated. A negative TST does not rule out TB in a child. Approximately 10% of otherwise normal children with culture-proven TB do not react to PPD initially. Most of these children have reactive skin tests during treatment, which suggests that TB contributes to the immunosuppression that prevented the skin reaction. The incidence of false-negative TST is higher in individuals who are tested soon after becoming infected with *M. tuberculosis* or who have debilitating or immunosuppressive illnesses.

The development of DTH responses to PPD can take up to 3 months, therefore a clinician cannot know immediately if a child has been exposed to *M. tuberculosis*. Unfortunately, in children under 5 years of age, severe TB, especially meningeal and disseminated disease, can occur in less than 3 months, before the TST becomes reactive. False-positive reactions to TST are often attributed to asymptomatic infection with environmental non-tubercular mycobacteria. Vaccination with *M. bovis* can cause transient reactivity in a subsequent TST, but the association is weak. Bacillus Calmette-Guerin (BCG) is the vaccine for TB that is still administered to children in many Western countries. Up to 90% of children who receive BCG as infants have a non-reactive TST at 5 years of age. Among older children or adolescents who receive BCG, most develop a reactive skin test initially; however, by 10 to 15 years post-vaccination, 80–90% have lost tuberculin reactivity. Many recipients of BCG have a reactive TST because they are infected with tuberculosis and are at risk of developing the disease, especially if they have had recent contact with an infectious TB patient. In general, TST reaction should be interpreted in the same manner for people who have received BCG and for unvaccinated people.

Granulomatous reaction

This type of DTH has the most severe consequences for the individual because of the presence of often extensive tissue damage. There are two types of granuloma: immune and foreign body granuloma. An immune granuloma usually results from the persistence within macrophages of micro-organisms or antigenic material which are resistant to macrophage-mediated destruction. A foreign body granuloma results from the persistence of other particles that are unable to be eliminated, e.g. silica. Immune granulomata consist of epithelioid cells and macrophages surrounded by lymphocytes. In contrast, lymphocytes are absent from foreign body granulomata.

The sensitization phase of a DTH response against *M. tuberculosis* leading to the development of an immune granuloma is thought to proceed as described above. During the activation phase of the response, the mycobacteria-specific CD4$^+$ T cells migrate to the site of the infection (usually the lungs), and release IFN-γ to activate the mycobacteria-infected macrophages at the site to destroy the intracellular bacteria. However, *M. tuberculosis* has evolved mechanisms that allow it to survive inside host macrophages. It blocks the fusion of mycobacteria-containing phagosomes with lysosomes and also prevents acidification of the phagosomes. Mycobacteria-infected macrophages are also less responsive to stimulation by IFN-γ. These evasion strategies allow *M. tuberculosis* to persist inside macrophages. The persistence of the mycobacteria leads to the accumulation and chronic stimulation of T cells at the infected site during the activation phase of the response. This in turn causes the differentiation of macrophages into epithelioid cells. Some of the macrophages also fuse to form multi-nucleated giant cells. The activated macrophages secrete cytokines that attract fibroblasts to the site. Fibroblast adhesion and proliferation are also promoted, e.g. by fibroblast

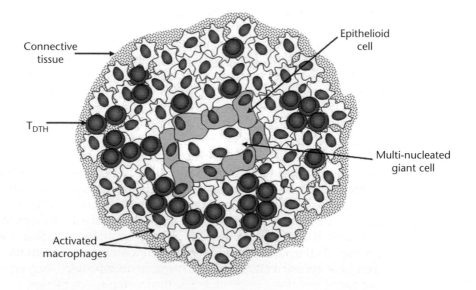

Figure 9.8
An immune granuloma is an impenetrable aggregation of cells, consisting largely of T cells and activated macrophages. Some of the macrophages fuse to become multi-nucleated giant cells while others differentiate into epithelioid cells. The mature granuloma is surrounded by a network of connective tissue.

growth factor (FGF). The final stage in granuloma formation is the production of collagen by the fibroblasts, which forms a mesh of strong connective tissue around the granuloma (see *Figure 9.8*). Once complete, the granuloma is impenetrable to other cells or molecules so the immune response is unable to clear it. Eventually the cells in the central area of the granuloma become necrotic. Despite this, viable organisms may remain and it is their reactivation, causing rupture of the granuloma, and spread to other tissues that can be devastating for the patient. The impairment of tissue function is caused by the presence of many tough granulomata which occupy the space of normal tissue and inhibit its function.

The development of a pro-inflammatory T_{DTH} response leading to the formation of granulomata is necessary for control of this infection. Studies in animal models have demonstrated that a Th2 response is unable to control mycobacterial infection but instead leads to the fatal disseminated form of the disease.

Over the past two decades, the incidence of TB in both developed and developing countries has increased dramatically. One of the major reasons for the rise in incidence of TB is the increase in the number of people with compromised immune systems due to HIV infections. For individuals with normal immune systems who are tuberculin positive, the risk of developing TB sometime during their lives is 10%. For people who are HIV positive, that risk is 50%. For over 40 years the standard drug for treating TB has been isoniazid. Studies have shown that it is 60–90% effective in preventing TB when it is taken over 6–12 months. However, isoniazid has significant drawbacks. It must be taken for a substantial length of time and, unfortunately, some strains of *M. tuberculosis* have become resistant to isoniazid and other first-line anti-TB drugs. This increased prevalence of multi-drug-resistant TB (MDR-TB) is of particular concern. Of the nine million new cases of TB reported every year, approximately 5% are MDR-TB cases. Recent reports from the World Health Organization have charted the emergence of extensively drug-resistant strains of *M. tuberculosis*, which cause a virtually untreatable form of TB.

Although cases among children represent a small percentage of all TB cases, infected children are a reservoir from which many adult cases will arise. TB diagnosis in children usually follows discovery of a case in an adult, and relies on tuberculin skin testing, chest radiograph, and clinical signs and symptoms. However, clinical symptoms are nonspecific, skin testing and chest radiographs can be difficult to interpret, and routine laboratory tests are not helpful. Although quicker and more sensitive laboratory testing, which takes into account recent advances in biomedical science, is being developed, the results have been disappointing. Better techniques would especially benefit children and infants in whom early diagnosis is imperative for preventing progressive TB. In developing countries, the risk for TB infection and disease is relatively uniform in the population. In industrialized countries, risk is more uneven and depends on the individual's past or present activities and their exposure to people at high risk for the disease.

The natural history of TB in children follows a continuum; however, it is useful to consider three basic stages: exposure, infection and disease. If a child is infected, it is usually because he/she was in close contact with an infected person. In adults, the distinction between TB infection and disease is usually clear because most disease is caused by reactivation of dormant organisms.

9.11 HYPERSENSITIVITY AND AUTOIMMUNE DISEASE

The prevalence of hypersensitivity reactions and associated disease has increased considerably in recent decades and, with the currently limited treatment regimens available, prevention appears to be the most logical approach. In some instances, however, this is not possible because the antigen that stimulates the hypersensitivity reaction is a self antigen. In these cases the hypersensitivity reaction gives rise to autoimmune disease. Both Type I and Type II hypersensitivity responses against proteins in the skin are thought to contribute to the development of lesions in the autoimmune skin disease bullous pemphigoid and Type II hypersensitivity responses also cause autoimmune thyroiditis, anaemia and nephritis. Type III reactions are important in the immunopathogenesis of rheumatoid arthritis, and a variety of chronic autoimmune diseases, including sarcoidosis and Crohn's disease, are caused by granulomatous Type IV reactions. The mechanisms responsible for the development of autoimmunity and autoimmune diseases will be discussed in the next chapter.

SUGGESTED FURTHER READING

Abler, G. and Kamradt, T. (2007) Regulation of protective and pathogenic Th17 responses. *Curr. Immunol. Rev.* **3**: 3–16.

Bischoff, S.C. (2008) Role of mast cells in allergic and non-allergic immune responses: comparison of human and murine data. *Nature Rev. Immunol.* **7**: 93–104.

Gould, H.J. and Sutton, B.J. (2008) IgE in allergy and asthma today. *Nature Rev. Immunol.* **8**: 205–217.

Holgate, S. and Polosa, R. (2008) Treatment strategies for allergy and asthma. *Nature Rev. Immunol.* **8**: 218–230.

Jancar, S. and Sánchez Crespo, M. (2005) Immune complex-mediated tissue injury: a multistep paradigm. *Trends Immunol.* **26**: 48–55.

Larché, M. (2007) Regulatory T cells in allergy and asthma. *Chest,* **132**: 1007–1014.

Saxon, A. and Diaz-Sanchez, D. (2005) Air pollution and allergy: you are what you breathe. Nature Immunol. **6**: 223–226.

Sokol, C.L., Barton, G.M., Farr, A.G. and Medzhitov, R. (2008) A mechanism for the initiation of allergen-induced T helper type 2 responses. *Nature Immunol.* **9**: 310–318.

Veldhoen, M., Hirota, K., Westendorf, A.M., *et al.* (2008) The aryl hydrocarbon receptor links TH17-cell-mediated autoimmunity to environmental toxins. *Nature,* **453**: 106–110.

Vercelli, D. (2008) Discovering susceptibility genes for allergy and asthma. *Nature Rev. Immunol.* **8**: 169–182.

SELF-ASSESSMENT QUESTIONS

1. Explain why FcεRI receptors can be specific for IgE.
2. What is an alternative name for Type I hypersensitivity and why is it appropriate?
3. What roles do histamine, prostaglandins, leukotrienes and proteases play in Type I hypersensitivity?
4. Why is adrenaline an effective treatment for anaphylactic shock?
5. Why is a Rh⁻ woman given small doses of anti-D antibody when she is known to be carrying a Rh⁺ baby?
6. When does hyperacute rejection occur?
7. List three conditions that may predispose to development of Type III hypersensitivity.
8. Which class of hypersensitivity is frequently referred to as immune complex disease and why?
9. Describe the two types of granuloma.
10. How does Benadryl® help ease the symptoms in Type I hypersensitivity responses?

Tolerance and autoimmune disease

Learning objectives
After studying this chapter you should confidently be able to:

■ **Discuss how immunological tolerance is maintained**
Immunological tolerance is maintained through the processes of central tolerance and peripheral tolerance. Central tolerance occurs during lymphocyte development in the primary lymphoid tissues. During central tolerance, autoreactive thymocytes are deleted. Autoreactive immature B cells may be deleted, rendered non-responsive, or may alter their antigen receptor so that it is no longer self-reactive. During peripheral tolerance, self-reactive T cells and B cells may be deleted or may be rendered non-responsive to antigen, either via anergy or via active suppression.

■ **Outline current concepts of the aetiologies of autoimmune diseases**
Most autoimmune diseases are polygenic diseases that require contributions from multiple genes to confer disease susceptibility. Not all individuals with a susceptible genetic make-up will develop autoimmune disease. Progression from susceptibility to overt autoimmune disease requires an environmental trigger. Likely environmental factors that may trigger autoimmune disease include infectious agents and environmental pollutants.

■ **Discuss the mechanisms responsible for tissue damage in autoimmune disease**
Tissue damage in autoimmune diseases is either predominantly cell-mediated or predominantly antibody-mediated, although in some diseases, especially later in disease, both of these mechanisms can be demonstrated. Cell-mediated damage is thought to be dependent on Th17 cells and there is evidence that these cells are involved in the pathogenesis of rheumatoid arthritis, multiple sclerosis and type I diabetes. Antibody-mediated damage normally proceeds via a Type II hypersensitivity mechanism, following binding of autoantibody to a tissue, or via a Type III hypersensitivity mechanism, following deposition of autoantibody–self antigen complexes in tissues.

■ **Describe current and potential therapies for autoimmune diseases**
Many of the current therapies for autoimmune diseases are palliative or anti-inflammatory. Biological drugs have now been developed that specifically target pro-inflammatory cytokines or cells that are important in the pathogenesis of particular autoimmune diseases. Several of these have already been used to effect in the treatment of rheumatoid arthritis, systemic lupus erythematosus and multiple sclerosis.

10.1 INTRODUCTION TO TOLERANCE AND AUTOIMMUNE DISEASE

A defining characteristic of adaptive immunity is its ability to discriminate between self and non-self antigens. This is all the more remarkable when one considers that the mechanisms used to generate the antigen-specific receptors of T cells and B cells are largely random. The processes of immunoglobulin and TCR gene rearrangement are not biased towards generating receptors that will preferentially react against non-self antigens. Therefore the immune system must ensure that any self-reactive lymphocytes that arise during lymphocyte development are either killed off or are rendered non-responsive to antigenic stimulation. As a consequence, B cells and T cells of most individuals do not react strongly against self antigens. This phenomenon is called immunological self-tolerance.

Immunological tolerance against self antigens is usually efficiently maintained throughout life. In some instances, however, this protective mechanism breaks down and the body's immune system launches an attack on self tissues causing immunopathology. This is the basis of the group of disorders that are collectively termed autoimmune diseases. Any tissue in the body can be the target of an autoimmune attack and in some autoimmune diseases multiple tissues are affected. Unlike foreign antigen, self antigens cannot be eliminated and so autoimmune reactions can develop into chronic inflammatory responses. In this chapter the mechanisms whereby immunological tolerance is maintained will be introduced first and then the characteristics of some of these autoimmune diseases will be discussed.

10.2 MECHANISMS OF TOLERANCE INDUCTION

Immunological tolerance is due to the lack of response of lymphocytes when exposed to specific antigens. This lack of response may result from any of three mechanisms (see *Table 10.1*). First, following exposure to antigen the lymphocytes may receive a signal to die. This mechanism of tolerance is termed deletion. Secondly, exposure to the antigen may render the lympho-

Table 10.1 Mechanisms of tolerance induction

Mechanism	Examples
Deletion	Deletion of autoreactive lymphocytes during development Peripheral deletion of autoreactive lymphocytes
Non-responsiveness to antigenic stimulation	Anergy Suppression by T_{REG} cells
Ignorance	Non-immunogenic antigen Low zone tolerance

cyte non-responsive. Thirdly, the antigen may not be immunogenic, or may not be accessible to the immune system, and therefore would not stimulate a lymphocyte response. In this case the lymphocytes are said to ignore the antigen and this mechanism of tolerance induction is termed immunological ignorance.

Immunological tolerance may be induced during lymphocyte development in primary lymphoid organs, a process called central tolerance. Alternatively, tolerance may be induced after the lymphocytes have left the primary lymphoid organs via a process termed peripheral tolerance.

Central tolerance

Central tolerance refers to the process whereby B and T cells are rendered non-responsive to self antigens during development in the bone marrow (see *Section 3.3*) and thymus (see *Section 3.6*), respectively. Immature B cells which express BCRs that bind strongly to membrane-associated antigens of bone marrow cells, must modify their autoreactive BCR by receptor editing or they receive a signal to die. In contrast, immature B cells with a BCR that binds strongly to soluble antigens are rendered anergic. Similarly, thymocytes which express TCRs that bind strongly to self antigen + MHC are deleted during negative selection. Expression of the *Aire* gene product in thymic medullary epithelial cells (MECs) is crucial for central T cell tolerance. Aire is a transcriptional activator that permits promiscuous gene expression in MECs, enabling the negative selection of thymocytes that are reactive against non-thymic antigens.

Central tolerance is the major mechanism whereby autoreactive lymphocytes are removed or silenced so that they cannot attack self tissues. However, some lymphocytes escape central tolerance. These cells must be tolerized in the periphery.

Peripheral tolerance

Autoreactive lymphocytes which escape central tolerance are usually rendered non-responsive in the periphery by a process known as peripheral tolerance. Both T cells and B cells may be tolerized in the periphery; however, as most immune responses require CD4$^+$ T cell help, inactivation or deletion of autoreactive CD4$^+$ T cells may be sufficient to prevent autoimmune reactions. In contrast, a failure in CD4$^+$ T cell tolerance may lead to cell-mediated and antibody-mediated autoimmune responses. There are several mechanisms whereby peripheral tolerance can be induced.

Immunological ignorance

Not all antigens are immunogenic (see *Section 2.7*). This may be because of the form of the antigen or because the antigen is not present in sufficient concentration to stimulate lymphocytes. In such cases the lymphocyte 'ignores' the antigen and does not respond. Alternatively, the antigen may be immunogenic but may be sequestered at a site that is not readily accessible to the immune system due to anatomical barriers and lack of lymphatic drainage. These so-called immune-privileged sites include the brain, the anterior chamber of the eye, and the testes. It has become clear in recent years, however, that active suppressor mechanisms are crucial for preventing immune reactions at these sites.

Clonal anergy

Naïve T cells require two signals in order to become activated:

■ signal 1 transmitted via the TCR/CD3 complex after recognition of antigen
■ signal 2 delivered via CD28 after it binds to B7 on professional APCs

If a naïve T cell receives signal 1 in the absence of signal 2 then that T cell is rendered non-responsive, or anergic. This mechanism of peripheral tolerance induction is called clonal anergy. This ensures that T cells can only become activated by appropriately stimulated professional APCs, because these are the only cells that, under normal circumstances, express B7. Immature DCs that have not been exposed to inflammatory signals have low expression of B7 and are unable to provide signal 2 to naïve T cells. If a T cell recognizes an antigen presented by an immature DC then that T cell is rendered anergic. This means that the T cell does not respond to stimulation with this antigen even if the same antigen is subsequently presented to the T cell in the presence of co-stimulation. This is appropriate because immature DCs present self or harmless antigens. Only if the DC encounters a harmful antigen will it be stimulated via TLRs or pro-inflammatory cytokines to differentiate into a mature DC and to express high levels of B7 molecules on its surface.

The two-signal requirement for T cell activation also means that if a T cell specific for a pancreas-specific antigen, for example, escapes deletion in the thymus, this T cell could not become activated by a pancreatic cell expressing that antigen in the periphery. Again, this is because the pancreatic cell will not be able to deliver signal 2 to the T cell. Consequently, the T cell is rendered anergic. If, however, the pancreatic cell were induced to express B7 molecules, it would then be able to activate the autoreactive T cell, leading to immunopathology.

An alternative mechanism of clonal anergy involves the negative regulator of T cell activation CTLA-4. CTLA-4 (CD178) binds to B7 molecules with higher affinity than does CD28. Unlike CD28, however, binding of CTLA-4 to B7 sends a negative signal into the T cell, rendering it hyporesponsive to antigenic stimulation. Other receptors that play a role in induction of anergy are PD-1 (CD279) and BTLA (CD272) (see *Section 7.4*).

Like T cells, B cells also require two signals for activation. For responses against T-dependent antigens, signal 1 is transmitted via the BCR complex following binding of antigen, and signal 2 is transmitted via CD40 after binding to CD154 on the T cell (see *Section 6.8*). For T-independent antigens, signal 2 is usually transmitted through TLRs on the B cell after they bind to their cognate molecular pattern on the antigen. If a B cell receives signal 1 in the absence of signal 2 it is rendered anergic. For T-dependent responses, this means that efficient induction of CD4$^+$ T cell tolerance is usually sufficient to prevent expansion of autoantibody-producing B cells.

Peripheral deletion

Recent research has implicated a role for Aire in peripheral deletion of autoreactive T cells that have escaped central tolerance. Aire is not only expressed in MECs in the thymus, but is also expressed in lymph node stromal cells. This allows promiscuous expression of ectopic genes in these cells. As a result of this, stromal cells in lymph nodes are thought to be able to delete self-reactive T cells in a manner analogous to negative selection in the thymus.

Studies using Fas-deficient mice have demonstrated that Fas-mediated apoptosis is crucial for removing autoreactive B and T cells by a process called activation-induced cell death (AICD; see *Section 7.5*). Fas (CD95) is a member of the TNF family and is expressed on the surfaces of activated B and T cells. The ligand for Fas, FasL (CD178) is expressed on activated T cells and certain epithelial cells. When FasL binds to Fas, a signal is transmitted through Fas that induces the apoptotic death of the Fas-expressing cell. Mice that are deficient in either Fas or FasL are deficient in this form of AICD and accumulate large numbers of autoreactive lymphocytes in their spleens and lymph nodes.

Suppression

It is now evident that a major mechanism responsible for maintenance of self-tolerance in the periphery is active T cell-mediated immunosuppression. Several subsets of suppressor or regulatory T cells have been described (see *Section 7.6*) and their roles and mechanisms of action are presently areas of intense research. Data from studies on murine models of autoimmune diseases suggest that different regulatory T cell subsets may guard against autoimmune responses directed against different tissues. In addition to their role in preventing autoreactive immune responses, CD4$^+$CD25$^+$Foxp3$^+$ regulatory T cells are thought to be crucial for maintaining immunological tolerance to food antigens. It has also become apparent that the immune privilege of sites such as the testes and at the materno–foetal interface is also dependent on the suppressive activities of regulatory T cells.

10.3   BREAKDOWN OF TOLERANCE AND AUTOIMMUNITY

In the majority of individuals, the normal mechanisms responsible for induction and maintenance of immunological tolerance are sufficient to prevent self-directed immune responses. In some cases, however, immunological tolerance breaks down. Breakdown of tolerance is a prerequisite for the development of autoimmune diseases. In most cases, the mechanisms responsible for the breakdown in immunological tolerance are unclear; however, the elucidation of the molecular bases of three monogenic autoimmune syndromes (see *Box 10.1*) has highlighted the importance of specific mechanisms of tolerance induction in protection against autoimmune disease.

Box 10.1 Genetics of autoimmune diseases

Monogenic autoimmune diseases are diseases that are caused by mutation or deletion of a single gene. Susceptibility to most autoimmune diseases involves contributions from many genes, i.e. they are polygenic disorders.

Autoimmune polyendocrinopathy-candidiasis-ectodermal dystrophy (APECED) is an autoimmune disease that results from mutation of the *Aire* gene. As a result, individuals with APECED are compromised in their ability to negatively select self-reactive thymocytes during T cell development. The *Aire* gene is also important for the selection of natural T_{REG} cells (see *Section 3.6*), and therefore it is likely that development of these suppressor cells is compromised in APECED patients. The clinical phenotype of APECED and the age of individuals when they develop symptoms vary widely, reflecting the diversity of *Aire* mutations associated with the disease. Individuals with severely disrupted Aire function develop systemic autoimmune disease and frequently present with type I diabetes, adrenal hypoplasia and hypoparathyroidism. The breakdown in T cell tolerance allows the development of self-reactive antibody responses and APECED patients have high levels of multiple autoantibodies in their serum.

Mutation of the gene encoding the Foxp3 transcription factor results in the multi-system autoimmune disease called immune dysregulation, polyendocrinopathy, enteropathy X-linked syndrome (IPEX). Since Foxp3 is required for the generation of natural and inducible T_{REG} cells (see *Section 7.6*), Foxp3 mutations impact the development of both of these major subsets of suppressor T cells. Mutations that seriously compromise Foxp3 function result in severe disease that usually causes early death. The disease is characterized by autoimmune attack on multiple endocrine organs, allergic inflammation, haemolytic anaemia and thrombocytopaenia. The spectrum of autoimmune reactions in IPEX clearly illustrates the importance of T_{REG} cells in maintaining immunological tolerance to multiple self antigens. This is also evidenced by the multi-organ autoimmune disease associated with deficiency of CD25, a molecule that is essential for the development and function of CD4$^+$CD25$^+$ T_{REG} cells.

The failure to remove autoreactive lymphocytes via AICD leads to the development of autoimmune lymphoproliferative syndromes (ALPS) which are characterized by splenomegaly and lymphadenopathy, due to the accumulation of large numbers of CD4$^-$CD8$^-$ T cells, and also by autoimmune diseases such as autoimmune haemolytic anaemia, autoimmune thrombocytopaenic purpura and autoimmune neutropaenia. The major forms of ALPS are caused by mutations in the genes that encode Fas (ALPS1a), FasL (ALPS1b) or caspase 10, a molecule that is involved in the Fas-mediated apoptotic pathway (see *Section 7.5*).

Apart from the rare monogenic autoimmune diseases described above, the mechanisms responsible for the breakdown of immunological tolerance in most autoimmune diseases are poorly understood. Targets of autoantibodies and of autoreactive T cells that are associated with specific autoimmune diseases have been defined, but the events that precipitate development of these autoimmune diseases are unknown. It is believed that most autoimmune diseases result from the interaction between specific genetic and environmental factors.

10.4 GENETIC SUSCEPTIBILITY TO AUTOIMMUNE DISEASES

Genetic analyses of large numbers of affected individuals suggest that most autoimmune diseases are polygenic diseases, i.e. their development is linked to multiple genes. It is believed that susceptibility to a specific autoimmune disease requires the expression of several of these genetic risk factors. Apart from the genes that are mutated in rare monogenic autoimmune syndromes (see *Section 10.3*), the strongest genetic risk factors for development of autoimmune diseases are HLA alleles. Because HLA molecules present antigens to T cells, the association between HLA alleles and autoimmune diseases is not surprising. To put it simply, T cells will be unable to react against a self antigen if that self antigen cannot be presented by a HLA molecule. For any given disease and its associated HLA molecule, a relative risk (RR) may be calculated:

$$\text{RR} = \frac{\text{Risk of person with a particular MHC allele developing the disease}}{\text{Risk of person without that allele developing the disease}}$$

The RR is a measure of the increased risk of an individual with a particular HLA allele developing the disease compared with individuals who do not have that HLA allele (see *Table 10.2*). For most diseases the RR is modest, reinforcing the notion that these are polygenic diseases.

Induction of self tolerance in the thymus requires that self antigen is visible there to developing T cells. If a self antigen is expressed at low levels in the thymus it may not be available in sufficient quantity to induce tolerance. The *IDDM2* susceptibility locus for type I diabetes encodes the insulin A chain. This *IDDM2* allele of insulin is expressed at approximately fourfold lower levels in the thymus compared with alleles of insulin that are not associated with type I diabetes. Similarly, an allele of the acetylcholine receptor α (AChRα) chain that is poorly expressed in the thymus is associated with early onset myasthenia gravis. It has been hypothesized that the poor expression of these proteins in the thymus is insufficient for negative selection of thymocytes that are reactive against insulin or AChRα, autoantigens that are associated with the development of type 1 diabetes and myasthenia

Table 10.2 Association of HLA alleles with susceptibility to autoimmune diseases

Disease	Associated HLA allele(s)	Relative risk
Ankylosing spondylitis	B27	87.4
Goodpasture's syndrome	DR2	15.9
Graves' disease	DR3	3.7
Hashimoto's thyroiditis	DR5	3.2
Myasthenia gravis	DR3	2.5
Rheumatoid arthritis	DR4	4.2
Type 1 diabetes	DQw8	5.6
	DR3	3.3
Systemic lupus erythematosus	DR3	5.8

gravis, respectively. Alternatively, the poor thymic expression of these proteins may preclude the development of protective T_{REG} cells.

Genetic studies have identified a variety of other genes that are associated with susceptibility to autoimmune disease. The gene that encodes the MHC class II transactivator CIITA is associated with type 1 diabetes, rheumatoid arthritis and systemic lupus erythematosus (SLE). Since CIITA controls expression of MHC class II molecules, it has been proposed that disease-associated *CTIIA* alleles might cause dysregulated MHC class II expression and, consequently, dysregulated activation of CD4$^+$ T cells. The gene encoding CTLA-4 has been linked with several autoimmune diseases, but in particular with SLE, leading to the suggestion that aberrant T cell peripheral tolerance may contribute to the pathogenesis of this disease. Development of Crohn's disease is associated with mutations in the gene encoding the NOD2 pattern recognition receptor, suggesting that a dysregulated response against intestinal bacteria might give rise to this form of inflammatory bowel disease.

Current theories of the pathogenesis of autoimmune diseases propose that genetic risk factors, such as those outlined above, cooperate to confer disease susceptibility, but that progression to overt autoimmune disease requires an environmental factor.

10.5 ENVIRONMENTAL TRIGGERS OF AUTOIMMUNE DISEASE

Despite their appreciable genetic associations, for most polygenic autoimmune diseases there is substantial discordance in the incidence of disease between identical twins. This observation led to the suggestion that there must be environmental stimuli that cause susceptible individuals to develop autoimmune disease. The most commonly proposed environmental triggers of autoimmune disease are infections and environmental pollutants or toxins.

Infectious triggers of autoimmune disease

Microbial infections have long been proposed as stimuli for the development of autoimmune disease in susceptible individuals. A number of infectious agents have been suspected of causing multiple sclerosis (e.g. measles virus), but compelling evidence for this is lacking. One hypothesis, called molecular mimicry, proposes that an immune response generated against a pathogen may result in the expansion of lymphocytes that cross-react with a self antigen. Following elimination of the pathogen, the immune response targets the cross-reactive self antigen. A well-known example of a human disease often associated with a cross-reactive immune response is rheumatic fever. This disease begins with an infection, usually a throat infection, with a group A β-haemolytic streptococcus. After some time, generally several years, cardiac inflammation develops. T cells isolated from cardiac valvular tissue of patients react against streptococcal M protein as well as against human myosin and vimentin. Antibodies against streptococcal antigens that cross-react with myocardial cells have also been described in this disease. In addition, the link between *Chlamydia* infections and heart disease may be due to antibody cross-reactivity between a *Chlamydia* protein and cardiac myosin. In most cases, however, the evidence for a specific infectious trigger for autoimmune diseases is weak. This may be due to the difficulty in determining the initiating autoantigen because once the disease has begun, the associated tissue damage may reveal antigens that were previously sequestered from the immune system. In this way the immune response might spread from a response directed against the initiating antigen to a response directed against cryptic antigens that have been revealed as a result of the inflammatory process. This phenomenon is referred to as epitope spreading and it has been documented in several murine models of human autoimmune diseases.

Environmental pollutants and autoimmune disease

The increasing incidence of autoimmune disease in industrialized nations suggests that environmental pollutants may play a role in disease development. The recent discovery of the involvement of the aryl hydrocarbon receptor (AHR) in development of Th17 cells has suggested a possible mechanism whereby environmental toxins might promote autoimmune disease. The AHR is a ligand-dependent transcription factor that promotes the development of pro-inflammatory Th17 cells, the subset of T cells that is now believed to be critical for cell-mediated autoimmune diseases. In an animal model of multiple sclerosis, AHR-stimulation accelerated the onset of the disease and led to more severe symptoms. The AHR binds to a wide variety of ligands, including hormones, eicosanoids and UV light-induced conversion products of tryptophan. Given the wide range of ligands that it can bind, AHR-dependent expansion of Th17 cells might explain previous observations of the effects of gender, diet and exposure to sunlight on susceptibility to, or relapses of, autoimmune disease.

10.6 THE SPECTRUM OF AUTOIMMUNE DISEASES

Autoimmune diseases affect approximately 5–7% of adults in Europe and North America. In general, autoimmune diseases occur more commonly in females than in males. Diagnosis is usually based on evaluation of clinical symptoms together with specific laboratory tests. A diagnosis of auto-immune disease based on clinical and laboratory findings is strengthened by any of the following criteria:

■ other autoimmune diseases have been diagnosed in the same individual or the same family
■ the patient expresses an MHC haplotype for which there is a statistical association with an autoimmune disease
■ there is a favourable response to treatment by immunosuppression

Autoimmune diseases are frequently broadly divided into two classes (see *Table 10.3*). The first class constitutes the organ-specific autoimmune diseases where the disease is limited to a specific tissue. An example of this class is Hashimoto's thyroiditis in which the thyroid is solely affected. The second class of autoimmune diseases comprises the systemic (or non-organ-specific) autoimmune diseases in which the autoimmune attack is not confined to one tissue. An example of this class is SLE where the disease frequently affects the kidneys, skin and small blood vessels.

In reality, most autoimmune diseases fall between these two extremes. A more useful classification is based on whether the tissue damage associated with the disease is predominantly caused by the cell-mediated arm of the immune response or by antibody-dependent mechanisms. However, this is not always clear as many autoimmune diseases have evidence of cell-mediated and antibody-mediated pathology.

10.7 PREDOMINANTLY CELL-MEDIATED AUTOIMMUNE DISEASES

The discovery of Th17 cells has forced researchers to re-examine the mechanisms responsible for cell-mediated autoimmune diseases. Recent research

Table 10.3 Systemic and predominantly organ-specific autoimmune diseases

Systemic	Organ-specific
Scleroderma	Graves' disease
Sjögren's syndrome	Hashimoto's thyroiditis
Systemic lupus erythematosus	Myasthenia gravis
Rheumatoid arthritis	Multiple sclerosis
	Pernicious anaemia
	Type 1 diabetes

suggests that dysregulated Th17 activity or a deficiency in T_{REG} function is responsible for the chronic inflammation associated with these disorders.

The characteristic cytokines produced by Th17 cells are IL-17 and TNF-α. Important functions of IL-17 include the induction of granulopoiesis, and the activation and attraction of neutrophils to sites of inflammation. IL-17 itself is not a neutrophil chemoattractant, but it induces the expression of IL-8 by tissue cells. IL-17 also induces the production of GM-CSF and G-CSF by bone marrow stromal cells, which leads to an increase in neutrophil production. The actions of IL-17 and TNF-α contribute substantially to the pro-inflammatory properties of Th17 cells.

Research using animal models of human autoimmune diseases has provided compelling evidence that Th17 cells are the critical T cell subset involved in cell-mediated autoimmune responses. Mice deficient in IL-17 or IL-23, a cytokine that promotes the expansion of Th17 cells, are less susceptible to development of mouse models of multiple sclerosis, rheumatoid arthritis and inflammatory bowel disease than control mice. In addition, IL-17 and IL-23 are increased in synovial fluid of rheumatoid arthritis patients and in cerebrospinal fluid of multiple sclerosis patients, as well as in lesional plaques of individuals with psoriasis vulgaris. These data suggest that Th17 cells may be key players in the development of cell-mediated autoimmune diseases.

Rheumatoid arthritis

Rheumatoid arthritis is predominantly a disease of the small arthrodial joints and is characterized by immune-mediated inflammation of the synovium. It is often referred to as an inflammatory type arthritis. Although rheumatoid arthritis primarily affects the joints, susceptible individuals can also develop vasculitis or pericarditis, so rheumatoid arthritis is considered a systemic autoimmune disease. The predominant symptoms of rheumatoid arthritis are associated with the joints of the hands and feet, although other joints may also become involved. The joints tend to be involved in a symmetrical pattern, so if knuckles on the right hand are inflamed, those on the left hand will be inflamed as well. Patients may have symptoms such as morning stiffness or stiffness following periods of inactivity, fatigue and weight loss. Rheumatoid arthritis is a chronic inflammatory disease. Spontaneous remission rarely occurs and the disease normally leads to progressive immune-mediated destruction of joint tissue. In advanced cases this can result in joint deformity and severe disability.

The incidence of rheumatoid arthritis is approximately 3 cases per 10 000 population per annum. The disease shows a distinct gender bias with women affected about five times as often as men. It is four to five times more common in smokers than in non-smokers. Rheumatoid arthritis is strongly associated with HLA-DR4 (specifically DR0401 and 0404). The median age at onset of the disease is between 40 and 50 years. The incidence of rheumatoid arthritis increases with age such that it affects some 25% of patients over the age of seventy. The prevalence of rheumatoid arthritis

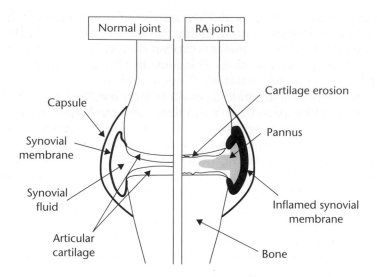

Figure 10.1

Comparison of normal and rheumatoid arthritis (RA) joints. Note the extensive synovial inflammation, pannus formation and erosion of articular cartilage in the rheumatoid arthritis joint.

among first degree relatives is 2–3% and disease genetic concordance in identical twins is approximately 15–20%.

The most common association with the onset of rheumatoid arthritis is the presence of IgM antibodies directed against antigenic determinants on the Fc portion of IgG. This autoantibody is known as rheumatoid factor and it is present in approximately 80% of patients with rheumatoid arthritis. The dilemma is that rheumatoid factor is not present in all rheumatoid arthritis patients and its level in the serum does not always correlate with disease severity. A finding of rheumatoid factor alone is not diagnostic because rheumatoid factor is frequently detected in other chronic inflammatory conditions, including chronic liver disease, sarcoidosis and chronic pulmonary disease. In addition, rheumatoid factor is detectable in sera of approximately 10% of the healthy population.

Histologically, there is a dense T cell-rich lymphocytic infiltrate into the synovium of the affected joints (see *Figure 10.1*). The synovial membrane thickens as its cells proliferate abnormally and enlarge in response to stimulation by inflammatory cytokines. Fibrin is deposited in the synovial fluid and also on the synovial membrane where it develops into granulation tissue called a pannus, which greatly reduces joint mobility.

Analysis of affected joints shows that large amounts of immune complexes are present in the joint fluid. These complexes may include both rheumatoid factor–IgG and collagen–anti-collagen; although a variety of other autoantigens have been identified in rheumatoid arthritis. The initiating factor leading to the production of autoantibodies in rheumatoid arthritis is unknown; however, high levels of BAFF and APRIL are detectable in synovial fluid of rheumatoid arthritis patients. BAFF and APRIL promote B cell survival (see *Section 3.3*) and might allow autoreactive B cells to escape deletion or anergy.

It is thought that the inflammatory response, leading to joint destruction, is initiated by immune complex deposition in the joints. As such, the initiation of rheumatoid arthritis proceeds via a mechanism similar to that described for Type III hypersensitivity (see *Section 9.9*). Some patients may show a systemic vasculitis (inflammation of blood vessel walls), with IgM, IgG and complement in vessel walls. Usually there are high levels of circulating immune complexes and apparent complement deficiency due to its constant activation and consumption. Analysis of blood from a patient with rheumatoid arthritis would often reveal lowered levels of complement proteins and such levels can often dictate treatment regimens.

The synovium of a rheumatoid arthritis joint contains large numbers of neutrophils, normally absent from joints. Detection of IL-17 and IL-23 in synovial fluid suggests the involvement of Th17 cells. IL-17 produced by these cells can stimulate IL-8 production by synovial fibroblasts, leading to further neutrophil accumulation. The neutrophils release degradative enzymes including elastase, cathepsins (which break down proteoglycan), glycosidases, and collagenases, leading to tissue damage. IL-17 will also promote degradation of extracellular matrix by stimulating the production of matrix metalloproteinases. In addition, IL-17 produced by Th17 cells induces the expression of receptor activator of nuclear factor (NF)-κB ligand (RANKL) on mesenchymal cells such as osteoblasts or synovial fibroblasts (see *Figure 10.2*). RANKL binds to its counter-receptor RANK on

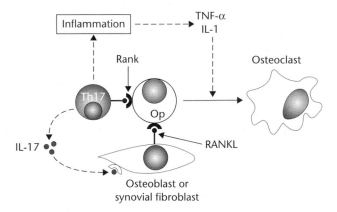

Figure 10.2

Th17 cells can promote the production of osteoclasts by secreting the cytokine IL-17 which induces the expression of RANKL on osteoblasts and synovial fibroblasts. RANKL binds to RANK on osteoclast precursor (Op) cells and stimulates them to differentiate into osteoclasts which digest bone. Th17 cells also express RANKL and so may directly stimulate Op cells to differentiate into osteoclasts. Osteoclast differentiation is promoted by pro-inflammatory cytokines such as TNF-α and IL-1.

the surface of osteoclast precursor cells and causes them to differentiate into osteoclasts. Th17 cells also express RANKL and can directly stimulate osteoclast production. Osteoclasts digest bone and are responsible for bone erosion associated with advanced rheumatoid arthritis.

Diagnosis of rheumatoid arthritis

A definitive diagnosis of rheumatoid arthritis often represents quite a difficult decision for any rheumatologist. Diagnosis of rheumatoid arthritis requires at least four of the following criteria to be met.

- Morning stiffness lasting for more than 1 hour most mornings for 6 weeks or more.
- Arthritis of more than three joints, present for 6 weeks or more.
- Arthritis of hand joints, present for 6 weeks or more.
- Symmetrical arthritis, present for 6 weeks or more.
- Subcutaneous rheumatoid nodules.
- Serum level of rheumatoid factor above the 95th percentile.
- Radiological changes consistent with joint erosion.

Treatment of rheumatoid arthritis

Currently there is no cure for rheumatoid arthritis but treatment in the past decade has certainly revolutionized the quality of life of sufferers. There are three main classes of drugs that may be used to alleviate the symptoms of the disease: non-steroidal anti-inflammatory drugs (NSAIDs); corticosteroids; and disease-modifying anti-rheumatic drugs (DMARDs). The three major goals in the treatment of rheumatoid arthritis are:

- reduction of inflammation and pain
- maintenance of joint function
- prevention of future joint destruction and deformity

NSAIDs can help reduce inflammation and pain. Treatment with DMARDs is designed to maintain joint function and prevent future deformity. DMARDs can take weeks or months to demonstrate a clinical response. DMARDs include antimalarials, gold salts, D-penicillamine and cyclosporine. New generation DMARDs include antibodies to block TNF-α (infliximab; Remicade®) and to deplete B cells (rituximab; Rituxan®) (see *Sections 10.9* and *14.4*) as well as recombinant proteins to neutralize IL-1 (anakinra; Kineret®). Often combinations of drugs are required to alleviate the disease process. For people with severely damaged hips or knees due to the disease process, total joint replacement can allow them to lead an independent life.

Multiple sclerosis

Multiple sclerosis is a chronic disease of the central nervous system (CNS) and one of the most common causes of chronic neurological disability in young adults. Clinically, multiple sclerosis is classified as either primary progressive or relapsing-remitting. The latter form of the disease can evolve into chronic progressive multiple sclerosis. The chronic-progressive form of the disease often leads to a complete loss of the ability to walk within 2 years of onset and total disability after 8–10 years. Symptoms of the disease include:

- weakness or paralysis in the limbs
- vertigo and incontinence
- muscle wasting
- progressive visual failure
- epilepsy and aphasia

In the population at large, the chance of developing multiple sclerosis is less than 0.1%. However, if one person in a family has the disease, that person's first-degree relatives have a 1–3% chance of also getting it. For identical twins, the likelihood that the second twin may develop multiple sclerosis if the first twin does is approximately 30%; for fraternal twins, the likelihood is similar to that for non-twin siblings, at about 4%. The fact that the incidence of identical twins both developing multiple sclerosis is significantly less than 100% indicates that the disease is not entirely genetically controlled and suggests that exposure to an environmental factor is necessary for disease development.

The underlying pathological basis of multiple sclerosis is thought to be the attack by autoreactive T cells and macrophages, or microglial cells, on Schwann cells in the white matter of the brain, leading to the destruction of the fatty myelin sheath that surrounds axons (see *Figure 10.3*). The demyelinated neurons can no longer effectively conduct nerve impulses. The areas of demyelination, also called plaques, are visible histologically and are

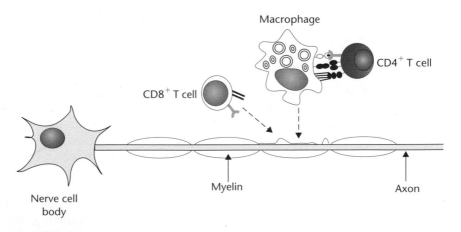

Figure 10.3

T cells may promote demyelination in multiple sclerosis either directly, via CD8$^+$ T cell-mediated destruction of myelin-producing cells, or indirectly, via CD4$^+$ T cell-dependent activation of macrophages and microglial cells.

characterized by infiltrates of CD4$^+$ and CD8$^+$ T cells. Deposition of IgG and complement can be detected in some lesions, suggesting that antibodies may contribute to tissue damage. A role for antibody in the pathogenesis of multiple sclerosis is supported by the common finding of increased intrathecally synthesized IgG in the cerebrospinal fluid (CSF) of multiple sclerosis patients. Symptoms of multiple sclerosis result from the cumulative effect of plaques in the brain and spinal cord.

Components of myelin such as myelin basic protein have been the focus of much research into candidate autoantigens in multiple sclerosis. When injected into laboratory animals myelin basic protein can induce experimental allergic encephalomyelitis (EAE), a chronic relapsing brain and spinal cord disease that resembles multiple sclerosis. The injected myelin may well stimulate the immune system to produce myelin-specific T cells that attack the animal's own myelin. The existence of autoreactive T cells or autoantibodies to myelin is not sufficient for multiple sclerosis to occur, as both may be detected in healthy individuals. It has been proposed that a critical event in the development of multiple sclerosis is breakdown of the blood–brain barrier, possibly as the result of an infection, allowing inflammatory cells to enter the CNS.

The initiating event in multiple sclerosis is unknown. Studies on EAE suggest that Th17 cells are involved in disease pathogenesis and this theory is strengthened by the detection of elevated levels of IL-17 and IL-23 in CSF of multiple sclerosis patients.

Treatment of multiple sclerosis

There is as yet no cure for multiple sclerosis. Many patients do well with no therapy at all and naturally occurring or spontaneous remissions make it difficult to determine therapeutic effects of experimental treatments. However, the use of medical resonance imaging (MRI) has allowed clinicians to chart the development of lesions. Treatment strategies aim to:

■ inhibit the disease process
■ promote remyelination
■ restore physical and neurological function

Until recently, the principal treatment for multiple sclerosis was NSAIDs; however, there is no strong evidence to support the use of these drugs to treat progressive forms of multiple sclerosis. Also, there is some indication that steroids may be more appropriate for people with movement, rather than sensory, symptoms. While steroids do not affect the course of multiple sclerosis over time, they can reduce the duration and severity of relapses in some patients.

Disease-modifying drugs may slow disease progression and help to reduce the frequency or severity of attacks. Disease-modifying drugs currently in use include IFN-β1a (Avonex® or Rebif®), IFN-β1b (Betaferon®) and glatiramer acetate (Copaxone®) injections. Glatiramer acetate is a myelin basic protein mimetic that can reduce the relapse rate of relapsing-remitting multiple sclerosis by almost one-third. Natalizumab (Tysabri®) is a monoclonal antibody against α4-integrin that has been shown to be effective in treatment of active relapsing-remitting multiple sclerosis and rapidly evolving severe relapsing-remitting multiple sclerosis.

Type 1 diabetes

Type 1 diabetes is also called insulin-dependent diabetes mellitus or early onset diabetes, as it usually occurs in children and in adults who are under 40 years of age. It is a chronic condition in which the pancreas makes little or no insulin because the β cells in the pancreatic islets of Langerhans have been destroyed by an autoimmune response. The inflammatory infiltrate is composed of both CD4$^+$ T cells and CD8$^+$ T cells. As with most autoimmune diseases, the initiating event that triggers the autoimmune attack in type 1 diabetes is unknown. Infections, especially with Coxsackie B virus, have been suggested to be triggering events but the evidence is inconclusive. Although the precise mechanisms responsible for β cell destruction are poorly understood, a variety of pro-inflammatory cytokines, such as TNF-α, and chemokines, such as CCL2, have been implicated in this process. Destruction of islet β cells in type 1 diabetes is promoted by Th17 cells. A range of autoantigens have been described in type 1 diabetes including glutamic acid decarboxylase 65, insulin and islet protein tyrosine phosphatase IA-2.

Type 1 diabetes symptoms often seem to appear abruptly, although damage to the β cells begins much earlier. The most common signs of type 1 diabetes include: continual thirst, hunger, frequent micturation (polyuria), and loss of weight. If untreated, type 1 diabetes can cause diabetic ketoacidosis, which can be fatal. To successfully control the disease, type I diabetics must inject insulin, follow a diet plan, exercise daily, and test blood glucose several times a day. Islet cell transplantation is now commonly used to treat type 1 diabetes. It is important to note that type 1 diabetes patients who receive islet cell transplants can destroy the transplanted β cells by the same process that initiated the diabetes.

10.8 PREDOMINANTLY ANTIBODY-MEDIATED AUTOIMMUNE DISEASES

Autoimmune diseases in which tissue damage is primarily antibody-mediated, frequently proceed via an immune complex-dependent Type III hypersensitivity mechanism (see *Section 9.9*), where complexes of antibody and self antigen are deposited in tissues. Alternatively these diseases may be initiated by antibody binding directly to the self antigen via a mechanism similar to a Type II hypersensitivity response (see *Section 9.8*). In most cases, however, production of high-affinity, class-switched antibody requires T cell help. Therefore, just as autoantibodies are a feature of many cell-mediated autoimmune diseases, autoreactive T cells are frequently found in patients with autoantibody-mediated autoimmune diseases.

Systemic lupus erythematosus

Systemic lupus erythematosus (SLE) is a chronic systemic autoimmune disease with many manifestations, and which can affect any of the body's organ systems. It derives its name 'lupus' (red wolf) from the characteristic red malar or papillonaceous (butterfly-shaped) facial rash that is an early symptom of the disease. Sun exposure may accentuate the malar rash as well as other symptoms of SLE. SLE can be distinguished from discoid lupus erythematosus (DLE) which affects sun-exposed regions of the skin and in severe cases causes a scarring rash in these sites. Only 1–5% of DLE patients develop SLE.

SLE is characterized by autoantibodies directed against a variety of nuclear antigens. Predominant autoantibodies are directed against double stranded (ds) DNA, DNA–chromatin complexes, RNA, and ribonucleo-proteins such as Sm/RNP. One model that has been proposed to explain the generation of autoantibodies in SLE suggests a delay in clearance of apoptotic cells from germinal centres by tingible body macrophages (see *Section 6.9*). The self nucleic acid–protein complexes released from these cells might then sequentially engage the BCR, in addition to TLR-7 or TLR-9 molecules on autoreactive B cells, leading to autoantibody production. Proliferation of these autoreactive B cells may be driven by BAFF, which is frequently elevated in SLE patients.

Accumulating evidence suggests an important role for type I IFN in development of SLE. Patients with SLE have elevated serum levels of type I IFN which, together with IL-6, stimulates plasma cell development, leading to high level antibody secretion. The main source of type I interferon is the plasmacytoid DC. Nucleoprotein complexes can bind to TLR-7 or TLR-9 on plasmacytoid DCs and stimulate the production of type I IFN. Type I IFN will trigger plasmacytoid DC maturation, allowing autoantigen-bearing DCs to activate naïve autoreactive T cells to provide help for autoreactive B cell responses. Recent studies using a murine model of SLE suggest that Th17 cells may promote development of autoreactive B cells, thus there may be a crucial cell-mediated component to this autoantibody-mediated auto-immune disease.

The production of autoantibodies leads to immune complex formation, i.e. a Type III hypersensitivity reaction (see *Section 9.9*). Immune complex deposition in many tissues leads to the manifestations of the disease. Many SLE patients develop renal complications because the immune complexes are often deposited in the renal glomeruli. A renal biopsy may be performed to determine the degree of involvement and determine therapy. Despite therapy, progression to chronic renal failure is common.

Synovial immune complexes can lead to joint pain, known as arthralgias. In fact, symmetrical arthritis and arthralgias are common features leading to SLE being confused with rheumatoid arthritis early in its course. Rheumatoid arthritis is therefore often referred to as an inflammatory-type arthritis, while arthralgias refers to joint pain with no associated inflammation. The presence of autoantibodies can usually be determined by antinuclear antibody (ANA) test performed using patient serum (see *Section 13.8*). The titre of the ANA gives a rough indication of the severity of the disease. Not all positive ANA tests indicate autoimmune disease, particularly when the titre is low, so after a positive screening ANA test, more specific tests for SLE are used, including detection of autoantibodies to dsDNA.

SLE can occur at all ages but a younger onset is associated with a more severe course and a higher incidence of immune complex-mediated nephritis and pericarditis. Females are more than nine times more likely to develop SLE than are males, with the disease presenting most often in young women.

Treatment of SLE

As SLE is exacerbated by exposure to sunlight, SLE patients are advised to use an effective sunblock as well as creams to treat the malar rash. NSAIDs are frequently used to treat the systemic symptoms of SLE, often in combination. The dose of drugs used must be carefully regulated, especially in patients who already have lupus nephritis. For people who fail conventional therapy, immunosuppressive drugs, such as cyclosporine, may be used. However, careful monitoring of renal function is critical with these agents as they can exhibit considerable nephrotoxicity. See the Case study in *Box 10.2*.

Box 10.2 Case study

Mary, a 28-year-old woman developed a red, symmetrical rash on her face and nose after an afternoon sunbathing on the beach. The rash persisted and was still apparent when she attended her physician 2 weeks later complaining of tiredness, swollen wrists and joint pain. Laboratory tests revealed that she had high levels of anti-nuclear antibodies in her serum. She was also severely deficient in serum albumin and had low serum levels of C3. Urinalysis showed 2 mg of protein ml^{-1} (normal range: 0–0.1 mg ml^{-1}).

1. What disorder is Mary likely to be suffering from?
2. Why does she have swollen, painful joints?
3. What is the significance of the decreased level of serum albumin?
4. Why are her serum levels of C3 depressed?

Answers are given alongside the answers to the self-assessment questions for *Chapter 10* at the back of the book.

Myasthenia gravis

Myasthenia gravis is a chronic neuromuscular disease characterized by abnormal weakness of voluntary muscles. The disease usually affects the extrinsic ocular muscles initially. In about 10% of patients the disease does not spread beyond these muscles. This form of the disease is called ocular myasthenia gravis. In most myasthenia gravis patients the disease spreads to involve other muscles. This form of the disease is called generalized myasthenia gravis. The disease may affect an individual of any race or age including newborn children; however, the disease is seen more frequently in young adult females and older males.

The symptoms of myasthenia gravis are caused by a reduced number of acetylcholine receptors (AChRs) on post-synaptic membranes at neuro-muscular junctions. These receptors are the normal binding-site of the neurotransmitter acetylcholine. The duration of the stimulus is limited by the enzyme acetylcholine esterase, which degrades the acetylcholine. In 80–90% of individuals with myasthenia gravis, autoantibodies are directed against the α chain of AChRs thereby making them unavailable to bind acetylcholine (see *Figure 10.4*). The autoimmune response may also cause other damage to the post-synaptic membrane. Approximately 10% of myasthenia gravis patients have autoantibodies directed against a muscle-specific tyrosine kinase (MuSK) that is associated with the AChR. In both cases, the outcome is that the nervous signal cannot pass to the muscle so motor function is impaired. The mechanisms responsible for autoantibody production in myasthenia gravis are unknown; however, studies have shown that there are reduced numbers of T_{REG} cells in myasthenia gravis patients.

Unlike disorders such as multiple sclerosis, myasthenia gravis usually causes no progressive damage to either the nervous system or to muscles.

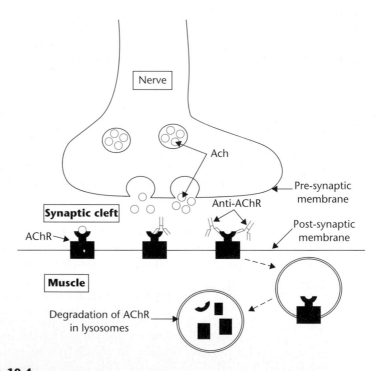

Figure 10.4
In myasthenia gravis, binding of antibodies to the acetycholine receptor (AChR) can inhibit binding of acetylcholine (Ach) to the receptor, thus inhibiting transmission of the nerve impulse. Antibody binding to the AChR can also lead to endocytosis and lysosomal degradation of the receptor, thus reducing the number of receptors available to bind to acetylcholine at the neuromuscular junction.

When the disease is treated and symptoms are in remission, the myasthenia gravis patient can expect normal muscle function.

Treatment of myasthenia gravis

The main treatment for myasthenia gravis is the use of acetylcholine esterase inhibitors. These prevent the degradation of unbound acetylcholine at the neuromuscular junction and so prolong the signal.

Goodpasture's syndrome

Goodpasture's syndrome (see *Box 10.3*) is a rare autoimmune disorder characterized by inflammation of the glomeruli of the kidneys (glomerulonephritis) and pulmonary haemorrhage. Symptoms of this disease include recurrent episodes of coughing up blood (haemoptysis), difficulty in breathing (dyspnoea), fatigue, chest pain and/or anaemia. In many cases, Goodpasture's syndrome may result in acute renal failure.

Box 10.3 Goodpasture's syndrome

Ernest Goodpasture is best known for his study of viruses. The method he developed for cultivating viruses made possible the production of vaccines against smallpox, chicken pox, and other viruses. In 1919 he first described the autoimmune kidney and lung disease that now bears his name.

The disorder is caused by an autoantibody directed against type IV collagen found in basement membranes. Although type IV collagen-containing basement membranes are found throughout the body, only the glomerular and alveolar basement membranes are affected in Goodpasture's syndrome. Pulmonary symptoms are not always exhibited because, in the absence of lung injury or inflammation, the alveolar endothelial cells usually prevent access of the autoantibodies to the alveolar basement membrane. In contrast, the glomerular endothelium is fenestrated, allowing ready access of autoantibodies to the underlying glomerular basement membrane (GBM). Goodpasture's syndrome is sometimes referred to as anti-GBM disease. The mechanism responsible for development of Goodpasture's syndrome is similar to a Type II hypersensitivity response. Binding of the autoantibody to the GBM results in complement activation, activation of Fc receptor-bearing cells and recruitment of neutrophils. This leads to severe tissue injury and, ultimately, loss of glomerular function. Most patients with this disorder progress to end-stage renal failure.

Graves' disease

Graves' disease, or Graves' hyperthyroidism, is caused by a generalized overactivity of the thyroid gland. It is also called diffuse toxic goitre; diffuse because the entire thyroid gland is involved in the disease process, toxic because the patient appears feverish as if due to an infection, and goitre because the thyroid gland enlarges in this condition. The incidence of Graves' disease increases steadily throughout the first decade of life and peaks during adolescence. Girls are affected 3–6 times more often than boys. Family histories are frequently positive for goitres, Graves' disease, or thyroiditis.

In Graves' disease, autoantibodies are produced against thyroid stimulating hormone (TSH) receptors on the surface of thyroid cells, stimulating those cells to overproduce thyroid hormones, mainly T3 and T4 (see *Figure 10.5*). Normally, thyroid hormone production is down-regulated by a feedback loop from the circulating levels of T3 and T4, which shuts down production of TSH by the pituitary gland. The anti-TSH receptor antibody produced in Graves' disease patients acts as a receptor agonist and stimulates production of thyroid hormones. Its action is unaffected by the T3/T4-dependent negative feedback and continues to stimulate the thyroid, even

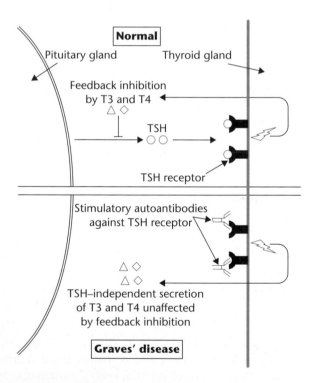

Figure 10.5
Graves' disease is caused by stimulatory autoantibodies directed against the thyroid stimulating hormone (TSH) receptor. These autoantibodies mimic the action of TSH and cause the thyroid to produce the thyroid hormones T3 and T4. Normally the production of T3 and T4 is suppressed by feedback inhibition which controls the production of TSH by the pituitary gland. Since the autoantibody-induced secretion of T3 and T4 is independent of TSH it is not susceptible to this feedback inhibition.

though TSH is absent. The main symptoms of Grave's disease are weight loss, trembling, muscle weakness of the upper arms and thighs, and insomnia.

Treatment of Graves' disease

Graves' disease may be treated using drugs such as methimazole (Tapazole®) that block the release of thyroid hormones. In more severe cases, radio-labelled iodine may be administered. Radio-labelled iodine is taken up by the thyroid and destroys thyroid cells. Thyroidectomy is the preferred treatment for patients with a large goitre or who are refractive to drug treatment.

Autoimmune thrombocytopaenic purpura

Thrombocytopaenic purpura is a condition characterized by low platelet count (thrombocytopaenia). Although most cases are asymptomatic, in instances where the platelet count is very low the affected individual is susceptible to bleeding (haemorrhage), frequently from the gums, nose and gastrointestinal tract. Patients frequently have a rash of small purplish spots on their skin (purpura) as a result of haemorrhage of small blood vessels in the skin. For many years the cause of the disease was unknown and the condition still is commonly called idiopathic thrombocytopaenic purpura (ITP). However, we now know that at least 65% of ITP patients have antibodies against surface antigens of platelets. These antibodies are usually of the IgG isotype and are most often directed against the platelet membrane glycoproteins (GP) IIb–IIIa or GPIb–IX. The autoantibodies bind to the platelets and target them for elimination by splenic macrophages. This disease, therefore, proceeds via a mechanism analogous to a Type II hypersensitivity reaction.

Treatment of autoimmune ITP

Treatment is necessary if the platelet count falls below 20 000 platelets ml^{-1} or if there is recurrent haemorrhaging. Patients with platelet counts below 10 000 platelets ml^{-1} risk fatal cerebral haemorrhage. Corticosteroid treatment is effective in most cases; however, in instances where the disease is refractory to steroid treatment, surgical removal of the spleen (splenectomy) is usually performed. Splenectomized individuals are susceptible to sepsis following infection with encapsulated bacteria such as *Haemophilus influenzae* and *Streptococcus pneumoniae* and should receive prophylactic antibiotics for life.

10.9 FUTURE THERAPIES FOR AUTOIMMUNE DISEASE

The incidence of autoimmune diseases is increasing in industrialized nations where they are now the third major cause of morbidity and mortality. Conventional therapies for these diseases consist largely of anti-inflammatory drugs and immunosuppressants. Recent years have seen the

Table 10.4 Selected biological drugs of potential use in therapy of autoimmune disease

Drug name	Formulation[a]	Disease
Anakinra®	IL-1RA	Rheumatoid arthritis Systemic lupus erythematosus
Etanercept®	Soluble TNF p75 receptor	Psoriasis Psoriatic arthritis Rheumatoid arthritis
Infliximab®	Anti-TNF-α	Crohn's disease Psoriasis Rheumatoid arthritis
Natalizumab®	Anti-α4-integrin	Crohn's disease Multiple sclerosis
Rituximab®	Anti-CD20	Rheumatoid arthritis Systemic lupus erythematosus Systemic vasculitis

[a] **Abbreviations**: IL-1RA, interleukin-1 receptor antagonist; TNF, tumour necrosis factor.

development of a variety of biological drugs that target key molecules or cells involved in the pathogenesis and progression of specific autoimmune diseases (see *Table 10.4*). Many of these biological drugs are designed to block the activities of pro-inflammatory cytokines and consist of:

■   soluble forms of receptors for those cytokines, e.g. etanercept, a soluble TNF-α receptor
■   antibodies directed against the cytokines, e.g. infliximab, a humanized anti-TNF-α antibody
■   recombinant cytokine receptor antagonists, e.g. anakinra, an IL-1 receptor antagonist

In addition, biologicals against cell surface molecules designed to alter cell function or to delete specific cell populations have also been developed. One of these, TGN1412, an antibody against CD28, showed the potential to induce T_{REG} function in studies in mice. Unfortunately, the phase I clinical trial of this drug in human volunteers had disastrous consequences. All six volunteers required hospitalization, with at least four of them developing systemic organ dysfunction, apparently due to overwhelming cytokine production by T cells.

Many other new generation biological drugs are undergoing clinical trials, but several have already made the transition to the clinic. Anti-TNF-α therapy has been shown to be effective in treatment of rheumatoid arthritis and its use has been extended to the treatment of other chronic inflammatory diseases; rituximab, a B cell-specific antibody that leads to B cell depletion *in vivo*, has been shown to be of benefit in treatment of SLE; and natalizumab, an anti-α4-integrin-specific antibody designed to inhibit leukocyte migration, is effective in treatment of multiple sclerosis. It is likely that these biological drugs will be of benefit in other autoimmune diseases.

SUGGESTED FURTHER READING

Afzali, B., Lombardi, G., Lechler, R.I. and Lord, G.M. (2007) The role of T helper 17 (Th17) and regulatory T cells (Treg) in human organ transplantation and autoimmune disease. *Clin. Exp. Immunol.* **148**: 32–46.

Atassi, Z. and Casali, P. (2008) Molecular mechanisms of autoimmunity. *Autoimmunity,* **41**: 123–132.

Chatenoud, L. (2006) Immune therapies of autoimmune diseases: are we approaching a real cure? *Curr. Opin. Immunol.* **18**: 710–717.

Christen, U. and von Herrath, M.G. (2004) Initiation of autoimmunity. *Curr. Opin. Immunol.* **16**: 759–767.

Conti-Fine, B.M., Milani, M. and Kaminski, H.J. (2006) Myasthenia gravis: past, present, and future. *J. Clin. Invest.* **116**: 2843–2854.

Firestein, G.S. (2003) Evolving concepts of rheumatoid arthritis. *Nature,* **423**: 356–361.

Jönsen, A., Bengtsson, A.A., Nived, O., Truedsson, L. and Sturfelt, G. (2007) Gene–environment interactions in the etiology of systemic lupus erythematosus. *Autoimmunity,* **40**: 613–617.

Klareskog, L., Padyukov, L., Rönnelid, J and Alfredsson, L. (2006) Genes, environment and immunity in the development of rheumatoid arthritis. *Curr. Opin. Immunol.* **18**: 650–655.

Kyewski, B and Klein, L. (2006) A central role for central tolerance. *Annu. Rev. Immunol.* **24**: 571–606.

Maier, L.M. and Wicker, L.S. (2005) Genetic susceptibility to type 1 diabetes. *Curr. Opin. Immunol.* **17**: 601–608.

Mackay, F., Silveira, P.A. and Brink, R. (2007) B cells and the BAFF/APRIL axis: fast-forward on autoimmunity and signaling. *Curr. Opin. Immunol.* **19**: 327–336.

McFarland, H.F. and Martin, R. (2007) Multiple sclerosis: a complicated picture of autoimmunity. *Nature Immunol.* **8**: 913–919.

Pascual, V., Farkas, L. and Banchereau, J. (2006) Systemic lupus erythematosus: all roads lead to type I interferons. *Curr. Opin. Immunol.* **18**: 676–682.

Ramanujam M. and Davidson A. (2008) Targeting of the immune system in systemic lupus erythematosus. *Expert. Rev. Mol. Med.* **10**: e2.

Sokol, C.L., Barton, G.M., Farr, A.G. and Medzhitov, R. (2008) A mechanism for the initiation of allergen-induced T helper type 2 responses. *Nature Immunol.* **9**: 310–318.

Tarlinton, D. (2008) IL-17 drives germinal center B cells. *Nature Immunol.* **9**: 124–126.

Ulmanen, I., Halonen, M., Imarinen, T. and Peltonen, L. (2005) Monogenic autoimmune diseases – lessons of self-tolerance. *Curr. Opin. Immunol.* **17**: 609–615.

Veldhoen, M., Hirota, K., Westendorf, A.M., *et al.* (2008) The aryl hydrocarbon receptor links T_H17-cell-mediated autoimmunity to environmental toxins. *Nature*, **453**: 106–110.

SELF-ASSESSMENT QUESTIONS

1. What is your understanding of the term tolerance?
2. What does polygenic disease imply when it describes an autoimmune disease?
3. What are the immunological mechanisms which may be responsible for tissue damage detected in an autoimmune disease?
4. Why does autoimmunity often result in chronic inflammation?
5. Describe mechanisms which may result in tolerance.
6. What is thought to be the strongest genetic risk factor for development of autoimmune diseases?
7. What are the environmental triggers of autoimmune disease thought to be?
8. What criteria strengthen the diagnosis of a condition as due to autoimmunity?
9. List 8 autoimmune conditions.
10. What are the three major goals in the treatment of RA?

<table>
<tr><td>CHAPTER
11</td></tr>
</table>

Transplantation and tumour immunology

Learning objectives
After studying this chapter you should confidently be able to:

■ **Understand the immunological challenge of transplanting cells, tissues and organs**
Transplants, including transfused blood cells, carry antigens from their donor that are regarded as foreign by the recipient of the transplant. These stimulate the recipient's immune system to mount responses capable of destroying, i.e. rejecting, the transplant. Some of the strongest rejection responses are induced by foreign MHC antigens. Rejection may occur very rapidly if antibodies against the donor's cells are already present in the recipient. If the transplant donor and recipient are genetically identical, rejection responses are not induced.

■ **Understand how tissue typing can help to minimize immune responses against transplants**
The pattern of MHC antigen expression, or haplotype, of an individual who needs to receive a transplant is determined by tissue typing. Serum antibodies from a potential recipient are tested to ensure that they do not react against donor cells. The best potential donor is the one whose MHC haplotype most closely matches that of the potential recipient.

■ **Discuss current approaches to suppressing immune responses against transplants**
Immunosupppression aims to diminish further any reactivity between donor and recipient that exists despite selection by tissue-typing. This allows transplants between a donor–recipient pair where the haplotypes are similar though not completely identical. Strategies include radiation to destroy potentially reactive leukocytes in the recipient, e.g. for bone marrow transplants, or drugs, e.g. cyclosporine, to diminish the potency of the recipient's immune responses.

■ **Discuss our current understanding of how cancer cells and tumours develop and survive despite the immune system**
Tumour cell strategies to avoid detection by the immune system include reduced expression of MHC antigens and tumour-associated antigens. Tumour cells frequently show genetic instability allowing the rapid evolution of weakly antigenic variants. Many tumours secrete substances that inhibit the generation of tumour-specific immune responses.

■ **Consider how manipulating the immune system might lead to effective treatments for cancer**
By identifying tumour-associated antigens, specific cellular or antibody-mediated immune responses can be targeted against the tumour cells. Cancer therapies, in particular the activation of cytolytic T cells, and cancer vaccines (cancer prevention) are being explored.

11.1 INTRODUCTION TO TRANSPLANTATION AND TUMOUR IMMUNOLOGY

Previous chapters have discussed how immune responses against foreign antigens are induced. In general, these responses are beneficial and they protect the integrity of the host. However, medical advances have resulted in situations where immune responses against certain foreign antigens are undesirable. During the twentieth century, surgical techniques had advanced sufficiently to allow diseased or damaged tissues to be replaced by transplantation of tissues taken, usually immediately post-mortem, from organ donors. This surgical procedure, called tissue transplantation or organ transplantation, has greatly enhanced the quality of life of individuals suffering from life-threatening major organ failure. In the vast majority of cases, the donor and recipient are not genetically identical so the transplanted tissue is treated as a foreign antigen by the recipient's immune system. Without intervention, the recipient's immune system will attack and reject the transplanted tissue. The goal of transplantation immunology is to prevent the recipient's immune system from rejecting the foreign tissue transplant.

Tumour immunologists face a different, yet equally challenging problem. Tumours arise from normal 'self' cells that have become transformed. In some cases cell transformation is a result of infection with certain tumour viruses, for example HTLV-1, the causative agent of adult T cell leukaemia. In most cases, however, the generation of tumour cells, termed tumourigenesis, results from mutation of cellular genes. The challenge of tumour immunology is to induce the immune system to attack tumourigenic 'self' cells.

This chapter discusses the approaches used by transplantation immunologists and tumour immunologists to encourage the immune system to ignore foreign tissues and cells or to attack self cells, respectively.

11.2 TISSUE TRANSPLANTATION

The earliest documented case of tissue transplantation dates to the second century BC, when the Indian surgeon Sushruta grafted skin from a patient's forehead to his nose to aid healing after the nose had been partially amputated. Today this procedure is called rhinoplasty. In the procedure performed by Sushruta, the donor and recipient were the same person. This means that the graft was an autograft (see *Box 11.1*). Autografting of skin on to a variety of sites has been practised for many centuries, and has generally been successful. In contrast, if the skin donor and skin graft recipient were different people then the allograft was usually rapidly rejected. Although skin grafting has been practised for many centuries, transplantation of internal organs was not possible until the early 1900s when techniques were developed that allowed vascular anastomosis (joining of blood vessels). Early experiments in solid organ transplantation also demonstrated that allografts were rapidly rejected.

Box 11.1 Different types of transplants

Autologous transplants – patients receive their own cells
Syngeneic transplants – patients receive cells from a genetically identical person, i.e. an identical twin
Allogeneic transplants – patients receive cells from a genetically similar, but not identical, person
Xenogeneic transplants – patients receive cells from a member of a different species

---

A major advance in our understanding of transplant rejection came from research performed in the 1930s by Peter Gorer and George Snell using genetically characterized strains of mice. Their work defined the major genes responsible for controlling transplant rejection. These genes are now referred to as MHC genes. Up until this point, the mechanisms responsible for graft rejection were unknown. In 1943, Peter Medawar (see *Box 11.2*) provided the first evidence that allografts were rejected by the immune system. Consequently, progress in allotransplantation required an appreciation of immunological tolerance (see *Box 11.3*). The recognition that the rejection of transplanted allografts is immune-mediated prompted the search for immunosuppressive treatments that would promote acceptance of the graft. Most of the early treatments were either unsuccessful or were too toxic to be used in patients. In the 1960s, azathioprine was the first immunosuppressive drug to be used successfully without exhibiting major side effects. This drug, together with prednisone, formed the mainstay of treatment for transplant patients until the advent of cyclosporine in the 1980s (see *Section 11.5*).

Box 11.2 The development of transplantation

Sir Peter Medawar, Nobel Prizewinner in 1960 (jointly with Sir Macfarlane Burnet, also an immunologist) pioneered the development of transplantation. His experiments on skin transplantation in animals were prompted by attempts to save Battle of Britain pilots in World War II who were very badly burned. His observations contributed to the understanding of histocompatibility and immunological tolerance.

Box 11.3 Immunological tolerance

The critical observation that led to our current understanding of immunological tolerance was made in 1945 by Ray Owen who was studying dizygotic (fraternal) cattle twins. These share the same placenta (a natural anastomosis) and therefore there is free exchange of blood (including haematopoietic stem cells) between the developing twins. Owen found that each twin grew to contain, in addition to its own blood cells, blood cells derived from its twin partner. Because both sets of genetically non-identical cells co-existed in the same animal, Owen recognized this to be an example of immunological tolerance, or acceptance, of an allograft (in this case blood cells). Several years later, Medawar and his co-workers demonstrated that skin allografts between dizygotic calves were also not rejected, and that exposure of animals to antigens during neonatal development resulted in a state of immunological tolerance to these antigens.

Today, transplantation immunology is a complex, rapidly developing and clinically important area of immunology. Bone marrow transplantation is the treatment of choice for a variety of haematological disorders, and transplantation of many solid organs has become commonplace. The choice of bone marrow or tissue donor is crucial if the transplanted tissue, referred to as a graft, is to be accepted. As indicated above, it is mainly MHC molecules, the molecules that allow our T cells to respond so effectively against foreign antigens, which serve as targets during transplant rejection.

For successful transplantation of tissues from one person to another a series of conditions must be satisfied.

- The pattern of MHC molecules expressed on the graft must be as similar as possible to the pattern of MHC molecules expressed by the recipient; in other words the tissue donor and tissue recipient must be closely MHC-matched.
- As a perfect match between MHC antigens of donor and recipient is virtually impossible (except between identical twins), an appropriate strategy must be employed to minimize the potential of the immune system to mount responses against the transplanted tissue.
- The cells or tissues to be transplanted must be maintained in the best possible living condition.
- Correct surgical and/or transfusion techniques must be used.

As a general rule, the closer the MHC-match between donor and recipient, the more likely the transplant will be accepted. If the donor and recipient are totally MHC-mismatched, then the recipient will mount a strong cellular immune response against the transplanted tissue and the tissue will be rejected. The potential match between the recipient's tissues and the donor's tissues is assessed using a method called tissue typing, sometimes referred to as HLA typing.

11.3 TISSUE TYPING

Tissue typing results determine whether a transplant procedure involving a particular recipient and a particular donor should, or should not, go ahead.

The tissue type of the potential recipient is determined, and potential donors are also typed to develop a panel. From the panel the one whose tissue type is the most similar to that of the potential recipient is selected, provided that his/her tissue type fulfils certain criteria that determine a 'good match'.

As discussed in *Section 5.6*, the MHC genes are very highly polymorphic. This means that within the population a large number of different MHC alleles exist from which a large number of different MHC antigens can be expressed. Some individuals may express MHC alleles that occur only with low frequency in the population within which they are living, so finding a suitable potential organ donor may be difficult. Frequently the best potential donor will be a close relative; if a person has no or few close relatives the chances of finding a good potential donor are reduced. Similarly, certain ethnic populations have a relatively higher expression of certain MHC alleles. If a member of that group migrates to a country with a very different ethnic composition, the chances of finding a good tissue match may be low. In general, very large cities are good places to seek transplants – 'all human life' as well as all possible MHC alleles are there. Therefore the chances of finding a close match by chance, rather than through family connections, are increased.

Although PCR-based assays are increasingly being used in HLA typing, most tissue typing is still performed using serological techniques. Leukocytes from the potential recipient are incubated with a panel of antibodies that react against defined MHC molecules (see *Figure 11.1*). A positive reaction indicates the presence on the subject's cells of the specific MHC antigen against which the antibodies are directed. The products of six different MHC genetic loci are usually tested. Binding of the antibodies to the cells can be assessed by flow cytometry (see *Section 13.10*). Alternatively, if antibodies of the appropriate isotype are used, antibody binding to the recipient's cells will render them susceptible to lysis following the addition of complement. The degree of cell lysis can be determined colourimetrically and may be used to determine if the recipient's cells express particular MHC molecules. Cells from potential donors are also tested to determine their pattern of MHC expression. When the results for a potential recipient and potential donor are closely matched, the chance of the recipient rejecting the donor's tissues is substantially reduced.

It is also important to determine if the recipient's serum contains alloantibodies, i.e. antibodies against non-self human antigens. This can happen following exposure to alloantigens during, for example, pregnancy (see the discussion of erythroblastosis fetalis in *Section 9.8*), blood transfusion or a previous tissue transplant. If present, these alloantibodies can cause hyperacute rejection of transplanted tissues (see *Section 11.5*). The presence of alloantibodies in patient sera is commonly assessed using the panel reactive antibody test (sometimes referred to as percent reactive antibody, because the result is expressed as a percentage), or PRA test. In this test the potential recipient's serum is added to samples of cells taken from a large pool of different individuals (potential donors). Antibody binding to the cells can be determined as described above. A high PRA value means that the

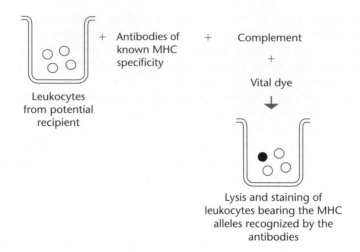

Figure 11.1
Serological detection of HLA alleles. The MHC allele-specific antibodies bind to cells that express that MHC allele but not to cells that do not express that allele. If complement is added, then any cells that have bound antibody will activate complement via the classical pathway. This results in the formation of pores in the cell membrane due to assembly of the membrane attack complex (see *Section 4.3*). These cells are unable to exclude vital dyes such as trypan blue and can easily be visualized by light microscopy.

recipient's serum contains antibodies that are reactive against a high percentage of the potential donor population. Consequently, patients with high PRA values usually spend much longer on transplant waiting lists.

For many types of transplants there is a dependence on deceased (cadaveric) donors. Cadaveric donors draw from a more random gene pool, at least compared to that of a recipient who has potential donors within a family. Unfortunately cadaveric donors still provide the largest source for kidneys and of course are the only source for heart transplants. Nonetheless very close matches are quite common.

A six-out-of-six HLA match with no PRA reactivity is the best possible result. This means that potential donor and potential recipient have identical antigens at six MHC loci and the recipient does not contain preformed antibodies capable of recognizing the donor's cells. Five-out-of-six matches and four-out-of-six matches are more common and are considered good matches. Depending upon the rarity of the blood group and the specific MHC antigens, matches that are theoretically 'less perfect' are frequently made and, with modern immunosuppressive drug therapy, are very often long-term successes.

Nonetheless, tissues donated by living relatives are still the most likely to be tolerated long-term. Factors contributing to this may relate to techniques of tissue removal and storage (i.e. the care in taking an organ from a living person as opposed to a cadaver). A wide variety of powerful vascular mediators are released in the presence of severe brain injury. As a consequence of this 'catecholamine storm', hearts and lungs from cadaveric donors may manifest such severe deterioration in function that they become too damaged to transplant. All cadaveric organs sustain this type of injury, some to a greater degree than others. In kidney transplantation this effect appears stronger than the effect of MHC matching, as the success rates for kidneys transplanted from spousal donors, where a close genetic match is highly unlikely, are superior to the success rates for kidneys transplanted from cadaveric donors with the same degree of MHC matching. However, with improvements in drug therapy, the success rates of transplants from cadaveric donors are increasing.

Tissue typing is a complex process, and this section really only provides an outline of the major steps in recipient/donor matching. A large portion of this matching must be done accurately and rapidly in the last hours before transplantation (speed being especially important in the case of organs from cadaveric donors). Fortunately, the technology exists to make possible quick, precise tissue typing for optimal transplant results.

11.4 TARGET ANTIGENS OF IMMUNE-MEDIATED GRAFT REJECTION

Despite careful tissue typing of donors and recipients, graft rejection does occur. A variety of antigens can serve as targets for the host immune response during rejection of transplanted tissues.

Major histocompatibility molecules

As discussed above, MHC molecules are the primary determinants of whether a tissue transplant is accepted or rejected by the recipient. If the organ donor and recipient are MHC-mismatched then, in the absence of any immunosuppression, the transplant will rapidly be rejected by the recipient. The recipient's immune system recognizes the donor MHC molecules as foreign and mounts an immune response against them. This type of rejection can be mediated by either antibodies or by T cells.

MHC-specific, antibody-mediated rejection (see *Section 11.5, Hyperacute rejection* below) is normally directed against MHC class I antigens. It occurs due to preformed IgG antibodies in the recipient that react against MHC class I antigens on the transplanted tissue. Generation of such antibodies may result from exposure to foreign MHC class I during a previous blood transfusion, organ transplantation, or pregnancy.

Recipient T cells can also recognize donor MHC molecules and react against them. These alloreactive T cells can directly react against foreign MHC molecules on donor APCs (direct recognition). Alternatively, non-self MHC molecules can be treated in the same way as any other foreign antigen and be processed and presented to recipient T cells on self MHC molecules (indirect recognition).

Minor histocompatibility antigens

Minor histocompatibility antigens were originally defined in transplantation experiments using inbred mouse strains. It was found that if donor and recipient animals differed at specific genetic loci, then the transplant would be rejected, but not as rapidly as in the case where donor and recipient were MHC-mismatched. We now know that these minor histocompatibility antigens are non-self proteins that are presented by MHC molecules to recipient T cells, resulting in an inflammatory response.

Blood group antigens

Human blood is generally classified into four groups depending on the presence or absence of antigens, called A and B antigens. It should be noted that these antigens are also present on other cells of the body, especially on vascular endothelial cells. Antibodies are either produced or not produced to the A and B antigens depending upon their genetically determined presence or absence. Natural antibodies are produced to these antigens, probably as a result of cross-reactivity with carbohydrate antigens of bacteria. Blood groups A and B are dominant over O (see *Table 11.1*).

Table 11.1 The human ABO blood group system

Phenotype	Genotype	Antigen expressed	Serum antibody
A	AA, AO	A	Anti-B
B	BB, BO	B	Anti-A
O	OO	H (no A or B antigen)	Anti-A and anti-B
AB	AB	A and B	No anti-A or anti-B

Species-specific carbohydrate antigens

These antigens are analogous to the blood group antigens described above and are expressed on vascular endothelium. Pre-existing antibodies against these antigens have significantly hindered progress in xenotransplantation. Like the blood group antigens, it is thought that antibodies to these antigens result from cross-reactivity with bacterial antigens. These preformed antibodies are present in the sera of most species and react to the vascular carbohydrate antigens of most other species.

Advances in gene targeting technology have prompted efforts to delete the genes responsible for the expression of these antigens from pigs in the hope that organs from these genetically manipulated animals might be suitable for transplantation into humans.

11.5 MECHANISMS OF GRAFT REJECTION

Following transplantation, the transplant may be accepted or it may be rejected. Rejection is invariably accompanied by fever, flu-like symptoms, oedema, and hypertension. Three main types of rejection are currently recognized: hyperacute, acute, and chronic.

Hyperacute rejection

This form of rejection occurs within minutes to days following transplantation. It occurs due to pre-existing antibodies in the recipient reacting with antigens expressed by the transplant. The main target of hyperacute rejection is the vascular endothelium of the transplant, and the most common antigens recognized are MHC class I and blood group antigens. In theory, preformed antibodies against foreign MHC class II could also give rise to this form of rejection but MHC class II molecules are normally expressed only at a low level on vascular endothelium. Preformed antibodies against species-specific carbohydrate antigens can cause hyperacute rejection of xenotransplants.

The antibodies that cause hyperacute rejection activate complement resulting in the initiation of inflammation. This results in the activation of the coagulation and fibrinolytic systems. Pathological changes include thrombosis and oedema with neutrophil infiltration. There is little or no mononuclear cell infiltration.

Serological screening, in particular PRA testing, prior to transplantation has dramatically reduced the incidence of hyperacute rejection.

Acute rejection

This is the most common form of rejection. It usually occurs within the first 6 months following transplantation and is mediated by T cells. Recent research suggests that Th17 cells (see *Section 6.5*) participate in acute graft rejection. The major target antigens during acute rejection are MHC molecules and minor histocompatibility antigens. Immunosuppressive therapy is the most effective way of preventing acute rejection.

There are two main mechanisms responsible for T cell-mediated acute graft rejection (see *Figure 11.2*).

Direct presentation

After transplantation, DCs present in the donor graft can migrate to the host lymph nodes, where they can present antigenic peptide on the donor MHC molecules to recipient T cells. The activated T cells then migrate back to the graft, causing inflammation.

Indirect presentation

After transplantation, DCs from the host can migrate into the transplant, where they can take up peptides and proteins from the graft, including

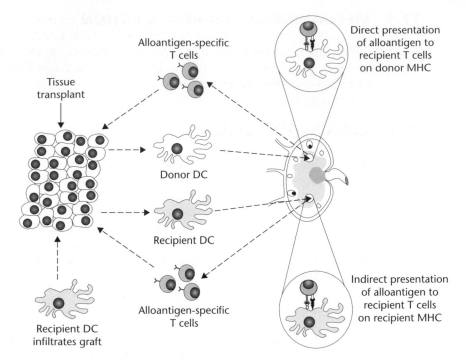

Figure 11.2
T cells can respond against alloantigens in two ways. In direct presentation, donor-derived DCs from the transplant migrate to the draining lymph node and present alloantigen on donor MHC molecules to recipient T cells. In indirect presentation, recipient DCs infiltrate the transplant and acquire alloantigen. They then migrate to the draining lymph node and present the alloantigen on recipient MHC molecules to recipient T cells. In each case, the activated T cells leave the lymph node and attack the transplanted tissue.

donor MHC and transplant-specific antigens. The host DCs then travel to lymph nodes, where they present peptides to host T cells on host MHC molecules. Again, the activated T cells migrate back to the graft, causing inflammation.

In addition, the transplantation procedure itself may cause local trauma, resulting in chemokine production by resident cells. The chemokines will attract macrophages which will release cytokines such as IL-1, TNF-α and IFN-γ, which attract and activate other immune cells. These cells also release several molecules that are directly cytotoxic, including oxygen radicals and nitric oxide.

Chronic rejection

Transplanted tissues can remain in place for considerable periods, yet rejection is underway and eventually the graft fails or has to be removed. If more than 12 months have passed this is known as chronic rejection. This is the most poorly understood form of rejection. It results in gradual deterioration of the graft. The tissue will show features of chronic inflammation, e.g. infiltrates of mononuclear leukocytes and smooth muscle cell proliferation. It is a major complication affecting most long-term transplant survivors. It is likely that both cellular and humoral immune effector mechanisms contribute to chronic graft rejection.

11.6 IMMUNOSUPPRESSION

The chances of a person who needs a transplant having an identical twin who can be a donor are extremely slim. Therefore virtually every transplant recipient must undergo therapies that aim to minimize the immune responses that their bodies will mount against the life-saving transplanted cells or tissues that they are to receive. These therapies induce immunosuppression. Therefore a very fine balance must be established between the ability of the individual to mount immune responses against pathogens, while allowing the foreign transplanted tissues to establish themselves successfully. This balance is extremely difficult to achieve and therefore for most transplant recipients a varying drug regimen becomes a life-long reality.

Unfortunately, current strategies to achieve immune suppression tend more towards a general state of diminished immune responsiveness. If the transplant recipient exhibits symptoms of an infection the medical advice is to reduce the level of immune suppression. When the infection has passed the normal level of immune suppression is resumed. All current immuno-suppressive drugs cause significant side-effects (see *Table 11.2*) so a major treatment goal is to reduce the recipient's dose of drugs to the lowest possible level at which rejection still does not occur. Currently a variety of immunosuppressive drugs are used, usually in combination, to prolong transplant survival.

Table 11.2 Side-effects of frequently used immunosuppressive drugs

Drug	Principal side-effect
Cyclosporine	Dysfunction of renal system, gastrointestinal tract and central nervous system; hypertension; diabetes
Corticosteroids	Hypertension; diabetes; poor wound healing; bone destruction; features of Cushing's syndrome (results from over-production of steroid hormones)

Azathioprine

Azathioprine belongs to the class of drugs known as mitotic inhibitors. When taken up by cells, azathioprine is converted to 6-mercaptopurine (6MP). 6MP inhibits production of the nucleotides AMP and GMP and, consequently, slows cell proliferation. Since lymphocytes are rapidly dividing cells they are preferentially, but not exclusively, targeted by this drug.

Corticosteroids

Prednisone and dexamethasone are general anti-inflammatory substances. They have been used in transplantation since the early 1960s. Prednisone is often administered together with azathioprine to prevent acute graft-versus-host disease (see *Section 11.11*). Most transplant patients are maintained on low dose corticosteroids for the life of the transplant.

Cyclosporine, FK506, and rapamycin

These are potent immunosuppressive drugs derived from fungi. Their effects are more restricted to inhibition of T cell activation than are the effects of the drugs mentioned above. Cyclosporine and FK506 inhibit the transcription of the genes encoding IL-2 and the IL-2 receptor, which are essential for T cell activation. Rapamycin also inhibits T cell activation, but at a later stage than cyclosporine and FK506.

The introduction of cyclosporine treatment in the 1980s dramatically improved transplant survival. The major drawback with this drug is its nephrotoxicity – in some cases this can lead to drug-induced kidney failure. The immunosuppressive activities of FK506 and rapamycin are 10–100 times more potent than that of cyclosporine, so lower doses of these drugs can be used to achieve the same level of immunosuppression. Regardless, it is important to monitor serum levels of these drugs in patients to ensure: (1) that therapeutic levels of the drugs are being achieved, and (2) that nephrotoxic levels of the drugs are being avoided.

See *Box 11.4* for a case study.

11.7 FUTURE DIRECTIONS IN TRANSPLANTATION

The development of more selective immunosuppressive treatments, coupled with careful screening to allow selection of appropriate donors, has greatly advanced the field of tissue/organ transplantation. Successful transplants have now been achieved with the many solid organs including kidney, liver, lung, heart, and combined heart and lung. Scarcity of organ donors is a major problem, and each year many patients die while waiting for a suitable organ donor to be found. Currently, there are more than 7000 individuals awaiting transplant in the UK alone. This has led researchers to investigate the feasibility of xenotransplantation, although there are immunological barriers to xenotransplantation that have yet to be overcome. In addition, there are concerns that transplant of organs from other animals into humans might enable dissemination of non-human pathogens to man. The potential use of embryonic stem cells to 'grow' tissues for transplantation is currently a matter of hot debate. The recent successful generation of tracheal cells for transplantation from adult stem cells (see *Box 11.5*) indicates that for *in vitro* growth of some tissues at least, adult stem cells may offer excit-

Box 11.4 Case study

Mrs Graham (45 years old) visited her GP complaining of blood in her urine periodically over a period of a few weeks. She also complained that she felt swollen and was feeling generally unwell and was concerned that she was passing less urine than usual. Extensive examination revealed no diabetes and no tumours, but showed high levels of salts and urea in serum with raised blood pressure, resulting in a diagnosis of rapidly progressive glomerulonephritis (kidney disease). Despite the use of medications the condition progressed to renal failure and haemodialysis was required. In preparation for potential renal transplant, she was HLA-typed. A suitable cross-match for tissue and blood was sought and found.

The transplantation operation was followed with prescribed prednisolone, cyclosporine and azathioprine. Initially urine output increased, blood pressure moved towards normal, and urea levels in serum dropped toward normal. Twelve days after the operation Mrs Graham felt unwell with a raised temperature, the swelling had returned and blood pressure started to rise again. There was no infection and no obstruction, therefore a biopsy of the kidney was taken and revealed a large number of mononuclear cells. A diagnosis of acute grade II rejection was given and only when an anti-lymphocyte monoclonal antibody against CD3 on T cells was given did her condition improve. She was discharged on cyclosporine.

1. Why was the rejection termed 'acute'?
2. What is your understanding of 'a suitable cross-match'?
3. Mrs Graham was discharged on cyclosporine. What is this and how does it work?
4. Why did the anti-lymphocyte monoclonal antibody against CD3 treatment improve Mrs Graham's condition?

Box 11.5 Stem cell-derived tissue transplant

A major milestone in adult stem cell research is the recent report of a successful trachea transplant, with 4 month follow-up, using a trachea that was partially generated within a laboratory using stem cells[1]. Donor cells were eliminated from the human donor trachea by scraping, and epithelial cells and mesenchymal stem cell-derived chondrocytes, cultured from recipient bone marrow, were added to the resultant trachea 'scaffold'. By adding a small number of mucosal cells from the recipient's throat, a functional human trachea composed mostly from only recipient cells was made. The success of the surgery offers hope for patients awaiting transplants, although more complex organs such as heart, kidney or liver may prove more difficult to grow within the laboratory. The major advantage of this stem cell-facilitated transplant surgery was that the recipient did not require the use of immunosuppressive drugs. This represents a significant scientific development in terms of personalized medicine and transplant research.

[1] Macchiarini P., Jungebluth P., Go T., *et al.* (2008) Clinical transplantation of a tissue-engineered airway. *The Lancet*, **372**: 2023–2030.

ing possibilities. The advantage of adult stem cells is that if they can be isolated from the proposed transplant recipient, any tissue that they can be stimulated to develop into *in vitro* will be a total MHC-match with the recipient, eliminating the need for immunosuppressants post-transplantation. This is the holy grail of transplantation immunology: to achieve transplant-specific tolerance for all tissue transplants. If this could be achieved, then the need for immunosuppressive drugs, together with the risk of chronic infection that the use of such drugs poses to patients, could be eliminated. Another exciting immunological discovery of the past few years has been the characterization of T_{REG} cells. T_{REG} cells play an important role in maintenance of immunological tolerance (see *Sections 7.6* and *10.2*). Researchers are attempting to find ways to generate large numbers of these suppressor T_{REG} cells *in vitro* for use in therapy of autoimmune diseases and in transplantation.

11.8   IMMUNE RESPONSES AGAINST TUMOURS

There is considerable evidence to suggest that the immune system is active against tumours. Lymphocytic infiltration of certain, but not all, cancers is associated with better prognosis, suggesting participation of anti-tumour immune responses in control of tumour development. In addition, some cancers can regress spontaneously in people with fully functional immune systems, and immunocompromised patients (e.g. those with immunodefi-ciencies associated with HIV infection and AIDS) have a higher frequency of cancers than do healthy people. Cancer is also primarily a disease of older people where systemic immunodeficiency is well-recognized. Finally, exper-iments in mice have directly demonstrated a role for T cells in elimination of tumours. It seems likely, therefore, that immune surveillance destroys many of the malignant cells that arise and reduces significantly the likeli-hood that cancer will develop.

The main mechanism responsible for immune-mediated control of cancer is $CD8^+$ CTL-mediated killing of tumour cells. It is unclear whether $CD4^+$ T cells are directly involved in tumour eradication; however, animal studies have demonstrated that $CD4^+$ T cell help is important for optimal $CD8^+$ T cell-mediated anti-tumour immunity. The antigens that are recog-nized by tumour-specific T cells are called tumour-associated antigens (TAAs). Some TAAs may also be expressed by normal cells, but they are usually expressed at much higher levels by tumour cells. Major TAAs include:

- overexpressed self proteins such as the melanoma-associated antigens MAGE, BAGE and GAGE, and carcino-embryonic antigen on colon, breast, lung and gastric cancers
- mutated oncogenes, e.g. *Bcr/Abl*, or mutated tumour suppressor gene products, e.g. mutated p53
- antigens expressed by tumourigenic viruses, e.g. HTLV-1

TAAs can be taken up by DCs, processed and presented to $CD8^+$ T cells via the cross-presentation pathway (see *Section 5.10*). The activated $CD8^+$ T cells then migrate to the site of tumour growth and attack the tumour cells (see *Figure 11.3*).

Unfortunately, many TAAs are only weakly immunogenic and do not stimulate sufficiently strong T cell responses to prevent tumour outgrowth. This has prompted intense research into vaccination strategies designed to enhance tumour-specific immune responses. The efficacy of the vaccine

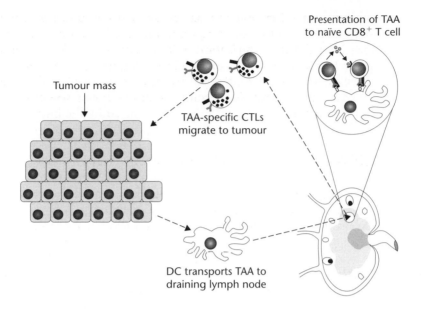

Figure 11.3
DCs infiltrate the tumour mass and acquire tumour-associated antigen (TAA). They carry the TAA to lymph nodes where they present the TAA to CD8⁺ T cells. With help from CD4⁺ T cells (see *Section 6.12*), the naïve CD8⁺ cells differentiate into TAA-specific cytotoxic T lymphocytes (CTLs). The TAA-specific CTLs leave the lymph node and attack the tumour cells.

against cervical cancer (see *Section 8.8*) provides hope that vaccination against other forms of human cancer might also be possible.

Adoptive T cell immunotherapy has been used successfully to treat EBV-associated post-transplant lymphoma. In this strategy, autologous EBV-specific T cells are expanded *in vitro* prior to infusion into the patient. The infused virus-specific CTLs kill the EBV⁺ tumour cells. Adoptive T cell immunotherapy, however, has proven less successful in treating non-viral tumours.

11.9 IMMUNE EVASION BY TUMOURS

Cancer cells that survive to proliferate and, depending on their original cell types, form solid tumours, must exert some influence that allows them to escape recognition and/or destruction by the immune system.

A range of different strategies can be seen to exist that allow cancer cells and tumours to evade T cell recognition. Some cancers attempt to remain undetected by reducing their expression of MHC class I antigens. Although NK cells specifically target cells with reduced MHC class I expression, T cell recognition of these cells is diminished. Certain tumour cells can directly inhibit immune responses (see *Section 12.7*) by secreting immunosuppressive factors such as TGF-β, IL-10, and PGE_2. Studies in animal models also indicate that transplanted tumours can cause the accumulation of tolerigenic DCs and T_{REG} cells in tumour-draining lymph nodes, thus inhibiting the induction of tumour-specific responses in the draining node.

The immune response against the tumour may select for the outgrowth of tumour cells that are no longer recognized by the immune system. These antigen-loss variants can grow rapidly in the absence of an effective anti-tumour response. There is also evidence that chronic inflammatory responses can promote tumour outgrowth. In particular, IL-23 inhibits the infiltration of $CD8^+$ T cells into the tumour environment and promotes the growth of new blood vessels (angiogenesis), a process that promotes growth of solid tumours. Thus the detection of leukocytes in a tumour does not always indicate a beneficial immune response.

11.10   MULTIPLE MYELOMA

Multiple myeloma is a form of cancer that involves malignant proliferation of the B cell-derived plasma cells responsible for the secretion of immunoglobulin. The tumours are called plasmacytomas and usually form in the bone marrow. On X-rays the presence of a plasmacytoma is indicated by a clear area where there would normally be shadow due to the intact bone marrow. Other indications that may lead to a diagnosis of multiple myeloma include anaemia, leukopaenia (lower than normal numbers of circulating leukocytes) leading to recurrent infections and, possibly, clotting difficulties due to decreased platelet numbers. In advanced disease bone destruction is common.

Although the malignant plasma cells produce antibodies, these are not beneficial to the host. The antibodies are termed myeloma proteins and, because they are not produced in response to infection, they are not of the specificity required to interact with foreign antigens. On laboratory analysis it is possible to differentiate between antibodies produced in response to infection and myeloma proteins. During infection, a normal immune response results in the production of antibodies specific for many different antigens on the infecting pathogen. The antibodies result from many different plasma cells and are said to be polyclonal. In multiple myeloma all antibodies result from proliferation of a single plasma cell so are monoclonal. Electrophoresis – recording the different patterns of movement of different proteins in a gel – readily differentiates between polyclonal and monoclonal antibody production (see *Figure 11.4*) thereby contributing to the diagnosis of multiple myeloma. Treatment for patients with multiple myeloma usually aims to decrease the burden of immunoglobulin proteins in circulation as these can cause kidney damage. Removal of the circulating myeloma proteins by the process of plasmapheresis – cleansing of the blood plasma in a procedure similar to renal dialysis – provides temporary respite. Chemotherapy or radiation therapy may destroy the malignant cells, though the duration of effective treatment may be limited. Bone marrow trans-

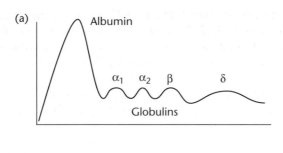

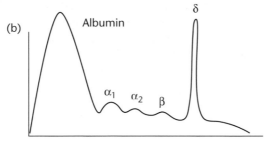

Figure 11.4
Protein electrophoresis of a normal serum sample (a) and of a serum sample from a patient with multiple myeloma showing elevated levels of protein in the gammaglobulin fraction (b).

plantation following high dose treatment to destroy the patient's bone marrow entirely is another potentially curative strategy.

11.11 BONE MARROW TRANSPLANTATION

In the treatment of diseases, most usually in the case of cancers of blood or immune cells, i.e. leukaemia or lymphoma, the chemotherapy or radiotherapy treatments given to destroy the cancer cells also destroy the bone marrow cells from which cells of the immune system arise. Other cells in the circulation, i.e. haematopoietic (blood) cells, are also produced by the bone marrow and their production may also be stopped following cancer treatment. To allow recovery the patient then receives a transplant of bone marrow cells or of peripheral blood stem cells that have the ability to regenerate immune and blood systems. Before receiving the bone marrow transplant the recipient is prepared by complete destruction of any remaining bone marrow using either high dose chemotherapy drugs or whole body irradiation.

For the transplant, bone marrow cells are usually obtained (harvested) from the marrow of the pelvic bones, although sometimes marrow from the sternum may be used. The marrow is drawn out through a special needle, processed, e.g. to remove any fragments of bone, and infused into the recipient's circulation. The marrow cells that will give rise to new immune and blood cells then localize to the recipient's bone marrow cavities. It is possible to store the extracted marrow by cryopreservation for use at a later stage.

In the case of stem cell transplantation, stem cells can be extracted from a donor's peripheral blood and either infused immediately into the recipient or cryopreserved. Blood found in the umbilical cord of newborn babies is another rich source of stem cells.

For some patients autologous bone marrow or stem cell transplantation may be possible (see *Box 11.1*). In that case the cells to be transplanted are harvested before the person undergoes chemotherapy or radiotherapy. If the patient has cancer it is essential that all cancer cells are removed, or purged, so that they cannot be re-introduced in the transplant procedure. Suitable purging methodologies include the use of tumour-specific monoclonal antibodies combined with complement. The antibody recognizes the cancer cells and opsonizes them, allowing their destruction by complement (see *Sections 2.9* and *4.3*).

Following the transplant procedure, re-establishment of the patient's immune system is monitored by frequent measurement of the numbers of peripheral blood cells through routine laboratory procedures. With autologous transplantation, the re-establishment of functional immunity usually occurs over a period of several months, though this is faster than with syngeneic or allogeneic transplants where complete restoration of immunity may take from one to two years. During this time patients are highly susceptible to infection and even common infectious agents may prove fatal. Patients are usually given antibiotics, and transfusions of blood, or its components, may be necessary to prevent anaemia or clotting deficiencies if platelet numbers are low. The period of recovery and establishment of a functional transplant is known as engraftment. In the post-engraftment phase, i.e. 1–2 years after engraftment, the patient may be re-immunized with the protective vaccines that he/she had received previously, predominantly during childhood. This enables the 'new' immune system developed by the transplanted marrow to confer the same level of protective immunity as it did prior to the destruction of immune cells by chemotherapy or radiation. Because transplant recipients are highly likely to continue receiving immunosuppressive drugs, they should not receive any live vaccines because of the significant risk of contracting serious, or fatal, disease even from the low dose administered in the vaccine. Should a bone marrow transplant prove not to be successful, either through failure to engraft, rejection or re-appearance of the cancer, the procedure may be repeated.

Graft-versus-host disease

Graft-versus-host disease (GvHD) is a particular complication affecting 50–70% of bone marrow transplant recipients. GvHD occurs if immune cells from the donor were included in the transplanted tissue (the graft). Bone marrow contains large numbers of T cells that migrate there as part of their function of immune surveillance. Following transplantation, these cells become activated by alloantigens in the recipient, resulting in production of cytokines and in gastrointestinal, hepatic, and dermal inflammation. Severe GvHD can lead to gastrointestinal haemorrhage and liver failure.

GvHD may either be acute or chronic and its prevention is by immunosuppression. Generally this is non-specific, e.g. using corticosteroids, so it may further complicate the patient's recovery. Ideally GvHD should be avoided by removing mature immune cells from the cell preparation prior to its infusion into the patient; however, complete removal may prove difficult. Current regimens to minimize GvHD include partial elimination of T cells from donor bone marrow using T cell-specific antibodies, combined with immunosuppression of the recipient to prevent graft rejection. The first appearance of GvHD in a patient is usually several weeks after transplantation, when the dosage of immunosuppressive drugs is being decreased and recovery is under way, i.e. during engraftment. A beneficial aspect of GvHD is graft-versus-leukaemia (GvL), where the immunocompetent cells in the graft recognize cancer cells that may remain, or re-appear, in the recipient and destroy them.

SUGGESTED FURTHER READING

Apte, R.N. and Voronov, E. (2008) Is interleukin-1 a good or bad 'guy' in tumour immunobiology and immunotherapy? *Immunol. Rev.* **222**: 222–241.

Harding, AJ. (2005) A brief history of blood transfusion. *Biomed. Sci.* **49**: 1147–1151.

Higgins, C. (2007) Multiple myeloma and serum free light chain measurement. *Biomed. Sci.***51**: 4128–4130.

Langowski, J.L., Zhang, X., Wu, L., *et al.* (2006) IL-23 promotes tumour incidence and growth. *Nature,* **442**: 461–465.

Lollini, P.-L. and Forni, G. (2002) Cancer immunoprevention: tracking down persistent tumour antigens. *Trends Immunol.* **24**: 62–66.

Mantovani, A., Sozzani, S., Locati, M., Allavena, P. and Sica, A. (2002) Macrophage: polarization: tumour-associated macrophages as a paradigm for polarized M mononuclear phagocytes. *Trends Immunol.* **23**: 549–555.

Martinez, O.M. and Rosen, H.R. (2005) Basic concepts in transplantation immunology. *Liver Transpl.* **11**: 370–381.

Munn, D.H. and Mellor, A.L. (2006) The tumour-draining lymph node as an immune–privileged site. *Immunol. Rev.* **213**: 146–158.

Rabinovich, G.A., Gabrilovich, D. and Sotomayor, E. (2007) Immunosuppressive strategies that are mediated by tumour cells. *Annu. Rev. Immunol.* **25**: 267–296.

Rosen, H.R. (2008) Transplantation immunology: what the clinician needs to know for immunotherapy. *Gastroenterology,* **134**: 1789–1801.

SELF-ASSESSMENT QUESTIONS

1. What causes hyperacute rejection of transplanted cells, tissues or organs?
2. What is the principal laboratory technique used to select the best donor for a person who needs a transplant?
3. Why are transplant recipients highly likely to be susceptible to infections?
4. How can transplant procedures go ahead even though donor and recipient do not express identical MHC alleles?
5. What is the purpose of the whole body radiation that may be given to a patient prior to receiving a bone marrow transplant?
6. What is graft-versus-host disease?
7. Give four reasons why immune responses may not destroy tumours.
8. If leukocytes are visible on a section of tumour tissue, does this indicate that the tumour will be destroyed by an immune response?
9. What are tumour-associated antigens?
10. What are myeloma proteins?

CHAPTER

12

Immunodeficiencies

Learning objectives
After studying this chapter you should confidently be able to:

- **Discuss the origins of primary and secondary immunodeficiencies**
  Primary immunodeficiencies arise from defects that are intrinsic to the immune system. Most often these defects are mutations in signalling or effector molecules that are critical for the function of the immune system. Secondary immunodeficiencies usually arise as a consequence of other conditions such as malnutrition or medical treatment, e.g. chemotherapy. With the exception of selective IgA deficiency, primary immuno-deficiencies are rare disorders whereas secondary immunodeficiencies are a major cause of morbidity and mortality worldwide. The secondary immunodeficiency AIDS claimed approximately 2.1 million lives in 2007 alone.

- **Describe the consequences for an individual of having impaired immune responses**
  The consequences of impaired immune responses range from mild to severe, depending on the component of the immune system that is defective. In instances where affected individuals are overtly immunodeficient they will usually present with recurrent infections. The nature of the infections is usually indicative of which element of the immune system is compromised. Recurrent infections with encapsulated bacteria are characteristic of immunoglobulin deficiencies. T cell deficiencies frequently result in recurrent viral, fungal or protozoan infections. Recurrent infections with pyogenic bacteria are suggestive of complement or phagocyte deficiencies. Severe immunodeficiencies require urgent medical intervention as they normally result in death due to overwhelming infections if untreated.

- **Discuss current approaches to the treatment of immune deficiencies**
  Many of the less severe immunoglobulin deficiencies are treated by administration of intravenous immunoglobulin together with the judicious use of antibiotics. Combined immunodeficiencies are frequently treated by bone marrow transplantation. Medical treatments that can cause immunosuppression, e.g. immunosuppressants to prevent transplant rejection or chemotherapy, must be carefully monitored to ensure that they do not lead to iatrogenic immunodeficiency. Infection with HIV is most effectively controlled using highly active antiretroviral therapy.

■ **Describe the clinical course of HIV infection**
During the acute stage, HIV infects CD4$^+$ cells and replicates to high levels causing viraemia. Virus-specific CTLs (CD8$^+$ T cells) attack and kill virus-infected cells. This, together with the cytopathic effect of virus replication leads to a precipitous drop in the number of CD4$^+$ T cells in peripheral blood. As the viral titre is reduced by the CTLs, the CD4$^+$ T cell count recovers somewhat. Infected macrophages and dendritic cells serve as a reservoir of infectious virus and transport the virus to secondary lymphoid tissues. During this stage the infected individual usually generates HIV-specific antibodies. The acute stage is either asymptomatic or the infected individual may present with flu-like symptoms. The next stage of the infection, called the latent stage, is a prolonged battle between the immune system and the virus. HIV reactivates from latency in secondary lymphoid tissues and is rapidly controlled by virus-specific CTLs. The CTLs do not eliminate the virus, partly due to the high mutation rate of HIV, which generates viral variants that are not recognized by the virus-specific CTLs that were generated during the acute stage. The latent stage is asymptomatic but is associated with a gradual decrease in CD4$^+$ T cell numbers. This stage of the infection may last for many years until the T cell numbers decline sufficiently so that cell-mediated immune responses are lost. At this stage the infected individual enters the third and final stage of infection and progresses to AIDS. This stage is characterized by opportunistic infections and often the development of unusual malignancies.

12.1 INTRODUCTION TO IMMUNODEFICIENCIES

The immune system is a tightly regulated, multi-component system of inter-acting cells and molecules. A malfunction of one or more of these components, or of the control mechanisms, may cause the system, or part of the system, to fail to respond. When this occurs the resulting disorder is called an immunodeficiency. Immunodeficiencies are a heterogeneous group of diseases that are caused by dysfunction of control or effector mechanisms of the immune system. Fortunately, there is substantial redundancy in the immune system, i.e. some components in the system are able to compensate for loss or malfunction of others. In contrast, deficiencies in other components of the immune system can lead to such overwhelming infections that the affected individual may die in infancy.

Recurrent infections are characteristic of immunodeficiency. Frequently the type of recurrent infection will indicate which component of the immune system is defective. Recurrent infections with bacterial pathogens such as *Haemophilus influenzae* or *Streptococcus pneumoniae* suggest a failure of immunoglobulin responses. Individuals with compromised cell-mediated immunity frequently present with recurrent viral, fungal or protozoan infections. Recurrent infections with pyogenic (pus-forming) bacteria might suggest complement or phagocyte deficiencies. Regardless of the deficiency, early diagnosis and treatment of immunodeficiencies is essential to minimize tissue damage.

Immunodeficiencies are usually classified as either primary or secondary immunodeficiencies.

12.2 PRIMARY IMMUNODEFICIENCIES

Primary immunodeficiencies are diseases where the defect is intrinsic to the immune system. These diseases are congenital and usually present early in life. Consequently, primary immunodeficiencies are frequently termed congenital immunodeficiencies. However, in certain instances, for example, in common variable immunodeficiency, the deficiency may not manifest until later in life. With few exceptions, the incidence of primary immunodeficiencies is low; approximately 1 in 10 000.

Primary immunodeficiencies may impact on either the innate or the adaptive immune system. Approximately 50% of the primary immunodeficiencies that have been described are deficiencies of the humoral arm of the immune system, whereas only 10% are defects of cell-mediated immunity alone. However, about 20% of immunodeficiencies affect both cell-mediated immunity and humoral immunity. In several of these 'combined' disorders the defect is intrinsic to the cell-mediated arm of the immune response, but the cell-mediated response is so severely impaired that T cell help for immunoglobulin responses is deficient. Of the remaining primary immunodeficiencies, approximately 18% are defects of phagocyte function and 2% are complement deficiencies.

12.3 PRIMARY IMMUNODEFICIENCIES OF INNATE IMMUNITY

The cells and molecules of the innate immune response constitute an effective initial barrier against microbial invasion. Because of this, deficiencies of one or more of these components can have serious consequences in terms of increased susceptibility to infection. Deficiencies in a variety of components of innate immunity have been identified (see *Table 12.1*). It is important to note that defects of these components may have knock-on effects on adaptive immune responses. For example, because of the role of complement activation products in regulating B cell and T cell responses (see *Section 7.7*), deficiency of complement components can lead to dysregulated humoral and cell-mediated immune responses.

Complement deficiencies

Deficiencies in all of the components of the complement cascade have been described. The central component of complement is C3, which is present in serum at a concentration of about 1 mg ml^{-1}. C3 lies at the pivotal point in the classical, alternative, and lectin pathways of complement activation (see *Section 4.3*). If C3 is deficient, all components downstream of C3 in the complement cascade, including C3a, C3b, C5a and the membrane attack

Table 12.1 Primary deficiencies of innate immunity[a]

Disease	Defect	Inheritance	Phenotype
Complement deficiency	C2, C4	AR	Immune complex disease
	C3	AR	Increased susceptibility to severe infections; usually lethal
	C5-C9	AR	Recurrent *Neisseria* infections
CGD	gp91^{phox}	X	Increased susceptibility to severe bacterial and fungal infections
	p47^{phox}	AR	
	p67^{phox}	AR	
CHS	*LYST*	AR	Albinism; increased susceptibility to bacterial, fungal and viral infections
Griscelli syndrome (type II)	Rab27A	AR	Albinism; increased susceptibility to bacterial, fungal and viral infections
LAD I	CD18	AR	Increased susceptibility to severe bacterial and fungal infections
LAD II	Fucose transporter	AR	Increased susceptibility to infections; psychological and growth retardation
NK deficiency	Unknown gene on chromosome 8	AR	Increased susceptibility to viral infections especially herpes viruses

[a]**Abbreviations**: AR, autosomal recessive; CGD, chronic granulomatous disease; CHS, Chédiak–Higashi syndrome; NK, natural killer cell; X, X-linked.

complex (MAC), are also affected. Consequently, the acute inflammatory response and neutrophil-mediated phagocytosis are severely impaired in C3-deficient individuals. Inherited deficiency of C3 is rare, but when it occurs it is associated with severe recurrent bacterial infections in infancy and is usually lethal (see *Box 12.1*).

Box 12.1 Treatment of complement deficiencies

Due to the high turnover rate of soluble components of the complement system, replacement therapy is not feasible as this would require daily injections of purified complement proteins. Treatment relies on immunization of affected individuals and prophylactic antibiotic treatment.

Deficiencies of early components (C1, C2, C4) of the classical pathway are normally associated with susceptibility to immune complex diseases like immune complex-mediated glomerulonephritis due to a deficiency in clearing immune complexes. In contrast, deficiencies of the late components of complement (C5–C9), which lead to formation of the MAC in the membranes of susceptible bacteria, are associated with recurrent infections with *Neisseria meningitidis* and *N. gonorrhea*.

The traditional method for assaying complement activity is called the total haemolytic assay (see *Section 13.11*). This assay measures the ability of a serum sample to lyse 50% of a standardized suspension of sheep red blood cells (SRBC) that have been coated with anti-SRBC antibody. This assay is usually referred to as a CH50 assay. It measures classical pathway activation as well as the terminal components that lead to the formation of the MAC. This test is frequently used in initial screening for complement deficiencies.

Chronic granulomatous disease

Chronic granulomatous disease (CGD) is an inherited disorder character- ized by the presence of neutrophils, which are unable to kill certain micro- organisms. Approximately 75% of patients develop the disease through an X-linked form of inheritance. These patients have a defect in a gene on the X chromosome that encodes the gp91^{phox} protein, a subunit of the cytochrome b$_{245}$ component of the NADPH oxidase complex (see *Figure 12.1*). The remaining 25% of affected individuals inherit the disease through an autosomal recessive pattern, with the affected genes encoding other components of NADPH oxidase such as p47^{phox} and p67^{phox}. As a conse- quence, CGD is much more common in males, with female patients accounting for only approximately 15% of cases. The incidence of CGD is approximately 1 in 200 000.

In phagocytes from CGD patients, the respiratory burst does not occur due to the failure to assemble, or due to defective function of, the NADPH oxidase complex. So although the neutrophils from CGD patients will migrate and ingest micro-organisms in response to inflammatory stimuli, they cannot kill the ingested organisms. More phagocytes are recruited to

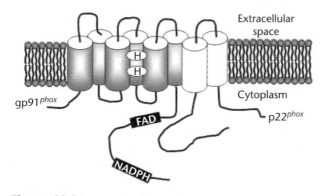

Figure 12.1
The gene that is most frequently mutated in chronic granulomatous disease encodes gp91^{phox}, which together with p22^{phox} forms the cytochrome b$_{245}$ component of NADPH oxidase. The binding sites for FAD, NADPH and haem (H) are indicated.

try to combat the infection and this leads to the formation of a granuloma (see *Section 9.10*). Patients with CGD have an increased susceptibility to recurrent serious infections by bacteria and fungi, necessitating prolonged antibiotic treatment. Fewer than 30% of children with CGD have infectious problems before 3 months of age. However, problems begin to surface soon after, with about 80% developing unusually frequent or severe infections before the age of 2 years. In addition to antibiotics to combat bacterial infections, IFN-γ is now a standard treatment for certain forms of CGD. IFN-γ increases the expression of NADPH oxidase by neutrophils.

Chédiak–Higashi syndrome

Chédiak–Higashi syndrome is a rare autosomal recessive immunodeficiency that presents with partial albinism and photophobia, and is characterized by the presence of large lysosomal granules in leukocytes and giant melanosomes in melanocytes. The disease is caused by a mutation in the *LYST* gene that encodes a lysosomal trafficking regulator protein. Chédiak–Higashi syndrome is sometimes called lysosomal storage disease. Neutrophils from affected individuals exhibit depressed bactericidal activity due to a failure in phago-lysosome formation. NK cells and CTLs from Chédiak–Higashi syndrome patients also are deficient in killing activity because their cytoplasmic granules fail to fuse with the plasma membrane. Fusion of these granules with the plasma membrane is a prerequisite for degranulation of NK cells and CTLs, and for subsequent release of perforin and granzymes from these cells.

Defects in leukocyte extravasation

To allow them to eliminate microbial infections in tissues, leukocytes must extravasate from the circulation across the blood vessel wall into the infected site (see *Section 4.5*). The first step of this process is the adhesion of leukocytes to the endothelial cells lining walls of the blood vessel. If this does not occur, the leukocytes will be swept along in the circulation away from the site of infection. Leukocyte adhesion deficiency (LAD) is a rare disorder in which leukocytes are unable to make strong adhesive contacts with vascular endothelial cells (see *Box 12.2*). Currently three different forms of LAD are recognized.

Box 12.2 Treatment of LAD

Treatment of LAD is focused on control of infections with antibiotic therapy. Severe LAD I has successfully been treated by bone marrow transplantation. Since the genetic defect in LAD I is known, it may one day be possible to correct this disorder by gene therapy.

LAD I

LAD I is the most common form of leukocyte adhesion deficiency. In this disorder there is a mutation in the β_2 integrin molecule CD18, a subunit of the leukocyte adhesion molecules LFA-1 ($\alpha_L\beta_2$ integrin) and Mac-1 ($\alpha_M\beta_2$ integrin). As a result of this mutation, the integrins cannot bind to their counter receptors on endothelial cells, ICAM-1 and ICAM-2. Firm adhesion between these integrins and their counter receptors is required to induce leukocyte arrest on the blood vessel wall. In LAD I the leukocytes fail to adhere tightly to the vascular endothelium and so cannot enter the infected tissue. As the major constituent of pus is dead neutrophils, LAD I is characterized by a lack of pus at sites of infection. LAD I patients present with recurrent bacterial infections from birth. The severity of the disorder is directly related to the degree of expression of CD18 on patients' cells. Severely affected individuals have less than 1% of normal expression of CD18 on their cells and usually die in infancy.

LAD II

LAD II results from a defect in the gene that encodes the golgi GDP-fucose transporter. As a result, the supply of fucose into the golgi apparatus is disrupted and fucosylation of glycoproteins cannot take place. The initial step in leukocyte extravasation into tissues involves the binding of P-selectin and E-selectin on activated endothelial cells to their fucosylated ligand on leukocytes, sialyl-Lewis^X (CD15). Since CD15 is not fucosylated in LAD II, the initial adhesive interaction between the selectins and CD15 cannot occur and leukocyte extravasation is impaired. The frequency and severity of infections in LAD II are less than those observed in LAD I. LAD II patients also suffer severe psychological and growth retardation.

LAD III

This is the most recently described form of leukocyte adhesion deficiency, and results from an inability of integrins to become activated. As a consequence, the integrins remain in their low affinity state and cannot form the tight adhesive interactions with their counter receptors, e.g. ICAM-1 and ICAM-2, which are required for leukocyte extravasation into tissues. The molecular defect(s) in LAD III are unknown.

12.4 PRIMARY IMMUNOGLOBULIN DEFICIENCY SYNDROMES

Primary immunoglobulin deficiency syndromes are disorders characterized by abnormally low levels of one or more immunoglobulin isotypes (see *Table 12.2*). These disorders do not present until after 6 months of age, as an infant is protected from infections by maternal IgG until that time (see *Figure 12.2*). In the normal healthy child, maternal immunoglobulin is sufficient to provide protection until the baby's own immune system is able to produce sufficient immunoglobulin. The last trimester of pregnancy is critical for the transfer of maternal IgG to the fetus. This is augmented by IgA

Table 12.2 Primary immunoglobulin deficiency syndromes[a]

Disease	Defect	Inheritance	Phenotype
Agammaglobulinaemia	Btk	X	Lack of peripheral B cells, deficiency of all immunoglobulin isotypes.
	μ heavy chain	AR	
	CD79a/CD79b	AR	
	BLNK	AR	
	VpreB/λ_5		
Hyper-IgM syndrome	CD40L	X	Elevated serum levels of IgM and low serum levels of all other isotypes.
	CD40	AR	
	AID	AR	
Common variable immunodeficiency	TACI	AR	Deficiency of IgG and IgA. IgM levels also depressed in some patients. Normal peripheral B cell numbers.
	ICOS	AR	
Selective IgA deficiency[b]	TACI	AR	Deficiency of IgA with other isotypes unaffected
	IgA heavy chain genes	AR	
IgG subclass deficiency[b]	IgG heavy chain genes	AR	Deficiency of one or more of the IgG subclasses

[a]**Abbreviations:** AID, activation-induced cytidine deaminase; AR, autosomal recessive; BLNK, B cell linker; ICOS, inducible T cell co-stimulator; TACI, transmembrane activator and CAML interactor; X, X-linked.

[b]The molecular bases of the majority of cases of selective IgA deficiency and of IgG subclass deficiency are unknown.

that is present in the mother's milk, especially in colostrum, the first milk produced. Not all immunoglobulin deficiencies are irreversible. Many children may have transient hypogammaglobulinaemia, but this reverses as soon as the child's immune system becomes sufficiently mature to generate its own immunoglobulin.

The underlying cause of primary immunoglobulin deficiencies can be an intrinsic defect of B cells as in the case of X-linked agammaglobulinaemia. However, because most B cell responses are dependent on T cell help, defective T cell function may also lead to immunoglobulin deficiency, e.g. X-linked hyper-IgM syndrome. In this section clinical features and mechanisms responsible for some of the better-understood primary immunoglobulin deficiencies will be discussed.

X-linked agammaglobulinaemia

X-linked agammaglobulinaemia (XLA), often called Bruton's disease, is a heritable, recessive immunodeficiency disease. This was one of the earliest immunodeficiencies to be described (see *Box 12.3*). It is caused by mutations

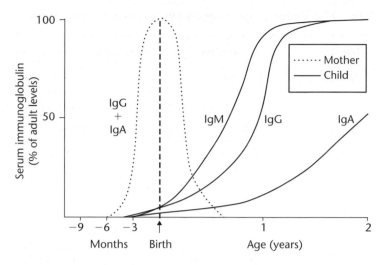

Figure 12.2
The development of immunoglobulin production during infancy takes place over a period of approximately 2 years. Protection by maternal antibodies is critical and lasts for several months after birth.

in the gene that encodes a cytosolic protein tyrosine kinase, Bruton's tyrosine kinase (Btk). *Btk* is localized to the central region of the long arm of the X chromosome at band Xq21.3 to Xq22. More than 340 unique mutations in this gene that result in XLA have been identified. Most of these mutations result in a truncated (incomplete) form of the Btk enzyme. Because males only have one copy of the X chromosome, XLA is much more common in males than in females. Females, however, can be carriers of this disease and may transmit it to their male offspring. The incidence of XLA is approximately 1 in 200 000 male births.

Box 12.3 X-linked agammaglobulinaemia

Dr Ogden Bruton first described XLA, sometimes called Bruton's agammaglobulinaemia, in 1952. The gene that is affected in XLA was discovered in 1993 and was named Bruton's tyrosine kinase, or Btk, in honour of Dr Bruton.

Btk function is required for the proliferation and the differentiation of B cells. It is critical for proper signal transduction in B cells during their development in the bone marrow (see *Figure 12.3*), and in its absence B cells do not develop past the pre-B cell stage. Depending on how completely the specific mutation impairs the function of Btk, affected individuals may have some B cells in the bone marrow and circulation, but their numbers may be reduced 100-fold or more relative to normal (see *Box 12.4*). XLA patients do not have germinal centres in secondary lymphoid tissues and may also lack tonsils and adenoids, which are B cell-rich lymphoid organs. Most cases

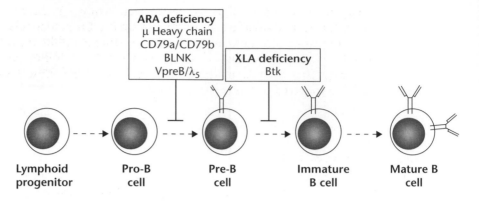

Figure 12.3
X-linked agammaglobulinaemia (XLA) results from a block in B cell development at the pre-B cell stage. In contrast, autosomal recessive agammaglobulinaemia (ARA) results from a block in B cell development at the pro-B cell stage.

Box 12.4 Diagnostic features of XLA

These include extremely low levels (or absence) of serum immunoglobulins as well as the absence of mature B cells. The symptoms are variable, however, and some patients do have low levels of IgM and IgG. If an expectant mother has been identified as a carrier of XLA, amniocentesis can be performed to collect fetal lymphocytes, and the numbers of fetal B cells then can be determined by flow cytometry (see *Section 13.10*). The ultimate confirmation of a diagnosis of XLA would be to show that the patient's cells lack the Btk protein. As patients are usually B cell-deficient, this analysis would have to be performed on patient monocytes or platelets that also express Btk. Due to the large number of Btk mutations that can cause XLA, screening for mutated *Btk* in the patient's DNA would not be realistic.

---

of XLA are characterized by the virtual absence of B lymphocytes and plasma cells. As a result, individuals with XLA are essentially deficient in serum immunoglobulins (agammaglobulinaemic).

Due to the lack of antibodies, XLA patients have increased susceptibility to infections with relatively common extracellular bacterial pathogens such as *Haemophilus influenzae*, *Streptococcus pyogenes*, *S. pneumoniae*, and *Staphylococcus aureus*. These are pyogenic (or pus-forming) bacteria. This increased susceptibility arises because the normal immune response against this type of infection involves opsonization of the pyogenic bacteria by complement-fixing antibody (e.g. IgG2) and complement, followed by efficient phagocytosis of the opsonized bacteria by neutrophils. In the absence of antibody, non-specific phagocytosis by neutrophils is not sufficient to eliminate the bacteria rapidly. Even with antibiotic therapy, this inefficient neutrophil response can lead to chronic inflammation and associated tissue damage. This is particularly common in the lungs where bronchiectasis (widening and scarring of the bronchial tubes) may result. An *in vitro* test to measure the function of neutrophils from these patients would demonstrate that neutrophils were functioning 'normally'. Note, however, that because of the lack of IgG the patients' neutrophils will not be able to perform 'normally' *in vivo*.

Box 12.5 Treatment of XLA

There currently is no cure for XLA. However, since this disease results from mutation of a single gene, it is possible that it may, in the future, be cured by gene therapy. In addition to antibiotic treatment, when appropriate, the current treatment of choice for XLA is intravenous injection of gamma-globulin (IVIG) to maintain serum IgG levels above 5 mg ml^{-1}. This treatment is extremely effective. The gammaglobulin is prepared from a large pool of donors (1000 or more donors). This means that it is likely to contain antibodies against the common pyogenic bacteria. The disadvantages of this treatment are the weekly infusions of immunoglobulin, which is time consuming and can be very unpleasant, as well as the expense of the treatment due to the careful screening required prior to release of human blood products for therapeutic use.

If XLA patients do not receive treatment other than antibiotics, they eventually die from chronic lung disease (see *Box 12.5*). XLA patients may be susceptible to gastrointestinal infections, especially with the *Giardia lamblia* parasite. Although cellular immunity in XLA patients is generally intact, they are prone to certain viral infections (see *Box 12.6*), in particular to enteric and respiratory viruses, most likely due to the deficiency in IgA, the immunoglobulin isotype that protects against infection at mucosal surfaces. Resistance to many other common infections usually is normal.

XLA usually presents in infancy or early childhood, typically at 6–9 months of age, when the protection provided by maternal IgG antibodies has declined. Common infection sites are the inner ear, sinuses and respiratory tract, leading to such recurrent problems as sinusitis, conjunctivitis, otitis media, rhinitis, osteomyelitis, meningitis, septicaemia, bronchitis, and pneumonia. Recurrent gastrointestinal infections occur, occasionally resulting in diarrhoea. In rare cases, adults at the age of around 20 years can be diagnosed with a mild form of XLA. This is presumably because their particular *Btk* mutations do not totally impair Btk enzyme function.

Box 12.6 Live viral vaccines

Patients with serious immune deficiencies, like XLA, should never be given live viral vaccines, as they cannot generate protective antibody responses. XLA patients who received the live oral polio vaccine developed paralytic poliomyelitis.

Common variable immunodeficiency

This disorder shares several features with XLA. Unlike XLA, however, common variable immunodeficiency (CVID) is not X-linked and so affects males and females in equal numbers. It can occur later in life (except for rare cases, XLA always presents in infancy) and, although immunoglobulin levels are low or absent (like XLA), B cell numbers are usually normal in CVID (unlike XLA). It is thought that CVID consists of a heterogeneous group of disorders with distinct molecular bases whose common symptom is a deficiency in the humoral arm of the adaptive immune response, i.e. a common immunodeficiency of variable cause. It is also sometimes referred to as hypogammaglobulinaemia, adult onset agammaglobulinaemia, or late onset hypogammaglobulinaemia. The incidence of CVID in the Caucasian population is approximately 1 in 25 000.

CVID is characterized by a severe deficiency of antibody-producing plasma cells, lower than normal levels of most or all immunoglobulin isotypes (see *Table 2.7*), and recurrent bacterial infections (just like those seen in XLA). In most patients there are reduced serum levels of IgG and IgA, although some patients may have reduced levels of IgM as well. Most patients with CVID have normal numbers of B cells; however, these B cells are unable to secrete antibody or to differentiate into high-level antibody-secreting plasma cells. This, together with the observation of T cell dysfunction in some CVID patients, prompted investigations into whether defective T cell 'help' is responsible for the symptoms of CVID. It has recently been found that 10–20% of CVID patients have mutations in the *TNFRSF13B* gene. This gene encodes the TACI protein, a surface protein of B cells that, in response to its ligands BAFF and APRIL, induces isotype switching to IgG and IgA (see *Section 6.10*). Thus, mutations that impair TACI function could cause the symptoms of some cases of CVID. This hypothesis is supported by the observation that TACI-deficient mice develop autoantibodies, a feature that is also seen in some patients with CVID. It has also been reported that approximately 1% of CVID patients are deficient in ICOS (CD278), a molecule that is important for differentiation of T cells (see *Section 6.4*). The deficiency in ICOS could lead to a defect in T cell cytokine-dependent isotype-switching in these patients.

The majority of patients with CVID are not diagnosed until they are aged 30–40 years (see *Box 12.7*); however, approximately 20% of CVID patients

---

Box 12.7 Common variable immunodeficiency

The diagnosis of CVID in individuals presenting with recurrent infections is confirmed by the finding of low levels of serum immunoglobulins, including IgG, IgA and usually IgM, but normal numbers of B cells. Like XLA, treatment of CVID involves the appropriate use of antibotics and IVIG. This almost always provides clinical improvement; however, since gammaglobulin preparations contain little IgA and IgM, the total antibody deficiency is not replaced. It is not uncommon for CVID patients to present with intestinal giardiasis, but this is effectively treated with metronidazole.

are under the age of 16 years. Although patients with CVID are hypogammaglobulinaemic, some of the antibodies that they produce are autoantibodies, in particular autoantibodies directed against red blood cells or platelets. As many as 10–20% of individuals with CVID first present with anaemia or thrombocytopaenia.

Similar to XLA, frequently presenting problems in CVID are recurrent infections of the ears, sinuses, bronchi, and lungs. If these infections are both severe and repeatedly occurring, there may be permanent damage to the bronchi, resulting in bronchiectasis. Common bacteria that often cause infection in CVID are the same as those indicated above for XLA. Gastrointestinal complaints occur frequently in CVID and may include abdominal pain, bloating, nausea, vomiting, diarrhoea, or weight loss. These symptoms may be indicative of malabsorption of fat or certain sugars, or may be due to infection with the *Giardia lamblia* parasite. In some CVID patients, large numbers of activated B cells may accumulate in lymphoid tissue. These B cells have probably been stimulated by bacteria or other foreign antigens, but cannot differentiate further to antibody-secreting plasma cells. This accumulation of B cells causes marked peripheral lymph node and spleen enlargement, a clinical feature that is not seen in XLA patients. See *Box 12.8* for a Case Study.

Box 12.8 Case study

Bill is a 36-year-old man who is admitted to hospital with pneumonia and recurrent diarrhoea. This is his second episode of pneumonia in the last 18 months. During that time he has also had five episodes of sinusitis. A jejunal aspirate was found to contain *Giardia lamblia*. Four years ago he was treated for anaemia. Laboratory tests on a sample of Bill's serum revealed the following:

IgG – 1.8 mg ml^{-1}
IgM – 0.2 mg ml^{-1}
IgA – 0.25 mg ml^{-1}
CH50 – normal

In addition, Bill had normal numbers of B cells and T cells in his peripheral blood. His older brother is receiving treatment for selective IgA deficiency.

1. Does Bill have selective IgA deficiency? Explain your reasoning.
2. How may Bill's disorder be distinguished from X-linked agammaglobulinaemia?
3. What would be the most appropriate treatment for Bill's condition?

Selective IgA deficiency

This immune deficiency is characterized by the total absence or severe deficiency of IgA. The disorder is termed 'selective' because other serum Ig isotypes are present at normal or increased levels, and the functions of T cells, phagocytes and complement are also normal. This is a relatively common immune deficiency with an incidence as high as 1 in 400, although it has been reported that the incidence of selective IgA deficiency is considerably lower in persons of Japanese descent. The serum levels of IgA in individuals with IgA deficiency are usually found to be 0.05 mg ml^{-1} or less, whereas serum IgA in normal adults ranges from 0.8 to 4.5 mg ml^{-1}. IgA serves to protect from infections at mucosal surfaces, therefore the most common recurrent infections in IgA-deficient patients are bacterial or viral infections at these sites.

The clinical spectrum of IgA deficiency varies from asymptomatic to significant illness (see *Box 12.9*). Thus, some IgA-deficient people may be unaware of their antibody deficiency, succumbing to no more than the usual number of upper respiratory infections and/or occasional diarrhoea. The reason why some IgA-deficient patients have more illness than others is not clear, although some affected individuals also lack a fraction of their lgG2 and/or IgG4 immunoglobulin pool and this may contribute to disease severity. IgA deficiency does not become detectable until approximately 6 months of age. For those IgA-deficient patients with a history of recurrent infections, the most common problems are ear infections, sinusitis and pneumonia. Other infection sites can be the throat, gastrointestinal tract or eyes. These infections may become chronic and may be refractory to antibiotic treatment, necessitating prolonged antibiotic therapy.

IgA deficiency in these patients arises because their B cells are unable to make the isotype switch necessary to become IgA-producing plasma cells. The exact causes of IgA deficiency are still largely unknown although there is evidence of familial inheritance. IgA deficiency also occurs frequently in immediate relatives of persons with CVID, suggesting a similar cause for the two disorders. This is supported by the finding that, like some CVID patients, a subset of patients with IgA deficiency has mutations in the gene encoding TACI. These mutations could explain the failure to isotype switch to IgA in these patients. In rare cases, partial IgA deficiency has been linked to deletions of the *IGA1* or *IGA2* genes that encode the heavy chains of the two IgA subclasses.

Autoantibodies may be present in some 40% of cases of IgA deficiency and autoimmune diseases are a common clinical presentation of people with this disorder. The autoimmune diseases most frequently seen in IgA deficiency are rheumatoid arthritis, systemic lupus erythematosus, Sjögren's syndrome, thyroiditis, and haemolytic anaemia.

Allergies, usually asthma and food allergies, are another common problem with IgA deficiency and these may range from mild to severe. A

Box 12.9 IgA deficiency

The diagnosis of IgA deficiency in individuals presenting with recurrent infections is confirmed by the finding of selectively low levels of serum IgA, but normal or slightly elevated numbers of B cells. There is currently no cure for IgA deficiency. Treatment options for this disease are restricted to treating the infections when they arise. Immunoglobulin injections are of no use for this condition as the concentration of IgA in these preparations is very low. In addition, intravenously administered IgA is not efficiently transported to mucosal surfaces in individuals with IgA deficiency.

more unusual form of allergy that occurs in people who have a total absence of IgA is an allergic reaction to IgA. Exposure through blood products containing IgA causes IgA-deficient individuals to develop antibodies against this foreign protein. Consequently, administration of blood products to IgA-deficient patients may induce anaphylactic shock.

X-linked hyper-IgM syndrome

X-linked hyper-IgM syndrome (XHIM) is characterized by abnormally low serum levels of IgA and IgG, accompanied by abnormally high serum levels of IgM. The clinical course is like that of XLA except for a greater frequency of 'autoimmune' haematological disorders (neutropaenia, haemolytic anaemia, thrombocytopaenia). In contrast to XLA patients who lack tonsils, tonsillar hypertrophy may occur in hyper-IgM patients due to infiltration with IgM-containing plasma cells. Neutropaenia may also be present leading to gingivitis, ulcerative stomatitis, fever and weight loss (see *Box 12.10*).

The gene that is mutated in XHIM patients is the X chromosome-encoded CD154 (CD40L) gene. The disease is an X-linked recessive disorder and female carriers have normal serum levels of IgG and IgA. Patients with XHIM express functional CD40 and, *in vitro*, their B cells respond normally to wild type CD154. However, as a result of their mutations in CD154, antigen-specific T cells in affected individuals are unable to instruct B cells to class switch from IgM to IgG, IgA or IgE (see *Section 6.10*). Consequently, serum levels of IgA and IgG are severely deficient, whereas IgM is elevated.

Like XLA, XHIM presents in infancy. Also like XLA and CVID, XHIM patients are susceptible to recurrent respiratory infections, and sometimes to enteric infections. The common pathogens affecting individuals with XHIM are the same as those indicated above for XLA.

Box 12.10 X-linked hyper-IgM syndrome

The diagnosis of XHIM in individuals presenting with recurrent infections is confirmed by the finding of high levels of serum IgM, but with abnormally low levels of the other immunoglobulin isotypes. There is currently no cure for XHIM, but since the disease results from mutation of a single gene, it is possible that it may, in the future, be cured by gene therapy. Like XLA and CVID, the treatment of choice for XHIM is IVIG.

IgG subclass deficiency

This occurs when there is an imbalance of the IgG subclasses with one or more subclasses being deficient (see *Box 12.11*). Babies are protected by maternal IgG for the first 6 months of their lives. During that time they start to make their own IgG. In general, serum concentrations of IgG1 and IgG3

Box 12.11 IgG subclass deficiency

Diagnosis of IgG subclass deficiency should demonstrate that the level of total immunoglobulin in serum is normal or only slightly depressed but that there is a selective deficiency of one or more of the four IgG subclasses. Usually antibiotic treatment, together with the patient's largely intact adaptive response, is sufficient to control the recurring infections in affected patients. In more serious cases, for example when two or more IgG subclasses are absent, IVIG has been shown to be of benefit.

reach adult levels by approximately 6 years of age, whereas IgG2 and IgG4 do not attain adult levels until 10 years of age. However, the rate at which IgG subclasses attain adult levels can vary substantially between individuals, so if a child is diagnosed with IgG subclass deficiency, they should be monitored to check if the situation has changed. Many children with IgG subclass deficiency acquire normal levels of serum IgG subclasses later in life. Note that even if the total level of serum IgG is normal, individual subclass levels may be higher or lower than normal. Just like in selective IgA deficiency, some patients with IgG subclass deficiency develop autoimmunity. In a minority of cases, IgG subclass deficiency is associated with mutations or deletions in the gene segments that encode the constant region of particular IgG subclasses. It is likely that mutations that impact on the class switch recombination process are responsible for other cases of IgG subclass deficiency.

Individuals with IgG subclass deficiency have increased susceptibility to infection. This is particularly true of IgG2-deficient patients who frequently have a history of recurrent pyogenic infections from childhood. Patients can present with a history of frequent infections involving the respiratory tract such as sinusitis, bronchitis and pneumonia. The nature of the recurring infection is dependent on the major function of the IgG subclass that is absent. IgG2-deficient patients may have a poor response to some vaccines, such as pneumococcal, or *Haemophilus influenzae* vaccines.

12.5 PRIMARY DEFICIENCIES OF CELL-MEDIATED IMMUNITY

Unlike the rather lengthy list of primary immunoglobulin deficiency syndromes, there are relatively few primary deficiencies of cell-mediated immunity. It is not that they do not occur, rather that when they do occur the deficiencies are so severe that they impair immunoglobulin responses as well. As a result, many immunodeficiencies that result from an intrinsic defect of T cells are classified as combined immunodeficiencies (see *Section 12.6*).

Thymic aplasia

Thymic aplasia, or thymic hypoplasia, is characterized by the absence of, or severe reduction in, thymic tissue. Because T cells develop in the thymus, thymic aplasia can result in a marked reduction in the numbers of CD4$^+$ and CD8$^+$ T cells (see *Box 12.12*). Thymic aplasia is rare, but the most common of these disorders are DiGeorge syndrome and Nezelof's syndrome.

Box 12.12 DiGeorge and Nezelof's syndromes

For severely immunodeficient children with DiGeorge or Nezelof's syndrome, grafting of at least partially MHC-matched thymic tissue is sometimes performed. The majority of children with DiGeorge or Nezelof's syndrome that show signs of immunodeficiency have only a mild to moderate deficit in T cell numbers. These patients usually do not require transplantation.

DiGeorge syndrome

DiGeorge syndrome is a congenital immune disorder characterized by lack of embryonic development or underdevelopment of the third and fourth pharyngeal pouches, which normally develop into the thymus. The majority of patients with DiGeorge syndrome have a small deletion of part of chromosome 22 (at position 22q11.2). DiGeorge syndrome is now commonly referred to as Chromosome 22q11.2 deletion syndrome.

Complete absence of the thymus is rare. When it occurs, cell-mediated immune responses are undetectable and T cell areas of lymphoid tissues are sparsely populated. Humoral responses are also suboptimal, reflecting the need for T cell help for the majority of antibody responses. Because of the central role of T cells in adaptive immunity, these individuals are susceptible to a wide range of bacterial and viral infections. The most common form of this disorder is partial DiGeorge syndrome. In this disorder there is enough thymic tissue present to allow the development of sufficient numbers of T cells so that affected individuals are not overtly immunodeficient.

Other tissues also develop from the third and fourth pharyngeal pouches, so individuals with DiGeorge syndrome may have defects in several organs. Facial characteristics associated with this syndrome vary greatly, but may include underdeveloped chin, ear lobe abnormalities and cleft palate. Individuals with DiGeorge syndrome may also lack parathyroid glands and frequently have severe cardiovascular disorders.

Nezelof's syndrome

Nezelof's syndrome is an extremely rare immunodeficiency characterized by the lack of a thymus, or by a small or abnormal thymus. Unlike DiGeorge syndrome, the parathyroid gland is unaffected in Nezelof's syndrome. Cell-mediated immune responses of affected individuals are depressed or absent and they do not reject allogeneic skin grafts. Immunoglobulin responses appear normal except in cases of severe T cell deficiency when humoral responses are also depressed. The cause of Nezelof's syndrome is unknown; however, family studies suggest an autosomal recessive inheritance.

Bare lymphocyte syndrome

Bare lymphocyte syndrome (BLS) is an autosomal recessive disorder in which MHC molecules are absent from the surfaces of cells. In these diseases the MHC genes themselves are normal; however, there are mutations in genes whose products are required for expression of MHC molecules. BLS is subdivided into different groups depending on whether MHC class I, class II, or both class I and class II molecules are deficient.

BLS I

Several cases of BLS I have been described where the affected individuals have mutations in the genes encoding TAP-1, TAP-2 or tapasin. *TAP-1* or *TAP-2* mutations impair the function of the TAP complex so few peptides get into the ER to bind to MHC class I molecules (see *Section 5.10*). A defect in tapasin results in a peptide loading complex that will inefficiently transfer peptides from TAP to MHC class I molecules. As a result of these mutations, the levels of MHC class I molecules on the surfaces of cells in affected individuals is low. Because of the low expression of MHC class I in the thymus, there is poor selection of CD8$^+$ T cells and individuals with BLS I have decreased numbers of mature TCRα/β-expressing CD8$^+$ T cells. Surprisingly, most people with BLS I do not show an increased susceptibility to viral infections, suggesting that TAP-independent mechanisms of peptide presentation on MHC class I molecules are sufficient for control of viral infections in these individuals. Affected individuals are more susceptible to chronic bacterial infections of the respiratory tract.

BLS II

BLS II is a genetically heterogeneous disease resulting from mutations in several transcription factors that regulate the expression of MHC class II genes. BLS II is subdivided into four groups (A–D) depending on the identity of the mutated gene. The genes that are mutated in BLS II encode the MHC class II transactivator *CTIIA* (group A), and the components of the RFX transcription factor *RFXANK* (group B), *RFX5* (group C) and *RFXAP* (group D). Because of the low expression of MHC class II in the thymus, there is poor selection of CD4$^+$ T cells. Any CD4$^+$ T cells that do develop will be largely non-functional due to the poor expression of MHC class II on APCs in the periphery. Because of the central role of CD4$^+$ T cells in immunity, BLS II patients are severely deficient in cell-mediated and humoral immune responses. Consequently, BLS II is sometimes classified as a severe combined immunodeficiency (SCID), although unlike classic SCID (see *Section 12.6*), BLS II patients do exhibit some lymphocyte function, in particular CD8$^+$ T cell function. Affected individuals are much more susceptible to a wide range of infections and, if untreated, frequently die in childhood due to chronic diarrhoea and repeated bacterial and viral infections. Because the RFX transcription factor also regulates expression of MHC class I genes, individuals with groups B, C and D BLS II also have poor expression of MHC class I molecules on their cells. Some investigators refer to these three subsets of BLS II as BLS III.

Wiskott–Aldrich syndrome

Wiskott–Aldrich syndrome (WAS) is an X-linked recessive disorder. The symptoms of the disease vary greatly but affected individuals may present with severe eczema, thrombocytopaenia (see *Box 12.13*), bleeding, and immunodeficiency due to depressed T cell function and reduced T cell numbers. Affected individuals usually die from haemorrhaging or overwhelming infections during the first few years of life. The incidence of WAS is approximately 1 in 250 000.

Box 12.13 Treatment of WAS

The spleen is the main site of removal of platelets, therefore thrombocytopaenia associated with WAS may be treated by splenectomy. However, this should only be performed if the platelet count is severely depressed, as this procedure puts the patient at risk of infections with encapsulated bacteria (e.g. *S. pneumoniae* or *H. influenzae*). In such cases the patient would receive life-long prophylactic antibiotics.

WAS results from mutation of the gene encoding the Wiskott–Aldrich syndrome protein (WASP), which is only expressed in cells of the haematopoietic lineage. WASP binds to an intracellular GTPase called Cdc42, which regulates the organization of the actin cytoskeleton, and has been shown to be important for T cell–B cell interactions. To date, more than 100 different WASP mutations have been found in WAS patients. This explains the variability of the symptoms seen in this disease, because the nature of the WASP mutation will determine the severity of the disease. Seriously affected individuals are susceptible to a variety of bacterial and viral infections, in addition to bleeding. Less inactivating WASP mutations cause X-linked thrombocytopaenia with no overt immunodeficiency.

Approximately 10% of WAS patients develop malignancies, usually lymphoma or leukaemia. In addition, up to 70% of WAS patients also develop autoimmune disease. This may be explained by the recent observations that WASP is required for the development and function of T_{REG} cells which are known to be important in maintaining tolerance to self antigens (see *Sections 7.6* and *10.2*).

Type 2 familial haemophagocytic lymphohistiocytosis

Type 2 familial haemophagocytic lymphohistiocytosis (FHL2) is a rare disease characterized by fever, hepatosplenomegaly, haemophagocytosis (phagocytosis of erythrocytes, leukocytes, and platelets by macrophages) in bone marrow and lymphoid organs, dysregulated proliferation of $CD8^+$ T cells and infiltration of $CD8^+$ cells into multiple tissues. FHL2 is usually associated with infection with Epstein–Barr virus or other viruses.

FHL2 is caused by a mutation in the gene that encodes perforin so that the function of this protein is impaired in affected individuals. Because of this, $CD8^+$ T cells and NK cells in FHL2 patients are compromised in their ability to kill virus-infected cells. The viral antigen persists and stimulates prolonged expansion of T cells. In addition, the perforin-dependent down-regulation of the immune response (see *Section 7.5*) is also impaired in FHL2. As a result, the proliferation of T cells and macrophages is unchecked and this leads to a marked increase in the level of cytokines, including IFN-γ and TNF-α, in the blood. FHL2 is invariably lethal unless immunosuppressants are used to inhibit the progressive T cell-dependent inflammation.

X-linked lymphoproliferative disease

X-linked lymphoproliferative disease (XLP), also called Duncan's disease, is an extremely rare immunodeficiency with a frequency of less than 1 in a million. The disease can manifest in many forms. The three most common forms are fatal infectious mononucleosis, lymphoma, and hypogammaglob-ulinaemia. Symptoms can present as early as 6 months of age and nearly 75% of patients die before 10 years of age (see *Box 12.14*).

Box 12.14 Treatment of XLP

There is no cure for XLP; however, because the gene responsible for this disorder is known, the disease may be amenable to gene therapy in the future. Currently, bone marrow transplantation is the treatment of choice.

   In XLP patients, the gene that encodes the signal-transducing molecule called SLAM-associated protein (SAP) is mutated. SAP is an adaptor protein that regulates T cell and NK cell activation. The precise mechanism whereby SAP mutations give rise to XLP is unclear; however, it has been suggested that CTLs from XLP patients are unable to kill EBV-infected B cells *in vivo*. The persistence of viral antigen would lead to mononucleosis due to profound antigen-induced proliferation of EBV-specific T cells. Since EBV is a transforming virus of B cells, failure to control EBV infection can lead to development of B cell lymphoma.

12.6   SEVERE COMBINED IMMUNODEFICIENCY

Some of the most serious primary immunodeficiencies are those in which the development and/or functions of both B cells and T cells, and frequently of NK cells, are impaired. Collectively these disorders are termed combined immunodeficiencies (CID). The most serious of these are characterized by the absence of T cells and, as a consequence, lack of B cell function as well. This form of combined immunodeficiency is called severe combined immunodeficiency (SCID). SCID results in marked susceptibility to severe and complicated infections with bacterial, viral, fungal and protozoal pathogens. Exposure to the varicella zoster (chickenpox) virus, either through live vaccine or in the environment, can be life-threatening with infection of the lungs and/or brain. The relatively common cytomegalovirus (CMV), found in the salivary glands of many people, can cause fatal pneumonia in children with SCID. The onset of infection in SCID usually occurs in the first 6 months of life. If untreated, affected babies usually die within a year due to severe, recurrent opportunistic infections. Infants with SCID must receive a bone marrow transplant if they are to survive.

SCID is actually a group of disorders each with a distinct genetic basis (see *Table 12.3*), and there are a number of cases of SCID for which the genetic basis is unknown. There is disagreement in the scientific literature regarding the classification of CID disorders as SCID. For example, BLS II, as well as the diseases caused by deficiencies of the enzymes purine nucleotide phosphorylase or ZAP-70, are usually clinically less severe than classic SCID. Consequently many researchers do not consider them to fulfil the criteria to be categorized as SCID. In contrast, other researchers consider these diseases to belong to the spectrum of SCID disorders. Because of the variation in the classification of these disorders, estimates of the frequency of SCID vary between 1 in 100 000 and 1 in 500 000 live births.

The most common form of SCID is caused by a genetic mutation localized to the proximal part of the long arm of the X chromosome; however, there also are autosomal recessive forms of this disorder, the most predominant form being that caused by deficiency of the enzyme adenosine deaminase.

Table 12.3 Classification of severe combined immunodeficiencies[a]

Mechanism	Mutated gene product	Inheritance	Affected cells[b]
Defective cytokine signalling	γc (IL-2Rγ)	X	T, NK
	JAK3	AR	T, NK
	IL-7Rα	AR	T
Premature cell death	ADA	AR	T, B, NK
	PNP	AR	T
Defective V(D)J recombination	RAG-1/RAG-2	AR	T, B
	ARTEMIS	AR	T, B
Defective signalling	TCR CD3δ/ε/ζ	AR	T
	CD45	AR	T
	ZAP-70	AR	T subset[c]

[a]**Abbreviations:** ADA, adenosine deaminase; AR, autosomal recessive; γc, common γ chain; IL, interleukin; JAK, Janus kinase; PNP, purine nucleotide phosphorylase; RAG, recombination activating gene; ZAP-70, zeta-associated polypeptide of 70 kDa.

[b]In many forms of severe combined immunodeficiency B cell development is not affected. In these instances, however, B cell function is severely compromised due to the lack of T cell help.

[c]ZAP-70 deficiency is characterized by a lack of CD8+ T cells. CD4+ T cells are present but cannot respond to antigen.

X-linked SCID

The most common form of SCID (approximately 50% of SCID cases in the USA) is due to mutation of a gene that is located on the X chromosome (see *Box 12.15*). This gene, *IL2RG*, encodes the common γ chain of the receptors for the cytokines IL-2, IL-4, IL-7, IL-9, IL-15 and IL-21 (see *Figure 12.4*). Mutations that result in a non-functional γ chain lead to a block in T cell and NK cell development due to an inability of precursor cells to respond to IL-7 and IL-15, cytokines that are crucial for development of these cell types. Consequently, individuals with X-linked SCID (X-SCID) are deficient in T cells and NK cells. In contrast, B cells are present but are non-functional. Less inactivating mutations of the *IL2RG* gene cause a less severe disorder, which has been termed X-CID.

Box 12.15 The 'boy in the bubble'

David Vetter (21 September 1971–22 February 1984), the original 'boy in the bubble' was born with X-linked SCID. He was raised in a sterile plastic incubator designed to protect him from infections. At the age of 12 he received bone marrow from his sister in an attempt to reconstitute his immune system. Sadly, the donated marrow contained Epstein–Barr virus (EBV). David died a short time afterwards from EBV-induced lymphoma.

This disease is inherited in an X-linked recessive pattern. Since males have one X chromosome, all males who have a defective *IL2RG* gene will develop X-SCID. Since females have two X chromosomes, females with one defective and one normal copy of the gene will not develop SCID but will be carriers.

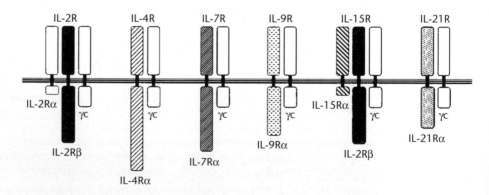

Figure 12.4
The IL-2 receptor (IL-2R) γ chain, or common γ chain (γc), is also a component of the receptors for IL-4, IL-7, IL-9, IL-15 and IL-21. In addition, the IL-15 receptor also contains the IL-2 receptor β chain.

Autosomal recessive SCID

Adenosine deaminase deficiency

Approximately 30% of children diagnosed with SCID are deficient in adenosine deaminase (ADA), an enzyme that is necessary for the breakdown of purines. Like all autosomal recessive disorders, if a child is to be affected they must inherit defective alleles of the gene from both parents. This form of SCID (ADA-SCID) results in a build up of deoxy-ATP (dATP) which inhibits the generation of deoxyribonucleotides in the cell. dATP accumulation is toxic to early lymphoid progenitor cells. Individuals with this form of SCID are largely deficient in T cells, B cells and NK cells.

Janus kinase 3 deficiency

Janus kinase 3 (JAK3) is an intracellular tyrosine kinase encoded on chromosome 19. JAK3 is required for transduction of intracellular signals from γ chain containing cytokine receptors. Consequently, mutations that disrupt JAK3 function cause a form of SCID that closely resembles X-SCID. Since this form of SCID is inherited in an autosomal recessive manner both boys and girls are affected. This disorder accounts for less than 10% of all cases of SCID.

Defects in V(D)J recombination

A rare autosomal recessive form of SCID has been described in which affected individuals fail to successfully recombine TCR and immunoglobulin genes. Genes found to be mutated in this form of SCID include the recombinase activating genes *RAG1* and *RAG2* as well as the gene that encodes the DNA repair factor ARTEMIS. As the products of these genes are required for successful V(D)J recombination (see *Section 3.2*), individuals with inactivating mutations in these genes lack mature T cells and B cells.

Treatment of SCID

The treatment of choice for children with SCID is bone marrow transplantation, ideally from a normal MHC-matched sibling donor. Prior to transplantation, the patient undergoes irradiation or chemotherapy to eliminate defective host bone marrow stem cells. In the absence of an MHC-matched donor, patients can be given a T cell depleted bone marrow transplant from a partially MHC-matched donor. T cell depletion is required to prevent GvHD (see *Section 11.11*). Without a bone marrow transplant, a child with SCID is at constant risk of severe or fatal infection and may be best kept in sterile isolation. Without treatment, survival beyond the first year of life is unusual. In ADA-SCID, if there is no suitable bone marrow donor the patient can receive regular injections of ADA that has been stabilized by the addition of polyethylene glycol.

There have been attempts to correct the defective gene in X-SCID and ADA-SCID patients by gene therapy. The results of these trials have suggested that this therapeutic approach is feasible. Unfortunately, in one trial of gene therapy for X-SCID, three of the patients developed acute lymphoblastic leukaemia due to the site of integration into the genome of the gene therapy vector. However, gene therapy is still the best hope of a cure for this disease. Additional gene therapy trials for ADA-SCID and X-SCID are ongoing.

12.7 SECONDARY IMMUNODEFICIENCIES

Secondary immunodeficiencies are not the result of intrinsic defects of components of the immune system but instead result from conditions that are acquired during life. They frequently occur as a result of a disease process or damage to some other body system, which then impacts upon the functions of the immune system. Unlike primary immunodeficiencies, which are rare disorders, secondary immunodeficiencies occur frequently and are a significant cause of morbidity and mortality worldwide. Causes of secondary immunodeficiencies include:

■ immunosuppressive drugs
■ irradiation and chemotherapy
■ malignancies
■ malnutrition
■ ageing
■ viral infections, e.g. measles virus, HIV

Infectious diseases may also be a serious complication in patients who have sustained serious burns, the principal reason being the significant amount of skin loss, with skin being the major barrier against invasion by pathogens. In addition, surgical procedures such as splenectomy can lead to increased susceptibility to infections. People undergoing splenectomy, e.g. for treatment of WAS (see *Box 12.13*), should receive prophylactic antibiotics for the rest of their lives as they will be at greater risk of infections with encapsulated bacteria.

Immunosuppressive drugs

To minimize the risk of graft rejection following tissue transplantation, the recipient is given immunosuppressive drugs (see *Section 11.6*). By definition these drugs counteract the immune response. Most transplant recipients need some level of immunosuppression for the rest of their lives to prevent transplant rejection. The balance between risk of rejection and risk from infectious disease is one that must be maintained through constant vigilance and clinical follow-up, and the dose of the immunosuppressive drugs adjusted accordingly. One way to overcome this problem would be to develop effective antigen-specific immunosuppressive therapies that would inhibit immune responses against the transplanted tissue, but would leave all other immune responses unhindered.

Irradiation and chemotherapy

Radiotherapy and chemotherapy are frequently used to treat malignancies. These treatments work by destroying rapidly proliferating cells such as malignant cells. However, they will also destroy other rapidly dividing cells such as precursor cells in the bone marrow and mature lymphocytes. This can lead to profound immunosuppression.

Malignancies

In animal models it has been found that during the later stages of tumour growth, immune responses against a variety of antigens are suppressed. For example, melanoma patients have depressed CTL responses against influenza A virus. Several mechanisms have been proposed to account for this tumour-induced immunosuppression (see *Figure 12.5*). Chief among

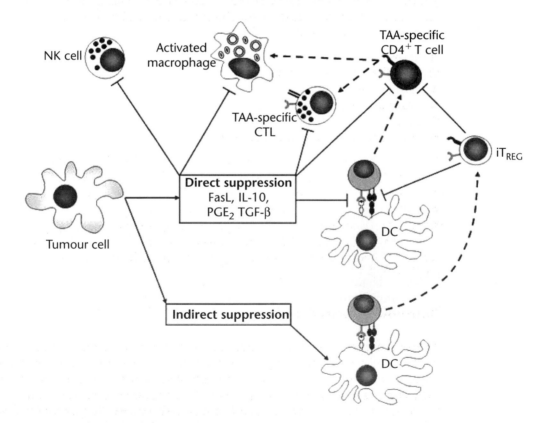

Figure 12.5
Molecules expressed by tumour cells have been shown to directly inhibit the activation and function of tumour-associated antigen (TAA)-specific CD4+ T cells and of macrophages, NK cells and CTLs, the main effector cells of anti-tumour immune responses. Tumour cells can also indirectly suppress anti-tumour immune responses by promoting the differentiation of inducible regulatory T cells (iT_REG cells).

these is the production of TGF-β by certain tumour cells. This immuno-suppressive cytokine inhibits T cell proliferation and suppresses the production of the pro-inflammatory cytokines IFN-γ and TNF-α. It may also bias T cell differentiation in favour of suppressor T_{REG} cells (see *Section 6.4*). Inhibition of TGF-β production *in vivo* has been demonstrated to alleviate tumour-associated immunosuppression.

Malnutrition

Malnutrition, in particular protein-calorie malnutrition, can cause extensive metabolic and hormonal changes and lead to generalized immunosuppression. Even modest systemic nutritional deficiency results in reduced DTH responses and decreased T cell numbers. Neutrophil function is reduced, and while phagocytosis is generally not affected, the ability to destroy ingested bacteria appears to decline. Malnutrition-associated immunosuppression is a major problem in many nations, and pathogens that generally only cause mild symptoms can cause serious disease and even death in malnourished individuals.

Ageing

In general, immune responses diminish with age. This phenomenon is termed immunosenescence. As a result, older people are afflicted by a large variety of infectious problems, which are accompanied by higher mortality rates than those seen in the younger population. The increase in some infections is dramatic, such as the strong association of herpes zoster (shingles) with increasing age. Others are more subtle, such as the increased risk of mortality due to influenza in the elderly. Skin testing with a panel of common antigens to which most individuals have become immune throughout life is a good measure of how well the immune system is responding. Unresponsiveness to antigens despite previous exposure is common in subjects over 65 years of age.

Many factors can contribute to immunosenescence. The ageing-associated thinning of skin and drying of skin and mucus membranes renders them more susceptible to injury or invasion by bacteria. Production of mature T cells may decrease as a result of the thymic involution that accompanies ageing. The number of mature $CD8^+$ T cells declines with age while $CD4^+$ T cells show little change in absolute number. Studies in mice and humans have found that there is an accumulation of memory T cells in aged individuals and a concomitant decrease in the numbers of naïve T cells. This means that in aged individuals there are fewer T cells to respond against pathogens that the immune system has not previously encountered.

The most prominent change in immune function associated with ageing is the decrease in lymphocyte proliferative responses. Lymphocyte proliferative responses decline gradually throughout life. This decrease in proliferative responses may be due to replicative senescence. This results from the progressive shortening of telomeres (see *Box 12.16*) during cell division.

Box 12.16 Telomeres

Telomeres are repetitive sequences of DNA found at the end of chromosomes. DNA replication cannot proceed all the way to the ends of the chromosomes so the telomeres protect against loss of coding sequence during cell division. Shortening of telomeres during mitosis limits the number of times that a cell can divide.

Nutritional abnormalities are common in the elderly and may compound immunosenescence. Undernourished elderly individuals are more likely than their well-nourished counterparts to die from infectious diseases.

Viral infection

Infections with certain viruses such as Epstein–Barr virus (EBV) and measles virus can cause generalized immunosuppression. In the case of the B cell-tropic virus EBV, this is partly due to the destruction of EBV-infected B cells by virus-specific CTLs. EBV-associated immunosuppression may also be due in part to the production of a viral homologue of the anti-inflammatory cytokine IL-10 (vIL-10) by EBV-infected cells, thus inhibiting cell-mediated immune responses. It has long been recognized that co-infection of *Mycobacterium tuberculosis*-infected individuals with measles virus results in disseminated tuberculosis. Immunosuppression by measles virus is still a cause for concern in countries where measles vaccine coverage is low. The host receptor for measles virus is CD46. Binding of the virus to CD46 on DCs and macrophages inhibits the production of IL-12 by these cells and, consequently, suppresses cell-mediated immune responses. Ligation of CD46 on T cells during T cell activation favours the development of suppressor Tr1 cells (see *Section 7.6*) and this may also contribute to measles-associated immunosuppression.

HIV infection and AIDS

The most devastating secondary immunodeficiency is acquired immune deficiency syndrome (AIDS), which is caused by the human immunodeficiency virus (HIV) (see *Box 12.17*). HIV is a retrovirus belonging to the lentivirus family. There are two species of HIV called HIV-1 and HIV-2. These species are closely related and both are believed to have originated in West-Central Africa. HIV-1 is thought to have evolved from the simian immunodeficiency virus SIV_{cpz} passing to humans from wild chimpanzees (*Pan troglodytes*). HIV-2 is thought to have evolved from a simian immunodeficiency virus that infects the Sooty Mangabey (*Cercocebus atys*). HIV-2 is primarily found in Western Africa, Mozambique and Angola, and is spreading in India. HIV-2 is less easily transmitted than the more virulent HIV-1, which is responsible for most cases of AIDS worldwide. AIDS is a global problem, with most cases occurring in sub-Saharan Africa, Asia, South

America, Eastern Europe and the USA. Currently, approximately 68% of all people who are infected with HIV live in sub-Saharan Africa.

Box 12.17 HIV

In the late 1970s and early 1980s young people, predominantly men, were seen to be presenting to hospitals and clinics in the USA with symptoms of infectious disease not normally seen in people of their age group in westernized countries. The virus responsible, HIV, was isolated and identified in 1983.

HIV can be transmitted by transfer of contaminated blood or blood products, semen, vaginal fluid, or breast milk, or by placental transfer. Mother to child transmission of HIV can occur at childbirth but such transmission of HIV-2 is rare. Rigorous screening of blood products for HIV contamination has mostly eliminated transfusion-mediated HIV infection in the developed world. HIV has been detected at low levels in saliva, urine and tears of HIV$^+$ individuals but the potential risk of viral transmission via these secretions is considered negligible. Consequently, the main mechanisms of transmission of HIV-1 are unprotected sexual intercourse, contaminated needles, breast-feeding by infected mothers, and mother to child transmission at childbirth.

Like all viruses, HIV-1 is an obligate intracellular parasite and can replicate only within nucleated cells. The primary receptor for HIV is the CD4 molecule. CD4 occurs in highest density on CD4$^+$ T cells, but also on DCs, macrophages and macrophage-like cells throughout the body, e.g. glial cells and astrocytes in the central nervous system. The immunodeficiency (AIDS) associated with late stage HIV infection results from the destruction of CD4$^+$ T cells and the resultant decline in cell-mediated immunity.

HIV-1 structure and replication

An HIV-1 particle consists of two identical RNA molecules contained within a proteinaceous nucleocapsid core composed of multimers of the p24 protein (see *Figure 12.6*). The nucleocapsid is surrounded by a matrix made up of p17 protein, which is surrounded by a lipid envelope that is derived from host cells. The major envelope glycoprotein, gp120, is attached to the lipid envelope by the gp41 protein. An infectious HIV particle also contains multiple copies of the viral protease, integrase and reverse transcriptase (RT) enzymes.

During infection of a cell, HIV-1 gp120 binds to CD4 and one of two co-receptors on the cell surface (see *Figure 12.7*). Macrophage-tropic (M-tropic) strains of HIV-1 use the chemokine receptor CCR5 as a co-receptor. Since CCR5 is expressed on macrophages, T cells and DCs, M-tropic HIV-1 can infect all of these cell types. Individuals with mutations in CCR5 appear to be less susceptible to infection with HIV-1, indicating that CCR5 may be

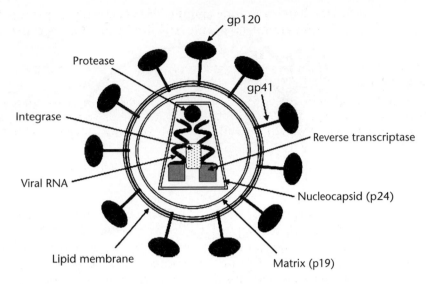

gp120

Protease

gp41

Integrase

Reverse transcriptase

Viral RNA

Nucleocapsid (p24)

Lipid membrane

Matrix (p19)

Figure 12.6
Structure of the human immunodeficiency virus (HIV)-1. In reality the virus particle contains many copies of the protease, integrase and reverse transcriptase enzymes.

the main co-receptor involved in establishing primary infection with HIV-1. HIV-1 may also infect DCs by binding to the C-type lectin DC-SIGN expressed on the surfaces of DCs. This pathway of infection may be particularly important as mucosal DCs are among the first cells encountered by HIV-1 following sexual transmission of the virus. Lymphotropic strains of HIV-1 use the chemokine receptor CXCR4 as a co-receptor for infection and these strains of HIV can also infect macrophages and T cells. HIV-1 strains that use the CCR5 or CXCR4 co-receptors are now commonly termed R5 or X4 viruses, respectively. During the course of infection the tropism of the virus can change enabling rapid viral spread, and some viral isolates are dual-tropic (R5X4).

Binding of gp120 to CD4 induces a conformational change in the gp120 molecule, revealing the binding site for the co-receptor. This stable attachment of HIV to the host cell enables the gp41 protein to initiate fusion of the viral envelope with the plasma membrane, which allows release of the viral nucleocapsid into the cytoplasm. Following uncoating by the viral protease, the RNA genome is transcribed into double-stranded DNA (dsDNA) by RT. This dsDNA is then integrated into the genomic DNA of the host cell by the HIV integrase enzyme. The integrated HIV DNA is called a provirus. The provirus may remain latent within an infected cell for years.

If the infected cell is activated to undergo gene transcription, e.g. during an immune response, this can also lead to activation of transcription of the proviral DNA resulting in production of HIV genomic RNA, as well as viral mRNA. The viral mRNA is translated into precursor polyproteins, which are

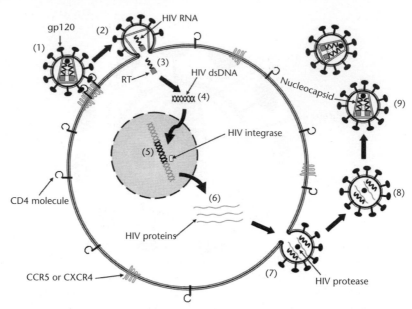

Figure 12.7
The infection cycle of HIV-1. (1) Viral gp120 binds to CD4 and either CCR5 or CXCR4 on the surface of a cell. (2) The virus fuses with the cell and (3) empties the contents of the nucleocapsid into the cell cytoplasm. (4) The viral reverse transcriptase (RT) enzyme converts the single stranded RNA genome into double stranded (ds) DNA which is shuttled to the nucleus of the cell and is (5) integrated into the genomic DNA of the cell by the HIV integrase enzyme. (6) When the infected cell is stimulated to divide, the viral genes are transcribed to generate viral genomic RNA as well as mRNA that is translated into precursor polyproteins. The precursor polyproteins are processed into mature viral proteins and (7) viral proteins and genomic RNA assemble at the cell membrane. (8) Virions bud off from the plasma membrane of the infected cell and (9) the remaining polyproteins are processed by the viral protease giving a mature HIV-1 virus particle.

cleaved (processed) to give mature viral proteins (see *Figure 12.8*). One of the precursor proteins, called gp160, is cleaved into gp41 and gp120, which are then inserted into the plasma membrane of the cell. Other viral proteins and viral RNA assemble at this point and immature virions containing the viral genome, HIV protease and as yet unprocessed viral polyproteins bud off from the plasma membrane. After release from the cell, HIV protease cleaves the unprocessed viral proteins resulting in the mature HIV virus particle.

Clinical course of HIV infection

Acute infection

Following HIV infection there is an initial incubation period of 2–3 weeks before symptoms, if any, appear. During this stage, HIV-1 infects and replicates in CD4$^+$ cells. This leads to high-level viraemia (see *Figure 12.9*). In

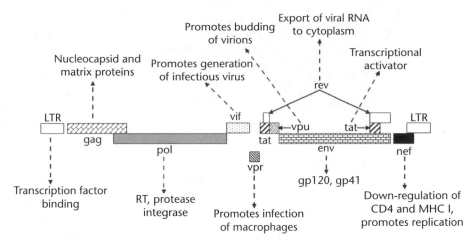

Figure 12.8
The HIV genome is flanked by two long terminal repeat (LTR) regions which are important for integration into the host genome as well as for binding of transcription factors during viral replication. The protein products of the remainder of the viral genome together with their known functions are indicated.

response to infection the immune system generates large numbers of HIV-specific CTLs. These CTLs kill HIV-infected cells, including CD4⁺ T cells that are infected with the virus. This, together with the cytopathic effects of virus production, leads to a dramatic decrease in the numbers of CD4⁺ T cells in peripheral blood. At this stage the HIV viral titre also drops as the CTL response attempts to control the infection. Towards the end of this stage many patients will also start to produce HIV-specific antibody (seroconversion) and most infected individuals will have seroconverted within 6 months following infection. The numbers of peripheral blood CD4⁺ T cells recover somewhat and the virus spreads to lymphoid tissues via infected DCs and macrophages. The acute stage of HIV infection may be asymptomatic or it may be associated with non-specific flu-like symptoms such as fever, muscle pain, sore throat and general malaise. These symptoms last for approximately 2 weeks before the infection enters clinical latency.

Clinical latency

During the latent stage of HIV infection, the CTL response maintains the viral titre in plasma at a very low level. During this stage HIV periodically reactivates from latency, and replicates within secondary lymphoid tissues where infected macrophages and DCs act as reservoirs of virus, but it is again rapidly controlled by CTLs. A strong HIV-specific CTL response is associated with slower disease progression and better prognosis, but the CTLs do not eliminate the virus. This is at least partly due to the high rate of mutation of HIV (approximately 3×10^{-5} per nucleotide per replicative

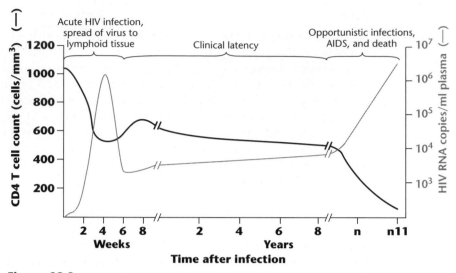

Figure 12.9
Correlation between CD4⁺ T cell numbers, HIV-1 viral load and the clinical stages of HIV infection.

cycle), which generates viral variants that are not recognized by the existing HIV-specific CTLs. In addition, persistent stimulation of HIV-specific CTLs due to the high viral burden induces anergy in the virus-specific CTLs via a PD-1-dependent mechanism (see *Section 7.4*). Follicular dendritic cells in germinal centres also become infected with HIV and, in addition, they present virus particles on their surfaces for recognition by B cells. Presentation of virus to T cells and B cells results in profound lymphocyte proliferation leading to lymphadenopathy.

The latent stage of HIV infection is asymptomatic and can last anywhere from weeks to approximately 20 years. More effective anti-HIV therapies are likely to extend the latent period further. This stage of HIV infection is characterized by a gradual decline in CD4⁺ T cell numbers, largely as a result of the cytopathic effects of virus replication as well as CTL-mediated killing of HIV-infected cells. During this stage, however, many non-infected CD4⁺ T cells are also killed. This is thought to be because soluble gp120 (produced by infected cells) binds to CD4 molecules on the surfaces of non-infected T cells. Anti-gp120 then binds to the gp120–CD4 complex and targets the T cells for elimination by ADCC. The numbers of the patient's peripheral blood T cells are monitored during this stage by flow cytometry (see *Section 13.10*). In non-infected individuals, the ratio of CD4⁺ T cells to CD8⁺ T cells in peripheral blood is approximately 2 to 1, but the CD4/CD8 ratio is reversed during this stage of HIV infection. If the numbers of CD4⁺ T cells decline sufficiently then cell-mediated immune responses will diminish to such an extent that the infected individual will present with opportunistic infections. At this point the patient has started to develop AIDS.

AIDS

With the decline in CD4$^+$ T cell numbers there is insufficient T cell help to maintain HIV-specific CTL function or HIV-specific immunoglobulin production. This leads to a further sharp increase in plasma titres of HIV. The decline in CD4$^+$ T cells also leads to a generalized immunodeficiency. This final phase of HIV infection is characterized by progression to AIDS (see *Table 12.4*). The symptoms of AIDS are largely due to opportunistic infections that are normally controlled by cell-mediated immune responses as well as to unusual malignancies such as Kaposi's sarcoma. In AIDS, the compromised immune system cannot control the opportunistic infections and such infections usually lead to death of the patient.

Increased susceptibility to *Candida* and *Mycobacterium tuberculosis* is common in AIDS patients and leads to the development of oral candidiasis (thrush) and tuberculosis (TB), respectively. TB is a major cause of death in AIDS patients, especially in sub-Saharan Africa, and the emergence of multi-drug resistant *M. tuberculosis* is a cause for concern worldwide. Pneumocystis pneumonia caused by the fungus *Pneumocystis jirovecii* (formerly *Pneumocystis carinii*) occurs rarely in immunocompetent people, but occurs frequently in HIV-infected individuals with CD4$^+$ T cell counts below 200 cells μl^{-1}. Pneumocystis pneumonia was a frequent cause of death amongst AIDS patients before the development of effective anti-fungal therapy. Reactivation of latent viral infections is also common in AIDS. Reactivation of the latent herpes viruses varicella zoster and EBV result in shingles and B cell lymphomas, respectively. Other herpes virus infections associated with AIDS are CMV which can cause blindness due to CMV retinitis, and human herpes virus-8 (HHV-8), the causative agent of Kaposi's sarcoma. Kaposi's sarcoma is the most common cancer in AIDS patients. Reactivation of latent infection with the JC polyomavirus causes progressive multifocal leukoencephalopathy, a normally fatal demyelinating disease of the central nervous system.

Other infections that may occur during AIDS are caused by the virus herpes simplex-1, the fungus *Cryptococcus neoformans* and the bacterium *Mycobacterium avium*.

Control of HIV infection

The AIDS pandemic has drastically reduced life expectancy in many countries. In eastern Zimbabwe, for example, the life expectancy of men and women decreased by 19 years and 22 years, respectively, between 1998 and 2005. As of November 2007, the World Health Organization estimated that AIDS had killed more than 27 million people since it was first recognized in December 1981. Approximately 33.2 million people (or 0.5% of the world's population) are infected with HIV. In 2007 alone, AIDS claimed in the region of 2.1 million lives, of which an estimated 330 000 were under the age of 15 years. Nearly 90% of all HIV-infected children live in sub-Saharan Africa where mother to child transmission of HIV is still prevalent. Without treatment, the rate of mother to child transmission of HIV is

Table 12.4 Clinical and laboratory indices leading to a diagnosis of AIDS

Laboratory index	Laboratory value
CD4$^+$ T cells	$\leq$ 200 cells/mm^3 of blood
Ratio of CD4$^+$:CD8$^+$ cells	$\leq$ 0.5
Level of HIV RNA in plasma	Sharply increased (usually > 10^5 copies/ml)

Clinical findings

In addition to the laboratory findings above, the patient has one of the following illnesses:

Infections

    Candidiasis of bronchi, trachea, lungs or oesophagus

    Extrapulmonary coccidiomycosis

    Extrapulmonary cryptococcosis,

    Chronic intestinal cryptosporidiosis,

    Atypical CMV infection

    HIV-related encephalopathy

    Chronic herpes simplex virus infection

    Extrapulmonary histoplasmosis

    Chronic intestinal isosporiasis

    Infection with *Mycobacterium avium* complex

    Extrapulmonary infections with other mycobacteria

    Pneumocystis pneumonia

    Progressive multifocal leukoencephalopathy

    Recurrent pneumonia

    Recurrent *Salmonella* septicaemia

    Toxoplasmosis of the brain

    Tuberculosis

Malignancies

    Kaposi's sarcoma

    Burkitt's lymphoma

    Invasive cervical cancer

Other

    HIV-associated wasting syndrome

approximately 25%. However, if the mother receives antiretroviral therapy and the child is delivered by caesarean section, the rate of mother to child transmission decreases to 1%. Unfortunately, in 2006, more than 95% of all new infections with HIV were in low- to middle-income countries where access to the most effective anti-HIV medications is not always available.

There is no cure for AIDS. The most effective protection against the disease is to avoid unprotected exposure to contaminated blood and body fluids. Testing of individuals potentially exposed to HIV is usually performed by antibody-based assays (see *Section 13.9*), which detect antibodies against the p24 protein and other HIV proteins. These tests will only detect antibody to virus in individuals following seroconversion.

Without treatment, progression from HIV infection to AIDS and death can occur within 1 year. The development of antiretroviral drugs has dramatically increased the median survival time of HIV-infected individuals. The antiretroviral drugs that are currently used to treat HIV infection inhibit the activities of reverse transcriptase (RT) and HIV protease; activities that are required for replication of the virus. There are two types of RT inhibitors in current use, nucleoside analogue RT inhibitors (NRTI), e.g. azidothymidine (AZT), and non-nucleoside RT inhibitors (NNRTI), e.g. nevirapine. HIV protease inhibitors include ritonavir and fosamprenavir. Due to the high rate of mutation of HIV, the virus can rapidly acquire mutations in RT or HIV protease that render it resistant to these drugs. Consequently, current treatment regimens consist of combinations of three drugs selected from at least two of the classes of antiretroviral drugs indicated above. This treatment is referred to as highly active antiretroviral therapy (HAART). Since the introduction of HAART, the survival time of people living with HIV has increased to greater than 20 years.

Not all individuals exhibit the same clinical course of HIV infection. Some individuals progress rapidly from infection to AIDS. Others, termed long-term non-progressors, develop strong HIV-specific immune responses and can remain asymptomatic for more than 12 years. This indication that a sufficiently strong immune response could control disease progression suggested that it might be possible to develop a vaccine against HIV. The development of an HIV vaccine has been an area of intense research for many years. Initial attempts at development of an HIV vaccine were unsuccessful. Currently, several candidate vaccines are undergoing clinical trials and some of these vaccines have been shown to induce cell-mediated immune responses against HIV.

In terms of mortality, the HIV pandemic is one of the worst in human history. The World Health Organization estimates that each day 6800 people become infected with HIV and approximately 5700 infected individuals die of AIDS. Although HAART has substantially improved the health of HIV-infected individuals, it is not a cure for HIV; HAART-resistant viral variants do arise. There is an urgent need to develop other drugs and therapies to combat this virus.

SUGGESTED FURTHER READING

Castigli, E. and Geha, R.S. (2006) Molecular basis of common variable immunodeficiency. *J. Allergy Clin. Immunol.* **117**: 740–746.

Cavazzana-Calvo, M. and Fischer, A. (2007) Gene therapy for severe combined immunodeficiency: are we there yet? *J. Clin. Invest.* **117**: 1456–1465.

Cerundolo, V. and de la Salle, H. (2006) Description of HLA class I- and CD8-deficient patients: Insights into the function of cytotoxic T lymphocytes and NK cells in host defense. *Semin. Immunol.* **18**: 330–336.

Maródi, L. and Notarangelo, L.D. (2007) Immunological and genetic bases of new primary immunodeficiencies. *Nature Rev. Immunol.* **7**: 851–861.

Munier, M.L. and Kelleher, A.D. (2007) Acutely dysregulated, chronically disabled by the enemy within: T-cell responses to HIV-1 infection. *Immunol. Cell Biol.* **85**: 6–15.

Woodland, D.L and Blackman, M.A. (2006) Immunity and age: living in the past? *Trends Immunol.* **27**: 303–307.

SELF-ASSESSMENT QUESTIONS

1. What is the difference between primary and secondary immunodeficiency?
2. A 6-month-old girl presents with severe bacterial, viral, and fungal infections. Laboratory tests indicate that she is deficient in all immunoglobulin isotypes. She also is deficient in T cells and NK cells. Which immunodeficiency is likely to be present? Explain your answer.
3. In which immunodeficiency are serum IgA levels selectively depressed?
4. What infections are common in individuals with deficiencies in complement components C6–C9?
5. In which condition is thymic deficiency found together with parathyroid abnormalities?
6. Why do immunoglobulin deficiencies usually not present within the first 5 months of life?
7. What protein is defective in X-linked chronic granulomatous disease patients and what cellular function is impaired as a consequence?
8. What are the main mechanisms responsible for depletion of CD4$^+$ T cells during HIV infection?
9. What is HAART?
10. What does the term *immunosenescence* refer to?

Immunology in practice

■ **Describe the application of immunology in a diagnostic or research laboratory setting**
Diagnostic immunology laboratories provide a wide repertoire of investigative techniques including: immunochemistry; autoantibody screening; allergy testing; immunophenotyping and molecular diagnostics. Immunological reagents also play important roles in clinical biochemistry, haematology, histology and virology diagnostic laboratories. Research laboratories also take advantage of immunological molecules through the use of immunoassays.

■ **Discuss the manipulation of immunological molecules, monoclonal and polyclonal antibodies and their use as diagnostic or research tools**
In practice, whether in a research or diagnostic setting, the most frequently used immunological molecule is the antibody. Antibodies are robust soluble proteins and so can be manipulated for use as reagents. Any given antibody will only bind to the antigen that stimulated its production. It is this key characteristic feature of the adaptive immune response, specificity, which makes immunodiagnostics possible.

■ **Outline a number of approaches to immunodiagnostics**
Diagnosis is possible through a number of methodologies:
  ■ detecting the causative agent
  ■ detecting antibodies against infectious agents
  ■ detecting the presence of antibodies to self antigens

■ **Discuss the current use of immunological reagents in the diagnosis of human disease related to the immune system**
A classical example of the use of antibody for diagnosis of an immune system-related disease, is the use of flow cytometry in routine immunology diagnostic laboratories for monitoring HIV infection and dictating HIV/AIDS therapy. Antibodies against CD4 and CD8 can quantify the number of CD4$^+$ T helper cells and CD8$^+$ cytotoxic T cells present in the blood of an HIV-infected patient. This helps monitor disease progression and drug effectiveness.

■ **Be aware of numerous applications of antibody-based methods for diagnosing various conditions**
Diagnosis of a number of conditions involves, in part, the detection of antibodies such as antinuclear antibodies (ANA) for systemic lupus

erythematosus and rheumatoid factor for rheumatoid arthritis. In addition, tests to detect HIV-specific antibody and HIV p24 protein are used in diagnosis of HIV infection, and home pregnancy tests make use of antibody to detect the hormone human chorionic gonadotropin.

13.1 INTRODUCTION TO PRACTICAL IMMUNOLOGY

The World Health Organization classifies the practice of immunology as 'clinical and laboratory endeavours that deal with diagnosis and management of diseases resulting from immune dysfunction or for conditions in which immunological manipulations play an important role in therapy'. Immunotherapy is discussed in greater detail in *Chapter 14*, while this chapter introduces basic immunological techniques that are commonly used in diagnostic and research laboratories.

A diagnostic immunology laboratory provides a wide range of investigative services such as:

- immunochemistry
- autoantibody screening
- allergy testing
- immunophenotyping
- molecular diagnostics

Immunological reagents also play important roles in clinical biochemistry, haematology, histology and virology laboratories. Such diagnostic laboratories also take advantage of immunological molecules and immunoassays to inform diagnoses of particular diseases and conditions. In addition, the exquisite specificity of antibodies for their target antigens has been exploited in research laboratories to study the localization and functions of a wide variety of biological molecules. Antibody-based purification techniques such as affinity chromatography are widely used in research laboratories and, on a larger scale, in pharmaceutical companies.

13.2 ANTIBODY AS A TOOL

Assays based upon the functions of cells or molecules of the immune system play a vital role in numerous diagnostic and research laboratories for investigations into various diseases. Assays which exploit either immune cells or molecules such as antibodies, are described as immunoassays. In practice, whether in a research or diagnostic setting, the most frequently used immunological molecule is the antibody.

The trigger for B lymphocytes to produce antibodies is the presence of an antigen. Each B lymphocyte is specific for one antigen and, upon stimulation, the cell divides and rapidly produces a clone of identical cells, all of which produce identical antibodies, highly specific for the original stimulating antigen (see *Sections 6.7–6.11*). These antibodies have high affinity for the antigen, resulting in strong binding between antibody and antigen, which is not easily broken. In addition, antibodies are relatively robust soluble proteins and so can be readily manipulated. Taken together, these characteristics of antibodies make them ideal reagents and this is why antibodies are used so frequently in immunoassays.

Antibody-based immunoassay is just one of the methodologies used in diagnostic laboratories. Allergies are sometimes diagnosed using the skin-prick test (see *Section 9.5*) which causes a cutaneous immediate hypersensitivity response in sensitized individuals. The skin test commonly used in schools for diagnosis of tuberculosis is based on reaction to purified protein derivative which, when injected below the skin, can produce a DTH response in individuals who have been exposed to *Mycobacterium tuberculosis* (see *Section 9.10*). In addition, many more recently emerging technologies, such as high-throughput real-time PCR, have greatly expanded the range of available diagnostic techniques.

13.3 DIAGNOSTIC TECHNIQUES

It is possible to diagnose an infection by measuring and comparing the levels of specific antibodies in acute (i.e. during illness) and convalescent serum. Exposure to infectious pathogens will normally result in an immune response that is characterized by the production of pathogen-specific antibodies and/or T cells. Consequently, the appearance of pathogen-specific antibodies in serum is a diagnostic sign of recent infection. The amount of antibody present in a serum sample is referred to as the titre. The antibody titre corresponds to the highest dilution at which that antibody can still be detected – a titre of 1/2450 indicates a higher amount of antibody present than a titre of 1/150 – and reflects the strength of the immune response an individual mounted against the pathogen.

Historically, examination of antibody titres was the routine approach for diagnosis of infections with viruses that were difficult or dangerous to cultivate. However, this approach is not suitable for diagnosis of serious infections where rapid therapeutic intervention may be necessary. It may be possible to detect infectious agents by immunoassay or by cultivation from patient samples followed by subsequent characterization, but the level of pathogen in the sample is not always sufficient to allow rapid diagnosis. Present day diagnostic virology and bacteriology laboratories have moved forward with the widespread application of real-time PCR, and in some cases quantitative multiplex real-time PCR, as an alternative diagnostic tool. These molecular techniques involve detecting nucleic acid specific to the causative agent.

A diagnostic virology laboratory receiving a swab from a patient suspected of having a herpes virus infection could, within 40 minutes, perform a multiplex real-time PCR assay on DNA extracted from the swab, and report on the presence of varicella zoster virus, and herpes simplex type 1 and type 2 viruses. This really is a remarkable advance compared to the slow and laborious method of inoculating embryonated chicken eggs with serum samples to cultivate and subsequently identify particular herpes viruses. High-throughput real-time PCR machines are now available which use robotics to enable hundreds of samples to be tested in one run, yielding diagnostic results within one hour.

Such advances in diagnosing infection are critical when the presence of a serious infection, such as meningitis or encephalitis, is under investigation. They can mean life or death for the patient in question, and the importance of the role of the highly skilled biomedical scientist or clinical scientist in achieving the diagnosis cannot be overstated. Doctors will use symptoms and patient history to narrow the search for the potential causative agent, but the biomedical scientist is required to confirm the definitive causative agent and ultimately inform appropriate treatment regimens.

Detection of serum antibodies to normal self antigens is important to aid diagnosis of autoimmune diseases. The initial step in laboratory confirmation of systemic lupus erythematosus is the detection of antinuclear antibodies (ANA) using immunofluorescence (see *Section 13.8*). Likewise, detection of rheumatoid factor aids diagnosis of rheumatoid arthritis. It is important to note that rheumatoid factor is not always present in a patient with RA and the levels can often fluctuate (see *Section 10.7*). Other examples include detection of antibody to heterogeneous nuclear ribonucleoprotein (hnRNP) in the diagnosis of mixed connective-tissue disease and detection of antibodies to thyroglobulin in the diagnosis of chronic lymphocytic thyroiditis.

Immunoassays are important tools in a variety of biomedical specialisms. In transplantation, tissue typing results dictate whether a transplant operation will be performed or not and most tissue typing relies on antibody-based characterization of the HLA molecules expressed by the potential recipient and donor (see *Section 11.3*). In addition, screening for donor-reactive antibodies in serum of transplant recipients is important to prevent hyperacute graft rejection (see *Sections 11.3* and *11.5*). An even more common immunoassay uses antibody to detect specific hormones, for example, commercially available home pregnancy tests are based on immunoassays that detect human chorionic gonadotrophin.

Flow cytometry is a useful technique which uses antibody–antigen interactions to characterize cells and particles. It can be used, for example, to monitor the progression of AIDS by measuring the numbers of $CD4^+$ T cells in blood. This information is important for planning patient treatment. Flow cytometry can also be used for leukaemia/lymphoma immunophenotyping and involves determining the precise characteristics of the cells that have proliferated due to malignancy (see *Section 13.10*).

The major constraint for any antibody-based immunoassay is the availability of the appropriate specific antibody. In general, two types of antibodies are used in immunoassays; polyclonal antibodies and monoclonal antibodies.

13.4 PRODUCTION OF POLYCLONAL ANTIBODIES

Animals such as rabbits, mice, goats or guinea pigs can be used to produce polyclonal antibodies for use in diagnostic and research laboratories. The animals usually receive regular injections of antigen in adjuvant (see *Box 13.1*) so that they develop high titres of specific antibody in their sera. After several rounds of immunization the animals are bled and the antibodies are purified from the serum. Antibody production in animals is a highly regulated procedure to ensure the highest standard of animal welfare.

Box 13.1 Immunological adjuvant

An immunological adjuvant is a substance that is used to enhance the immune response against an injected antigen. The most common adjuvants used to enhance the immune response against vaccines in humans are aluminium salts. Oil-based adjuvants are commonly used in animals.

The most important factor for generation of specific antibodies is a source of purified immunogen. A substance that is weakly immunogenic would not be particularly good at provoking the immune system to make antibodies against it, and use of an impure immunogen will result in the generation of antibodies against the contaminating substances. Immunogens are generally large molecules and contain a large number of different epitopes. The immunized animal's immune system will respond against many of these epitopes during an adaptive immune response. Consequently, during an immune response, many different B cells will produce antibodies that will react with the many different epitopes of the immunogen. This response is said to be polyclonal.

Polyclonal antibodies can be used for immunoassays, although they are not always ideal because of their broad specificity. As described above, polyclonal antibodies are produced when an injected antigen stimulates the proliferation and differentiation of B cells that have different epitope specificities. Each B cell proliferates and so any polyclonal antibody mixture (often called polyclonal antiserum) contains antibodies from more than one clone of B cells (see *Box 13.2*) capable of binding to different regions on the antigen (see *Figure 13.1*).

Box 13.2 Clone of cells

A clone consists of a single cell and all of the genetically identical progeny cells that it gives rise to when it divides.

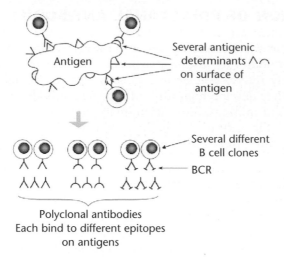

Figure 13.1
A polyclonal antiserum contains the products of many different B cell clones. Each antibody binds to a different antigenic determinant on the antigen which initiated the antibody response. Such diversity of antibodies is an advantage to a researcher as it allows multiple epitopes to be detected on a protein of interest.

A drawback of polyclonal antibodies is the potential for cross-reactivity. Cross-reactivity can occur when the antibodies produced react with epitopes that have similar amino acid sequences to epitopes of the injected protein. In addition, antibody preparations obtained from an animal using this methodology may also contain other naturally occurring antibodies. Often these do not cause problems, particularly if the antibody preparation can be used in an immunoassay at a relatively high dilution, i.e. diluting out many of those natural antibodies present at low concentration. However, there is always the potential that some of these unwanted contaminant antibodies could react non-specifically in immunoassays and result in false positive results. Ideally it would be advantageous to be able to obtain a homogeneous product, containing high concentrations of antibody specific to a single antigenic determinant. Such antibodies are called monoclonal antibodies.

13.5   PRODUCTION OF MONOCLONAL ANTIBODIES

Monoclonal antibodies are antibodies produced by a single B cell clone. All of the antibody molecules produced by a clone are identical and react against a single epitope. Monoclonal antibodies have many advantages over polyclonal antibodies:

■   they react with one epitope only, i.e. they are more specific for the antigen

- there is less cross-reactivity with other proteins
- a pure product can easily be obtained
- no contaminating antibody specificities are present

Monoclonal antibodies are produced using cell culture. B lymphocytes do not grow well in culture conditions outside the body, but technical advances made by Georges Köhler and César Milstein in 1975 allowed the production of a single antibody-secreting B cell (see *Box 13.3*). This was achieved by fusing an antibody-secreting B cell with a malignant lymphocytic cell (myeloma cell) which has lost the ability to secrete antibody. Such fusion results in a hybrid which, when cultured, produces a clone of identical immortal antibody-secreting cells. The clone is referred to as a hybridoma cell line and only those clones with a high percentage of cells secreting antibody are used. This guarantees a high yield of monoclonal antibody.

Box 13.3 Monoclonal antibodies

Köhler and Milstein were immunologists working on a fundamental question: they wanted to be able to prove whether single B cells produced antibody of only a single specificity. In order to do this they had to find a way to produce large quantities of antibody that would be the product of only a single B cell. Once they had achieved this goal, they realized that their work might have further application to techniques and procedures that required large quantities of specific antibody. They shared the Nobel Prize with Niels K. Jerne, another immunologist, in 1984.

The usual method used to produce a monoclonal antibody against an antigen involves immunization of animals with the antigen of interest. Although mice are used most often for the production of monoclonal antibodies, it is also possible to use rats, hamsters and rabbits. Usually different strains of mice are immunized with different doses of the antigen in adjuvant. Pre-immune and immune sera are assessed for the presence of antibodies. A single mouse that has generated a high titre of antibody is usually selected and receives a final injection of antigen. The spleen is removed from the mouse 3–4 days after the final injection of antigen. Spleen cells, which contain a high proportion of B cells, are prepared and fused with a myeloma cell line that is deficient in the enzyme hypoxanthine–guanine phosphoribosyl transferase (HPGRT). Cell fusion is usually accomplished by addition of polyethylene glycol.

Following fusion the cells are cultured in multiwell plates. The fused cells are propagated in selection medium containing hypoxanthine, aminopterin and thymidine (HAT). The HAT-containing medium causes death of any unfused HPGRT-deficient myeloma cells, as they are unable to produce purine nucleotides by the *de novo* or salvage pathway. Unfused B cells also die due to their short life span, and only B cell–myeloma hybrids (hybridomas) survive. The culture fluid is tested for the presence of antibody by ELISA (see *Section 13.9*) and positive wells are expanded and retested (see *Figure 13.2*). Hybridomas secreting monoclonal antibodies with the most

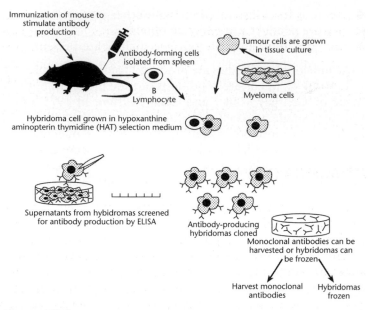

Figure 13.2
Outline of the conventional method used for the production of monoclonal antibodies (hybridoma technology).

desirable characteristics are selected. The selected hybridomas are cloned several times to increase the probability of monoclonality, and to ensure the production of high quality monoclonal antibodies.

13.6   MOLECULAR TECHNIQUES FOR ANTIBODY PRODUCTION

Phage display technology allows the expression of single chain variable fragments (scFv; see *Section 14.3*) of immunoglobulins on the surface of bacteriophages. Phage display libraries have been generated that contain $>10^{11}$ human scFvs. These libraries can be screened *in vitro* for the ability of the scFvs to bind to particular antigens. Bacteriophages containing scFvs with the desired characteristics can be propagated in bacteria and the selected scFvs can be produced *in vitro*.

In the past, a common barrier to generation of high quality antibodies was the lack of sufficient quantities of highly purified immunogen. This may be because the antigen of interest is present only at low levels, or the antigen may be labile and may be destroyed by conventional purification strategies. Nowadays, if the protein sequence is known, recombinant protein antigen can readily be produced following expression of the gene encoding the protein in bacteria. In this procedure an artificial 'tag' can be added to the recombinant protein to facilitate purification. The purified antigen can then be used as an immunogen to generate antibodies or to screen phage display libraries as described above. The very high purity of the recombinant protein overcomes the difficulties created when antibodies are raised against impure preparations of native proteins. A drawback of this technology is that not all proteins will adopt their native conformation following expression in bacteria. Antibodies induced following immunization with these misfolded proteins will, in general, not bind to the native protein. This can often be circumvented by producing the recombinant proteins in insect cells which allows eukaryotic proteins to adopt their correct conformations.

13.7   IMMUNOASSAYS

Any given immunoassay uses a known antibody to detect the presence of an antigen, whether it is a component of a tissue, on an isolated cell, or a soluble molecule. It is possible to use a known antibody to detect the presence of a substance giving a 'Yes' or 'No' answer for the presence of the target molecule. However, these qualitative tests give no indication of the amount of antigen detected. Through careful control of test conditions and with the use of known standards, it is possible to use immunoassays to measure how much of a target antigen or antibody is present. Such assays are known as quantitative tests.

Antibody-based immunoassays have many advantages over conventional biochemical tests such as:

■ increased specificity
■ increased sensitivity
■ increased flexibility

Immunoassays that are commonly encountered in diagnostic and research laboratories include immunochemistry, enzyme-linked immunosorbent assays (ELISA), and flow cytometry and fluorescence-activated cell sorting (FACS).

13.8   IMMUNOCHEMISTRY

The use of specific antibodies to probe for the presence of an antigen in a section of tissue is known as immunohistochemistry, while immunocytochemistry techniques probe for antigen in isolated cell populations. The principle underlying both techniques is identical and, in practice, the two terms are used interchangeably. In general they combine histological, immunological and biochemical techniques. They build upon, and can be used in a complementary manner to, conventional colorimetric staining techniques.

Conventional colorimetric staining techniques rely on the binding of chemical stains to a particular type of biochemical molecule and show a consistent pattern of staining wherever that particular biochemical molecule is present; a general stain for protein will produce a similar pattern regardless of the precise nature of the protein. The interpretation of conventional

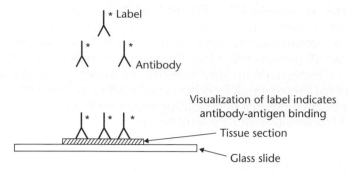

Figure 13.3
Cells or tissue fixed to a glass slide may or may not contain the antigen of interest. Specific antibody–antigen binding occurs and the presence of a label on the antibody allows the presence of antigen to be visualized and its location within the section determined.

histological staining patterns is a highly skilled task, requiring a great deal of experience combined with intuition and deduction. When immunological reagents are used, however, particular characteristics of different protein molecules can be highlighted so that they appear distinct. The presence of any antigen can be determined once an antibody reagent specific for that antigen is available. A technical challenge is that antigen–antibody binding is colourless and cannot be visualized. Specialized techniques must therefore be used to detect the antigen–antibody complex. This visualization is achieved by adding a marker, or label, to the reagent antibody that allows bound antibody to be detected (see *Figure 13.3*).

The most important consideration when preparing antibody-labelled molecules is that the labelling should not affect antibody binding activity. Typically the label is small compared to the size of the antibody, and the binding of the antibody to antigen is unaffected after the label is added, as long as the label does not attach to the antigen binding site. The most commonly used labels are fluorochromes (molecules that fluoresce at a particular wavelength when exposed to UV light) and enzymes. In addition, attachment of electron-dense labels to antibodies allows them to be used in immunoelectron microscopy (see *Box 13.4*). The two major types of immunostaining are direct and indirect immunostaining.

Box 13.4 Immunoelectron microscopy

Although one of the big advantages of enzyme-linked immunohistochemistry is that the results can be visualized under light microscopy, there is also the option of using an electron-dense label for electron microscopy. One material that is used in this way is colloidal gold. Under electron microscopy structures that have been stained with colloidal gold may be identified by the presence of distinct dark 'dots' at the sites of antibody binding.

Direct and indirect immunostaining

Direct immunostaining involves the detection of a target antigen, e.g. collagen, using a collagen-specific antibody that is 'directly' conjugated to a label such as an enzyme or fluorochrome (see *Figure 13.4*). The site where the antibody has bound is visualized as described below. The main disadvantage of this technique is that it is not sufficiently sensitive to detect antigens that are present at very low levels.

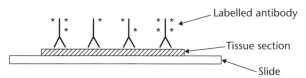

Labelled antibody

Tissue section

Slide

Figure 13.4
In direct immunostaining the label is directly attached to the antibody and amplification of the signal from antibody–antigen binding is achieved by attachment of multiple molecules of label to one antibody molecule. Methods which employ a fluorescent label refer to this as direct immunofluorescence.

With indirect immunostaining the antibody that is specific for the target antigen (the primary antibody) is not itself labelled. Following binding of the primary antibody to the target antigen, another antibody is added (the secondary antibody) that binds to the primary antibody. Use of a polyclonal secondary antibody allows many molecules of labelled secondary antibody to bind to the primary antibody (see *Figure 13.5*). As a result many molecules of the label become localized to the site of deposition of the primary antibody. This amplification step results in more intense staining compared with direct immunostaining.

Immunofluorescent staining

The fluorescent dye fluorescein is widely used to label antibodies and the resultant staining technique is termed immunofluorescent staining. The isothiocyanate derivative of fluorescein, known as fluorescein isothiocyanate (FITC) allows strong permanent covalent binding of the dye to amino acids of the antibody. Visualization requires the use of a specific fluorescence microscope with the ability to excite the fluorochrome with light at the appropriate wavelength (488 nm for FITC). Additionally, the signal is often light-sensitive and so care must be taken to keep specimens in the dark to avoid photobleaching. Other fluorescent dyes can be used including rhodamine and Texas red: both result in a red colour when viewed under the fluorescence microscope. The availability of fluorescent labels which result in different colours (due to differences in the wavelengths at which they emit light) allows for double labelling, whereby two antibodies labelled with different fluorescent labels are used at the same time, and their binding

(a)

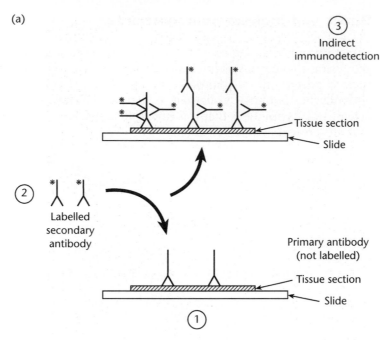

Figure 13.5
(a) In indirect immunostaining, the first antibody added is against the specific antigen to be detected and it is known as the primary antibody (1). Further amplification of an antigen–antibody binding signal is achieved using a secondary antibody with a label attached. This secondary antibody binds specifically to the primary antibody (2). More than one labelled secondary antibody can bind to each primary antibody and therefore the signal is increased, making this detection method more sensitive (3). Methods which employ a fluorescent label are termed indirect immunofluorescence. (b) Photomicrograph of human cells counterstained with PI to demonstrate the nuclei (red dots). The green fluorescent signal detected in the cytoplasmic region of the cells represents the presence of the antigen to which the primary antibody was specific for. Therefore, from the two images given it can be noted that the protein of interest is only expressed in cells which have a green signal; the other cells do not express this protein, so the antibody cannot bind and no green fluorescent signal is obtained.

to the different antigens is indicated by different colours of staining. Numerous dyes are available commercially, each with their own advantages depending on the immunoassay. Another type of dye, which is known as a counterstain, can also be added to highlight cellular structure and allow the fluorescent signal detected with antibody to be localized to a cell. Propidium iodide (PI) binds to nucleic acid by intercalating between the bases with little or no sequence preference, and its fluorescence is enhanced up to 30-fold upon binding. It therefore results in all nuclei appearing as red dots and allows cells to be visualized easily (see *Figure 13.5b*).

A common application of immunofluorescent staining is the anti-nuclear antibody (ANA) test. A positive ANA test is associated with several auto-immune disorders including systemic lupus erythematosus (see *Section 10.8*).

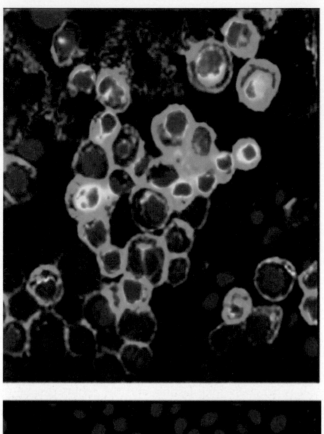

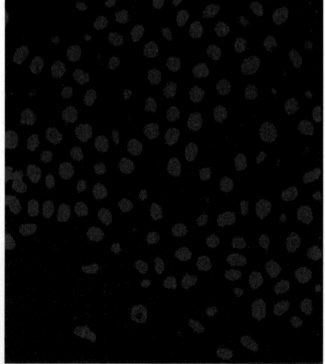

Figure 13.5 (b)

In the ANA test, dilutions of a patient's serum are added to commercially prepared microscope slides which have a sample of cells affixed to their surfaces. If the patient's serum contains ANAs, these will bind to the nuclei of the cells. After washing away unbound material, a fluorescently labelled antibody specific for human IgG is added. This labelled anti-human IgG will bind to any patient IgG that has bound to the cells. The slides can then be viewed using a fluorescence microscope to determine if the patient's serum contains ANAs and, if it does, to determine the ANA titre of the serum.

Enzyme-linked immunoassays

Enzyme-linked systems are common in immunohistochemistry. The principle of the technique is that an enzyme is conjugated (bound chemically) to an antibody. Consequently each site where an antibody binds will also contain the enzyme. When the enzyme substrate is added, the enzyme converts it to a coloured product which is deposited at the site where the antibody has bound. The location of the coloured product is indicative of antigen–antibody binding and the patterns observed are usually clear and distinct. Enzymes used extensively in immunohistochemistry include:

- horseradish peroxidase (usually used to produce a brown stain)
- alkaline phosphatase (usually used to produce a red stain)

The major advantages of enzyme-linked immunostaining methods are that the end result is generally long-lasting, and the results can be viewed by routine light microscopy. For detection of target antigens that are only expressed at low levels the avidin–biotin system provides greater signal amplification.

Avidin–biotin system

Avidin is a protein component of egg white that binds with extremely high affinity to biotin, a water-soluble vitamin (vitamin B_7). Their binding is stable at extremes of temperature, pH, etc. Avidin is a tetramer containing four identical binding sites for biotin. This allows multiple biotinylated (biotin-conjugated) ligands, e.g. biotinylated enzymes, to bind to one molecule of avidin resulting in substantial signal amplification. The avidin–biotin system is commonly used in indirect immunohistochemistry.

The avidin–biotin complex method uses a biotin-conjugated enzyme that is pre-incubated with avidin. This results in the formation of avidin–biotinylated enzyme complexes. These can then be incubated with a biotinylated secondary antibody, such as biotinylated rabbit anti-mouse IgG, to form large complexes containing avidin, biotinylated enzyme and biotinylated antibody. These complexes can be used to visualize the binding of a primary antibody to its target antigen. For example, binding of a mouse IgG primary antibody against collagen to a tissue section, could be revealed using a complex containing a biotinylated rabbit anti-mouse IgG secondary antibody. The secondary antibody (biotinylated rabbit anti-mouse IgG) would bind to the primary antibody (mouse IgG). Because avidin–biotinylated

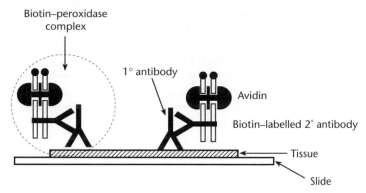

Figure 13.6
Overview of the avidin–biotin complex (ABC) detection method.

enzyme complexes are attached to the secondary antibody this results in local-ization of many enzyme molecules to the site on the tissue where the primary antibody has bound. Addition of the enzyme substrate leads to the deposi-tion of large amounts of coloured product at this site (see *Figure 13.6*). The main disadvantage of this method, apart from the additional steps that must be performed, is that it may be difficult for the large complexes to penetrate into tissues.

Additional refinements of enzyme-linked systems have involved the use of labelled 'tertiary' antibodies directed against the enzyme label. This additional 'layer' again leads to additional signal amplification. Examples of such a system include: peroxidise–anti-peroxidase; alkaline phosphatase–anti-alkaline phosphatase; and glucose oxidase–anti-glucose oxidase) (see *Box 13.5*).

Box 13.5
The avidin–biotin complex (ABC) method has been reported to be approximately 40 times more sensitive than other enzyme-linked methods, e.g. phosphatase–anti-phosphatase (PAP) and is also considerably faster to complete.

Sample preparation

Whichever immunohistochemical visualization method is used, there are some basic criteria that must be satisfied if the technique is to be effective:

■ morphology of the tissues and cells must be retained
■ antigenicity must be preserved
■ antigenic sites must be accessible

The most important aspect of sample preparation is chemical fixation. Correct fixation of the tissue or cell sample is essential because inappropri-ate fixation can lead to the destruction of antigenic sites or make the tissue impenetrable to the reagent antibody. Fixation is necessary because it arrests tissue activities such as diffusion of soluble components or enzymatic activity, it prevents tissue decomposition, and it gives the tissue some protection against the various stages in the immunostaining procedure. The ideal fixative differs from tissue to tissue and from antigen to antigen. Certain chemical fixatives may destroy some antigenic structures but leave others unaffected. Common fixatives include formaldehyde-based fixatives for paraffin-embedded tissues and cold acetone or methanol for fixation of frozen sections.

Despite careful sample preparation the target antigen may not be accessible to the antibody. In these cases it is sometimes possible to 'unmask' antigens within a tissue section. This can also help to remove unwanted background staining. Commonly used procedures that are used to 'unmask' tissue antigens include limited proteolytic digestion with enzymes such as chymotrypsin, trypsin and the use of heat-through steamers or microwaves.

A further consideration when using enzyme-labelling methods is the possible presence of endogenous enzyme activity within the tissue or cell sample. For example, horseradish peroxidase substrates can also be converted to product by the peroxidase activity of tissue haemoproteins and catalases. If these enzymes react with the substrate they produce a high level of non-specific background staining that is difficult to distinguish from the specific staining. Fortunately, it is possible to destroy the endogenous activity during the processing. Endogenous peroxidase can be destroyed by immersion in a solution containing 3% hydrogen peroxide. However, for tissues that are especially rich in peroxidase activity an alternative enzyme label should be used. If the avidin–biotin system is being used, care must be taken with tissues that are rich in biotin, e.g. liver, mammary gland, adipose tissue or kidney. The high background staining observed when using the avidin–biotin system with these tissues can be substantially reduced using commercially available avidin–biotin blocking reagents.

A common problem in immunostaining is non-specific binding of antibodies to protein binding sites. Prior to addition of antibody these non-specific binding sites must be blocked. This is usually done by incubating the sample in a 'blocking solution' that will adhere to protein-binding sites. Normal serum is frequently used as the blocking agent, although care must be taken to ensure that the species of origin of the serum will not cause further unwanted interactions with the primary or secondary antibody.

13.9 ENZYME-LINKED IMMUNOSORBENT ASSAY

Enzyme-linked immunosorbent assays (ELISAs) also exploit the specific interactions of antibodies with antigens. They differ from immunohistochemical techniques in that they are used to detect and quantify soluble molecules. The basic procedure for ELISA involves coating the wells of a microtitre plate with antibody specific for the target antigen (see *Figure 13.7*). After washing the wells to remove any unbound antibody, non-specific binding sites on the wells are blocked with a protein solution, usually a

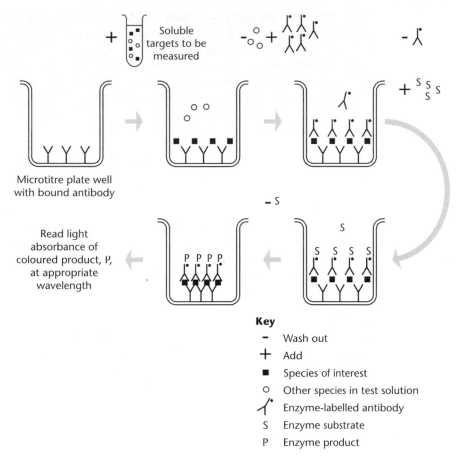

Key

−	Wash out
+	Add
■	Species of interest
o	Other species in test solution
⅄	Enzyme-labelled antibody
S	Enzyme substrate
P	Enzyme product

Figure 13.7
Overview of the procedure for a 'sandwich' ELISA.

solution of bovine serum albumin. After washing the wells again the test sample is added. If the target antigen is present in the test sample it will bind to the antibody that has coated the wells. The wells are again washed to remove unbound material and another antibody specific for the target antigen is added. This antibody is labelled with an enzyme and is chosen so that it binds to a different site on the antigen than does the 'coating antibody'. In practice this labelled antibody is usually a polyclonal antibody and so it will bind to multiple sites on the antigen allowing a greater signal to be obtained. After washing again to remove unbound labelled antibody, the enzyme substrate is added. The substrate is chosen so that the enzyme will convert it to a soluble product that can be quantified spectrophotometrically. By comparing the absorbance values of test wells with those of wells containing known quantities of target antigen, the amount of antigen in the test samples can be determined. This form of ELISA is called a 'sandwich' ELISA. Variations of this basic procedure include: direct ELISA where the target antigen is immobilized on to the plate; competitive ELISA where the concentration of antigen is calculated based on competition with a known amount of labelled antigen; and multiplex ELISA which allows the simultaneous detection of many different antigens in the same sample.

Microtitre plate ELISA uses very small quantities both of reagents and of samples and many of the steps in the assay can be automated through the use of automatic place washers, reagent dispensers and plate readers. Very high throughput of samples for a wide range of different tests has been made possible through the widespread availability and use of ELISA. Robotic ELISA is used in most routine diagnostic immunology laboratories for the testing of patient blood for the presence of IgE antibodies to allergens such as pollen, nuts, etc.

HIV testing

AIDS is a secondary immunodeficiency disorder, which is a result of acquiring HIV infection which then impacts upon the functions of the immune system (see *Section 12.7*). ELISA-based HIV tests are designed to detect anti-HIV antibody or HIV viral proteins in sera of potentially infected individuals. For most people HIV-specific antibodies take between 3 weeks and 6 months to develop following exposure to the virus. An ELISA to detect HIV p24 antigen allows diagnosis of HIV infection within 3 to 4 weeks of exposure. Many current tests for HIV infection detect both HIV-specific antibody as well as viral antigen, allowing reliable diagnosis of infection within 3 months of exposure to the virus. More rapid diagnosis (within 2 to 3 weeks of exposure) is possible using PCR-based tests on blood samples to detect the HIV genome. This test can also provide a measure of the amount of virus in the blood (the 'viral load'). However, as with all PCR assays, the high sensitivity of this test means that false positive results are common. All positive PCR tests for HIV should be confirmed with a test to detect HIV-specific antibody or HIV antigen.

Most commercial screening assays for HIV are designed to detect both HIV-1 and 2, but infections with HIV-2 must be distinguished, as the prognosis, epidemiology and treatment are different to HIV-1. Early knowledge of a positive result is a critical component in controlling the spread of HIV. Testing also allows the identification of HIV-negative people who may benefit from counselling about high-risk behaviour. HIV viral load assays are often used in clinical management in conjunction with clinical signs and symptoms and other laboratory markers of disease progression. Blood samples are never tested for the presence of HIV without a specific request from the doctor responsible for a patient's clinical management.

13.10 FLOW CYTOMETRY AND FLUORESCENCE-ACTIVATED CELL SORTING

The advent of flow cytometry has allowed the high throughput of samples that can be assessed with ELISA, to be extended to the analysis of cell populations. Conventionally, when fluorochrome-labelled antibodies bind to cells, their presence is detected visually with fluorescence microscopy. This is time-consuming and subject to operator-dependent error. Flow cytometry allows fluorescently labelled cell populations to be enumerated and, if desired, to be separated into individual populations by fluorescence-activated cell sorting for further study.

Flow cytometry is a technology that allows the characteristics of cells to be examined as they flow in a fluid stream through a focused beam of light (usually a laser beam). It is frequently referred to as multi-parameter flow cytometry because multiple characteristics of the cells can be detected and analysed simultaneously. These characteristics include cell size, granularity (or internal complexity), and relative fluorescence intensity. A common use of flow cytometry is analysis of cells based on the surface molecules they express. This is done using fluorescently conjugated antibodies that bind specifically to those surface molecules. The conjugated antibodies bound to the cells will be excited by light of the appropriate wavelength (the excitation wavelength) and emit light at a different wavelength (emission). This emitted light will be picked up by one of several light detectors.

Through the use of fluorochromes that are able to emit at different wavelengths, it is possible to detect multiple cell surface molecules simultaneously. For example, an antibody against CD4 cell surface marker labelled with a fluorochrome which emits at 488 nm, can be used in conjunction with an antibody against CD8 labelled with a fluorochrome which emits light at 594 nm. This would allow both CD4$^+$ cells and CD8$^+$ cells to be detected and analysed simultaneously in one sample.

A flow cytometer consists of five main components (see *Figure 13.8*).

- A flow cell: a device through which cells in sheath fluid flow in single file through the beam of light.
- A light source: modern flow cytometers have multiple light sources, including lasers, allowing a greater range of cellular characteristics to be detected.
- A detector and conversion system: these generate the signals to be analysed.

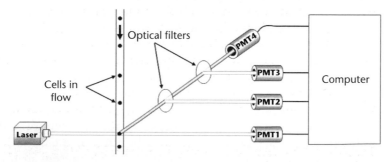

Figure 13.8
The basic elements of a flow cytometer consist of a flow cell through which cells pass to be analysed, a light source (laser), filters to direct light of particular wavelengths to photomultiplier tubes which detect, convert and amplify the light signal. The amplified signals are then analysed by computer.

■ An amplification system: this amplifies the signal.
■ A computer: this analyses the signals and generates data plots.

As the cells pass through the flow cell they are illuminated by a beam of light. Detectors in line with the point where the cells pass through the beam of light detect light that passes through the cells (forward scatter or FSC). FSC is an indication of relative cell size (or volume). Detectors perpendicular to the point where the cells pass through the beam of light detect light that is deflected by 90° (side scatter or SSC). SSC is an indication of the relative granularity of a cell.

Emitted fluorescence is detected by one of several fluorescence detectors, each designed to detect emitted light of different wavelengths, allowing the simultaneous detection of multiple fluorochromes. The detectors generate electronic signals that are proportional to the intensity of the light hitting them, so quantitative data regarding the physical characteristics of the cells may be obtained. The proportion of cells in a population showing a particular pattern of fluorescence can be enumerated and the data displayed (see *Figure 13.9*). Cell populations to be analysed can be incubated with multiple different antibodies, each labelled with different fluorochromes, in a single test, allowing the simultaneous acquisition of data on multiple cell populations.

Recent models of flow cytometers can analyse thousands of particles per second. In practice, any suspended particle or cell, including bacteria and intracellular organelles, ranging from 0.2 to 150 mm in size can be analysed by flow cytometry. Cells from solid tissue may also be analysed; however, the tissue must first be disaggregated to generate a single cell suspension.

A further application of flow cytometry is the detection and measurement of molecules inside a cell (intracellular antigens). To do this, the cells must first be fixed and permeabilized to allow the antibody access to the interior of the cell. One application of this technique is the measurement of cytokines produced by T cells following stimulation; this is termed intracellular cytokine staining.

Fluorescence-activated cell sorting (FACS) is an extension of flow cytometry that allows cells to be purified based on their physical characteristics. In this technology, the fluid carrying the cells is dispersed into droplets containing, on average, one cell per droplet. Droplets containing cells with the desired characteristics (e.g. $CD4^+$) are given an electric charge by a charging ring. This allows the droplet to be deflected away from the main stream and into a collecting vessel. FACS allows the isolation of highly purified minor cell populations for further analysis.

Flow cytometry is used in routine diagnostic immunology laboratories for monitoring and directing HIV/AIDS therapy. Fluorescent conjugated antibodies against CD4 and CD8 can be used to quantify the number of $CD4^+$ T helper cells and $CD8^+$ cytotoxic T cells present in the blood from a patient with HIV infection. This information is used to monitor disease progression and drug effectiveness. Clinicians and laboratory staff work closely to monitor the ratio of $CD4^+$:$CD8^+$ T cells as this will inform them if the helper T cell population is reduced due to HIV infection. Since the number of T helper cells present dictates drug therapy, patient blood is

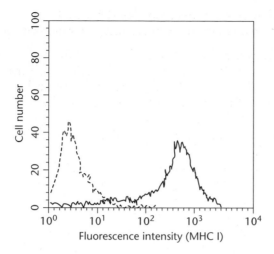

Figure 13.9
Flow histogram showing the expression of MHC class I on a lymphoid cell line (solid line). The dashed line indicates the level of staining using a control antibody.

constantly monitored using flow cytometry.

Flow cytometry can be applied in other diagnostic fields such as oncology or haematology and its application is limited only by the availability of the antibodies against the appropriate target antigens.

13.11 TOTAL HAEMOLYTIC ASSAY

The total haemolytic assay is usually referred to as a CH50 assay as it measures complement regulatory protein factor H. This is the traditional method for assaying complement activity in a patient's blood. The result is reported in haemolytic units or CH_{50} units as it measures the ability of the serum sample to lyse 50% of a standardized sample of antibody-coated sheep red blood cells (SRBC). The CH50 assay measures the classical pathway of complement activation as well as the terminal components that lead to the formation of the MAC. The assay is performed in a cold-water bath to control complement activity. Positive and negative control tubes are included in the assay to determine the maximum level of lysis of the SRBC sample as well as the level of spontaneous lysis of the SRBC sample. Following addition of serial dilutions of a patient's serum, the degree of lysis of the SRBC is measured spectrophotometrically. Quantification is achieved by comparing the degree of lysis in the test sample against a standard curve generated by using known amounts of complement.

Normal levels of total complement present in a healthy individual can range from 40 to 100 haemolytic units (CH_{50} units). Complement levels above the normal range can signal infection or inflammation, while levels below normal are associated with certain autoimmune disorders or immunodeficiencies (see *Section 12.3*). Depressed levels of C1, C2, and C4 complement components can often be found in RA or in SLE (see *Sections 10.7* and *10.8*) where a drop in levels sometimes precedes kidney inflammation. As well as being performed on serum, this assay can be carried out on synovial fluid. The CH50 assay is typically used in initial screening for detecting complement deficiencies or in monitoring treatment of some autoimmune disorders.

SUGGESTED FURTHER READING

Albitar, M. (2007) *Monoclonal Antibodies: Methods and Protocols.* Humana Press Inc., Totowa, USA.

Broides, A., Shubinsky, G., Yermiahu, T., *et al.* (2008) Flow cytometry and morphology analysis of bone marrow in a child with brucellosis and hematologic manifestations. *J. Pediatr. Hematol. Oncol.* **30**: 378–381.

Eyzaguirre, E. and Haque, A.K. (2008) Application of immunohistochemistry to infections. *Arch. Pathol. Lab. Med.* **132**: 424–431.

Jagirdar, J. (2008) Immunohistochemistry: then and now. *Arch. Pathol. Lab. Med.* **132**: 323–325.

Mackay, I.M. (2007) *Real-time PCR in Microbiology: From Diagnosis to Characterization.* Caister Academic Press, Wymondham, UK.

Parry, J.V., Mortimer, P.P., Perry, K.R., Pillay, D. and Zuckerman, M. (2003) Towards error free HIV diagnosis: guidelines on laboratory practice. *Commun. Dis. Public Health,* **6**: 334–350.

Rose, N.R. (1999) Genesis and evolution of diagnostic and clinical immunology. *Clin. Diag. Lab. Immunol.* **6**: 289–290.

SELF-ASSESSMENT QUESTIONS

1. Name four commonly used assays in present day research and/or diagnostic immunology laboratories.
2. Immunological reagents play an obvious, important role in an immunology diagnostic laboratory. Do they play a role in other laboratories within the area of biomedical science?
3. What is the most frequently used immunological reagent in diagnostic or research laboratories?
4. What advantages does indirect immunohistochemistry have over the direct method?
5. What does ELISA stand for and which routine diagnostic screening does it play a key role in?
6. What key characteristic of the adaptive immune response allows immunodiagnostics to work?
7. What role does flow cytometry play in the diagnosis of AIDS?
8. What is FITC?
9. What is FACS?
10. Name three enzyme-linked systems used in immunohistochemistry.

Immunotherapy

Learning objectives
After studying this chapter you should confidently be able to:

■ **Understand the concept of immunotherapy**
Immunotherapy is the use of immunological reagents such as antibody
and cytokines, or cells such as T cells, in an attempt to provide specific
and effective therapy for diseases such as inflammatory diseases, cancers
and autoimmune disorders.

■ **Understand the human anti-murine antibody response**
In practice, whether in a therapeutic, research or diagnostic setting, the
most frequently used immunological molecule is the antibody.
Unfortunately, the traditional method of producing antibodies in mice can
result in an unwanted immune response with the production of a human
anti-murine antibody response (HAMA). Attempts made to prevent this
unwanted reaction include humanization of antibodies and production of
single or poly-chain antibody fragments.

■ **Discuss the manipulation of immunological molecules: antibody
fragments and cytokines, and their use as therapeutic tools**
Humanization of antibodies and the production of single or poly-chain
antibody fragments are now commonly used in immunodiagnostics and
immunotherapy. Single chain variable fragment and Fab fragments have
many advantages over traditional monoclonal antibodies as carriers of
drugs and/or radio-isotopes to tumours, for *in vivo* diagnostic or
therapeutic purposes. Molecules called bi-specific T cell engagers can
induce the targeted destruction of tumour cells by CTLs. Fusion proteins
consisting of the Fc portion of an antibody molecule joined to the ligand
binding domain of a cytokine receptor can be used to neutralize cytokine
activity *in vivo*.

■ **Discuss the current use of immunological reagents in the treatment
of human diseases**
A classical example of immunotherapy is the administration of the anti-
rhesus antibody to prevent haemolytic disease of the newborn. Antibodies
against CD4 present on the surface of T lymphocytes can help in
preventing transplant rejection, and a plethora of antibodies or antibody
fragments against cytokines are used as therapeutic agents for
autoimmune disorders and cancers. Injection of a bladder tumour with
tuberculosis–BCG (Bacillus Calmette–Guerin), or the use of a genetically
modified *Listeria monocytogenes*, which secretes a molecule found on the
surface of cervical cancer cells, promotes an immune response against
tumour cells which results in tumour shrinkage. Auto-vaccination of

autologous T lymphocytes, grown *ex vivo* in the presence of the autoantigen known to be involved in disease process, can activate the immune system to selectively inhibit self-reactive T lymphocytes, with resultant inhibition of disease progression.

■ **Discuss and understand the limitations of immunological reagents in the treatment of human diseases using immunotherapy**
Success stories for immunotherapy include: Herceptin; Infliximab; Rituximab and anti-rhesus therapy. Alone, a potential immunotherapeutic has little chance of making substantial improvements to therapy for most diseases, but truly effective immunotherapy is benefiting from the development of multiple-component regimens.

14.1   INTRODUCTION TO IMMUNOTHERAPY

Immunotherapy is the beneficial manipulation of the immune response, and has been made possible by the availability of high quality immunological reagents such as monoclonal antibodies, recombinant cytokines and fusion proteins. When monoclonal antibodies were first developed, great interest and excitement was stimulated in their potential *in vivo* use. The hope was that such specific reagents could be used to target drug treatments to specific cells within the body and so avoid the side-effects associated with conventional treatments like radiotherapy and chemotherapy. The theory underlying such therapy required the conjugation of the drug of choice to a specific monoclonal antibody, which would then enable the product to function as a 'magic bullet', directing the attached drug to its proposed site of action. It was hoped that monoclonal antibody therapies such as this would revolutionize the treatment of cancer where side-effects have been a major limiting factor for most treatments. However, monoclonal antibody therapy has been slow to achieve its anticipated potential and there are a number of reasons for this:

■ the conjugation process altering the antibody specificity or reducing the effectiveness of the drug
■ the conjugation process not being sufficiently strong to ensure that the drug would not be released at inappropriate microenvironments within the body, e.g. where extremes of pH might overcome the conjugation
■ no definite tumour-specific antigens are known against which a specific monoclonal antibody can be raised – monoclonal antibodies against tumour-associated antigens (see *Section 11.8*) can also target non-cancerous cells
■ many tumour cells tend to shed their surface antigens more frequently than normal cells; when the antigens are re-expressed they may be different to the original

Even if a monoclonal antibody–drug conjugate reached the tumour site, its incorporation into the target tumour cell could not be guaranteed. Repeated administration of the antibody–drug conjugate would be required to induce an effective response. Because the monoclonal antibodies are generally raised in mice, they are murine proteins and so become targets of the human immune response; this human anti-mouse antibody (HAMA) response can destroy the antibody–drug conjugate and may lead to disorders in the patient, such as Type III hypersensitivity reactions (see *Section 9.9*), due to large amounts of immune complexes in the circulation.

14.2 HUMANIZATION OF ANTIBODIES

As outlined above, many antibodies are made in mice and, when they are used in humans as therapeutic or diagnostic reagents, repeated exposure can result in an unwanted immune response against the murine antibody, the HAMA response. Various strategies are available to reduce such a response, including recombining the DNA encoding the murine antibody variable domains (the region which dictates antibody–antigen binding specificity) with the DNA encoding human antibody constant domains, to produce a chimeric antibody (see *Figure 14.1*). This chimeric antibody reduces the HAMA response but retains high specificity for the target antigen. As a result of such 'humanization', antibodies can be given in multiple doses and tend to have a longer half-life, resulting in more effective immunotherapy.

Monoclonal antibodies (see *Section 13.5*) are also used as diagnostic aids in the visualization of tumours within the body, especially either prior to or following surgery for cancer. Antibodies raised against a tumour type can be labelled with a stable isotope, e.g. indium 111, and injected into the

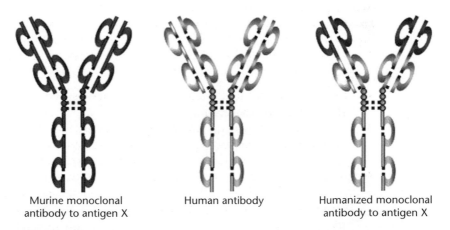

Murine monoclonal antibody to antigen X   Human antibody   Humanized monoclonal antibody to antigen X

Figure 14.1
Chimeric antibody products are achieved by antibody manipulation technologies which reduce the HAMA response: recombining the murine antibody variable domains (the region which dictates antibody–antigen binding specificity) with human antibody constant domains produces a chimeric antibody. This chimeric antibody retains high specificity for the antigen target.

patient. A large fraction of the labelled antibody localizes to the site of the tumour and can be visualized using an appropriate body scanner. This allows clinicians to see the location of a tumour relative to vital organs or tissues and decide whether or not surgery is appropriate or to establish if initial surgery had been successful and removed the tumour tissue. It also allows visualization of secondary tumours, which may be present some distance from the primary tumour.

The specificity and affinity with which antibodies bind to their target antigens offer great potential for use in targeted drug delivery to, and immunodiagnosis of, cancers. However, in some instances this potential is countered by the possibility of the antibody binding via its Fc portion to Fc receptors on non-cancerous cells. To circumvent this problem fragments of antibodies that lack the Fc portion are now frequently used.

14.3 IMMUNOGLOBULIN FRAGMENTS AND FUSION PROTEINS

An antibody is often referred to as a 'Y-shaped' molecule with binding sites for antigen at the end of each arm of the Y. Depending on the subtype of the antibody; IgM, IgA, IgD, IgG or IgE, varying numbers of binding sites are available. The arms are known as the antigen-binding region, Fab, while the stem is known as the Fc region. The Fc portion is the region of the antibody molecule that is responsible for activating complement and for binding to Fc receptors. Although these functions of the Fc region are crucial during an immune response, they can compromise the use of antibodies in targeted drug delivery and in immunodiagnosis. In addition, the size of antibody molecules can sometimes limit their ability to penetrate a tumour mass. To overcome these limitations, single or poly-chain antibody fragments are now commonly used in immunodiagnosis and immunotherapy.

Fab fragments

A Fab fragment consists of one 'arm' of the basic 'Y-shaped' immunoglobulin structure and contains an immunoglobulin light chain linked via a disulphide bond to the V_H-C_H1 fragment of the immunoglobulin heavy chain (see *Figure 2.7*). When a monoclonal antibody is available, enzymes such as papain can cleave the antibody to give two Fab fragments and one Fc fragment. Fab fragments can also be produced by cloning and expression of the DNA encoding the $V_H C_H1$ and $V_L C_L$ regions of the antibody of interest. Fab fragments can be used in both clinical and research settings.

scFv

A single chain variable fragment (scFv) consists of an immunoglobulin light chain variable region linked via a short peptide sequence to an immunoglobulin heavy chain variable region. This has many advantages over traditional monoclonal antibodies as carrier of drugs or radio-isotopes to tumours. Due to the smaller size, this molecule can achieve better tumour penetration and quicker blood clearance. The smaller size of scFv proteins also renders them less immunogenic than immunoglobulin or Fab molecules. scFvs can be made in several ways using modern protein expression technologies, e.g. from synthetic DNA using cloning and expression in *E. coli* or from genetically engineered eukaryotic cell lines.

Bi-specific T cell engagers

A bi-specific T cell engager (BiTE) is a fusion protein designed to direct the patient's T cells to eliminate the cancerous cells. BiTEs consist of two immunoglobulin variable regions linked together by a short peptide sequence. They are constructed so that one of the variable regions binds to an antigen on the tumour cell and the other variable region binds to a molecule on the surface of CTLs. BiTEs act as a 'bridge' between the CTL and the tumour cell and cause the CTL to release its cytolytic mediators towards the tumour cell. This results in the death of the tumour cell. This approach has been successfully used in treatment of non-Hodgkin's lymphoma, acute lymphoblastic leukaemia, certain lung cancers and malignant melanoma.

Immunoglobulin fusion proteins

In addition to the antibody-based molecules described above, immunotherapeutic reagents consisting of an immunoglobulin heavy chain connected to the ligand binding domain of, for example, cytokine receptors have been developed. These reagents have proved useful in the treatment of disorders in which particular cytokines are known to play important pathogenic roles (see *Section 14.5*).

14.4 APPLICATIONS OF IMMUNOTHERAPY

The production of mouse monoclonal antibodies or fragments, and the ability to humanize antibodies, allows opportunities for immunotherapy beyond those restricted to infectious diseases. Perhaps one of the best-known clinical uses of an antibody is the administration of the anti-rhesus (anti-Rh, or anti-D) antibody to prevent haemolytic disease of the newborn (see *Section 9.8*). Antibodies against CD4 found on T lymphocytes have been used to prevent transplant rejection, while a plethora of antibodies against cytokines are now evolving as potential therapeutic agents.

Manipulation of the cell-mediated arm of the immune response has also been used to treat disease. The induction of regulatory T cells (see *Section 7.6*) to inhibit the progression of autoimmune diseases has been an area of intense biomedical research. In auto-vaccination for treatment of rheumatoid arthritis patient blood lymphocytes are cultured *ex vivo* (as outlined in *Section 14.7*) in the presence of cartilage-associated antigens (autoantigens known to be involved in the disease process) followed by infusion of the patient with the resultant T lymphocyte population. Successful vaccination would result in immune-mediated, selective inactivation of the self-reactive T lymphocytes with resultant inhibition of disease progression. Other strategies designed to subvert autoimmune reactions include the induction of tolerance in autoreactive T cells using 'altered peptide ligands'. Altered peptide ligands are variants of the self-peptide recognized by the autoreactive T cells and induce anergy.

Induction of oral tolerance is another approach taken in immunotherapy. This involves a patient, usually a person with Type I hypersensitivity (allergy), taking increasingly large doses of the specific allergen. Successful oral vaccination causes the patient to become tolerant to the allergen. Currently large-scale recombinant allergens are being produced for use as edible vaccines and may well hold great promise for the future.

14.5 IMMUNOTHERAPY FOR RHEUMATOID ARTHRITIS

Rheumatoid arthritis (see *Section 10.7*) is an autoimmune disease characterized as an inflammatory-type arthrititis. It ranges greatly in severity, but can cause disability in approximately 75% of patients, with approximately 40% of sufferers unable to work within 5 years of onset and 50% within 10 years. In addition, many patients have a shortened life expectancy due to the eventual multi-organ nature of the disease. Rheumatoid arthritis can affect approximately 1% of the population with a higher incidence in women (ratio of 2.5:1).

Initial indicators of disease onset include pain, swelling, fatigue and stiffness of joints upon wakening, which can advance to loss of function. As discussed in *Section 10.7*, the immunological mechanisms responsible for this disease may be multifactorial and the absence of rheumatoid factor is not necessarily indicative of the absence of rheumatoid arthritis. Treatment with NSAIDs, analgesics and corticosteroids may reduce joint pain and swelling and improve function, but they play no role in controlling the disease and merely treat the symptoms. Additional drugs known as disease modifying anti-rheumatic drugs (DMARDs) are required to address the disease process. These include the anti-cancer drugs methotrexate, sulphalazine, leflunomide and inhibitors of the cytokine TNF. In some instances these drugs alone, or in combination, can help reduce joint damage and preserve joint integrity and function.

TNF inhibitors include etanercept and infliximab (see *Section 10.9*). Etanercept is a recombinant fusion protein designed to mimic soluble type II TNF receptors while infliximab is a chimeric anti-TNF-α monoclonal antibody containing a murine TNF-α binding region and a human IgG1 backbone. Infliximab, sold as Remicade®, neutralizes the biological activity of the TNF-α by binding soluble and transmembrane TNF-α, and preventing receptor binding. Infliximab has been approved for the treatment of numerous inflammatory disorders. When successful, these forms of immunotherapy can significantly reduce the clinical signs and symptoms of rheumatoid arthritis and other inflammatory conditions and slow disease progression.

Unfortunately, not all rheumatoid arthritis patients respond to anti-TNF therapies. These patients are known as non-responders and disease progression is not halted after treatment with anti-TNF drugs, whether alone or in combination with methothrexate. Current research is investigating the possibility of genetic analyses of patients in an attempt to predict if they will respond to anti-TNF treatment, i.e. personalizing treatment such that anti-TNF drugs are not administered to non-responders.

Non-responders are eligible for treatment with other types of immunotherapy such as rituximab. This chimeric monoclonal antibody, also known as Rituxan® and Mabthera®, specifically targets and depletes CD20-positive B cells and is therefore used to treat diseases characterized by having too many B cells or dysfunctional or overactive B cells, such as in non-Hodgkin's lymphoma, and rheumatoid arthritis. This B cell immunotherapy has been approved for the treatment of numerous malignancies, rheumatoid arthritis and a range of other autoimmune diseases, and transplant recipients. It has been administered to more than a million patients worldwide and it is the most successful immunotherapeutic agent used to date.

A new fully humanized monoclonal antibody, adalimumab, blocks the adverse effects of excess TNF-α. Recent reports of the use of adalimumab early in the course of rheumatoid arthritis indicate excellent rates of remission.

It is generally agreed that the best outcomes for patients with rheumatoid arthritis occur when treatment is started early. Usually, combinations of therapeutic agents are required for a response to be noted. Often the anti-cytokine therapies are administered in combination with anticancer drugs such as methotrexate. Methotrexate is an anti-metabolite and it works by interfering with how cells use essential nutrients, in particular folic acid, and ultimately it stops cells dividing. It therefore inhibits the activity of the cells of the immune system with resultant reduction in inflammation and reduced growth of cells in the synovial membrane of the affected joints. The use of methotrexate may have detrimental effects on fertility and its use in young females of childbearing age has been questioned.

As with any therapy which reduces the host defence mechanisms, complications can occur due to severe infections, and approximately 5% of rheumatoid arthritis patients undergoing active immunotherapy can be vunerable to such infections. As with any immunocompromised individual, precautionary measures such as vaccination against influenza are advised. Additionally, individuals taking methotrexate require full blood count monitoring as this drug may alter red blood cell development with resultant anaemia. Cell-mediated immunity is often reduced in rheumatoid arthritis patients and this would also reduce a patient's ability to fight infection. See the Case Study in *Box 14.1*.

Box 14.1 Case study

Jessica is a 35-year-old female who recently attended her GP expressing concern about a persistent cough and chest pain. Jessica first presented to the GP at the age of 28 years, after the birth of her first child, expressing concern over joint pain in both her hands. After each subsequent birth she reported decreased pain during pregnancy and peaks of pain post pregnancy. The GP tested Jessica's blood after the birth of her third child and reported that her blood was rheumatoid factor negative and tests were not conclusive. Jessica insisted on a referral to a consultant rheumatologist and subsequent testing revealed the following clinical picture indicative of rheumatoid arthritis:
1. rheumatoid factor negative
2. lowered serum levels of complement
3. erosions on finger joints of both hands, and on toe, wrist and knee joints evident upon MRI scanning

Jesicca declined treatment until she was aged 35 and after the birth of her fourth child. Initial treatments were not successful and only on the third attempt at a different treatment regimen did Jessica report any reduction in pain and tiredness. It was approximately 6 months after this that Jessica attended the GP reporting chest pain and persistent coughing.

1. Provide an overall diagnosis for Jessica.
2. Why, when Jessica originally presented at the age of 28, was this diagnosis not made?
3. Why did Jessica decline treatment when initially offered?
4. How do you propose Jessica's condition was treated and why did it take so many different attempts to get a treatment that worked for her?
5. What is the most likely cause of the symptoms Jessica presented to the GP with most recently?

14.6 CANCER IMMUNOTHERAPY

As far back as the 1850s it was suspected that the immune system could somehow be harnessed to help fight cancer. This stemmed from the observation by doctors that some tumours would shrink when the patient had an infection (see *Box 14.2*).

Box 14.2 Early cancer 'cure'

Infections with bacteria, fungi, viruses and protozoa have been observed to lead to spontaneous egression of tumours. William Coley developed a bacterial vaccine for cancer in the late 1800s. Coley's vaccines, known as Coley's Toxins, induced a fever in patients and this was associated with tumour regression. He claimed to have cured many patients with otherwise incurable cancer. The principal component of Coley's Toxin was the bacterium *Streptococcus pyogenes*.

Since that time many attempts have been made to treat cancer through immunotherapy. Immunotherapy may be local or systemic. Local immunotherapy attempts to deliver treatment directly to the affected area whereas systemic immunotherapy is generally used in cases in which cancer has spread. The cytokine IFN-α is often given systemically to shrink tumours.

An example of local immunotherapy is the injection of a bladder tumour with the tuberculosis vaccine BCG. The resultant immune response, to the live but weakened form of *Mycobacterium bovis*, causes tumour shrinkage. Advances in this area include the use of a genetically modified *Listeria monocytogenes* which secretes a molecule, HPV-E7, found on the surface of cervical cancer cells., Upon entering the body this modified *Listeria* enters monocytes and expresses this HPV-E7 on the cell surface. The monocytes are APCs and induce an immune response against HPV-E7-expressing cells which results in tumour shrinkage.

Chronic granulomatous disease (CGD) (see *Section 12.3*) is an uncommon inherited disorder of phagocytes in which the respiratory burst does not occur due to the failure of the NADPH oxidase enzyme system to assemble, or due to its defective function. Neutrophils from CGD patients can migrate and ingest micro-organisms in response to inflammatory stimuli, but they cannot kill the ingested organisms. More phagocytes are recruited to try to combat the infection and this leads to the formation of a granuloma (Type IV hypersensitivity, see *Section 9.10*). Patients with CGD have an increased susceptibility to recurrent, serious infections by bacteria and fungi, necessitating prolonged antibiotic treatment. In addition to antibiotics to combat bacterial infections, IFN-γ therapy is also known to be an effective treatment for reducing serious infections in patients with CGD, as IFN-γ increases the expression of NADPH oxidase by neutrophils. It is now a standard treatment for certain forms of CGD.

Targeted immunotherapy can make use of antibody-based therapies whereby antibodies against cancer cells attach and can:

■ stop the cancer cells growing by blocking the binding of certain growth factors
■ tag the cancer cell for destruction by the immune system
■ deliver attached drugs such as radio-isotopes specifically to the cancer cells
■ deliver an enzyme antibody complex to tumour cells in parallel with a chemical – this is known as antibody-directed enzyme/pro-drug therapy (ADEPT).

The breast cancer drug Herceptin® is one of the successes of the field of antibody-based cancer therapy. Herceptin® is also known as trastuzumab and is a selective monoclonal antibody therapy often used in combination with chemotherapy. This therapeutic approach has led to a considerable reduction in recurrence and mortality for breast cancer patients. Herceptin® can reduce or stop cancer cell growth in HER2-positive breast cancers. HER2 is a cell surface protein that is associated with poor prognosis of breast cancer. Approximately 25% of all breast cancers are HER2-positive and they are more aggressive than HER2-negative tumours. Herceptin® binds to and blocks the HER2 protein and thus alters growth; ultimately it helps shrink tumours and reduces the risk of tumours returning post surgery. Herceptin® is currently approved for use in patients with metastatic HER2-positive cancer, as a post-surgical treatment either alone or in combination with chemotherapy.

14.7 ADOPTIVE IMMUNOTHERAPY

Adoptive immunotherapy or adoptive cell therapy is a form of therapy in which autologous (i.e. self) tumour-infiltrating lymphocytes are transferred to patients with cancer. It is one of the most effective treatments for patients with metastatic melanoma and can lead to objective cancer regression in approximately 50% of patients. The immune cells are directed specifically towards the patient's tumour.

The initial phases of adoptive immunotherapy treatment involve the collection of leukocytes from the patient (leukopheresis) and *in vitro* culture of the leukocytes in the presence of high concentrations of the cytokine IL-2. The IL-2 treatment causes the leukocytes to proliferate through several cycles of replication and to differentiate into lymphokine-activated killer (LAK) cells. As well as possessing cytotoxic activity, the cells also express the IL-2 receptor and so will continue to replicate in the presence of IL-2. The expanded populations are re-infused into the patient from whom they were originally collected, together with the lowest possible maintenance dose of IL-2. Melanoma and renal carcinomas have been treated using adoptive immunotherapy. Perhaps the most effective use of this procedure is in post-surgery patients or in those where the disease is in the early stage of relapse. A number of complete or partial recoveries have been documented for tumours that had proved resistant to the conventional treatments of chemotherapy and radiotherapy.

There are many potential hazards in IL-2/LAK therapy. Some areas in which particular care is required include the following:

- Avoiding the risk of contamination of the leukocytes during collection, culture or re-infusion.
- The high toxicity of IL-2. Early treatments with IL-2 involved direct infusion of the cytokine into the patient; however, the toxicity was overwhelming due to the high doses required. The procedure has to be carried out in an intensive care unit. The symptoms of IL-2 toxicity include fever, diarrhoea, thrombocytopaenia, pulmonary oedema, confusion (sleepiness, disorientation, depression), insomnia and coma.
- The potential for the re-infused LAK cells to migrate to other body sites apart from the tumour, e.g. lung, liver and spleen and cause damage to these otherwise healthy tissues.

Refinements of LAK/IL-2 treatment include the use of tumour infiltrating lymphocytes (TIL) instead of circulating leukocytes. While this modification may increase the likelihood of the re-infused cells migrating to the tumour site, and allow the cells to respond specifically to the tumour cells to which they have previously been exposed, additional complications arise. There is the need to extract the viable TIL from the patient's excised tumour tissue and combinations of physical and enzymatic disruption of the tumour are used. The development of treatment protocols whereby IL-2 could be used to induce LAK *in vivo* would obviate this very troublesome stage. The ability to genetically engineer human lymphocytes and use them to mediate cancer regression in patients has recently been demonstrated, and this has created the possibility of extending this type of immunotherapy to patients with a wide variety of cancer types. This is a promising new approach to cancer treatment. This genetic engineering could include cytokines, which could then activate T cells in close proximity to the tumour. Complications due to the interaction of cytokines with normal cells or systemic toxicity would no longer occur.

Cytokines, e.g. TNF-α, clearly have the potential to kill tumour cells; however, this can be complicated by the accompanying inherent toxicity of the cytokine towards normal host cells. The condition known as cachexia is characteristic of advanced cancer, with muscle wasting and severe metabolic disturbance. Unfortunately, TNF-α treatment also induces this life-threatening condition. It has been an unfulfilled goal of immunologists to manipulate the TNF protein in such a way so as to retain its anti-tumour activity while deleting its cachectic function.

Numerous studies over the years have shown that the use of single cytokines for therapy is unlikely to be beneficial. Combinations of a number of cytokines that more closely resemble the *in vivo* situation may prove more effective; however, the precise constituents of such a cytokine cocktail or the optimal concentrations of each cytokine are as yet unknown.

The susceptibility of tumours to the induced immune responses may also be increased. Most tumour cells typically express very low numbers of MHC molecules so are less likely to be targets of T cells. Inducing the increased expression of MHC class I molecules on the tumour cells by cytokine treatment may render them more immunogenic.

IFN-α_2 used in combination with retinoids causes regression in some advanced squamous carcinomas of the skin and cervix. It inhibits vascular and endothelial cell proliferation and it may influence cell differentiation so it is a potential treatment for melanomas, hypernephromas and hemangiomas.

14.8 THE FUTURE FOR IMMUNOTHERAPY

Exploiting the specificity of the immune system holds great potential for cancer treatment; however, many limitations of this approach have been identified through years of trials and research. Until recently, despite significant and ongoing efforts to improve the quality of life and overall survival of cancer patients, or of patients with various other disorders, immunotherapy has achieved only modest improvements. It is likely that truly effective therapy of cancer and other diseases will require multiple immunotherapeutic regimens together with existing conventional drugs.

SUGGESTED FURTHER READING

Bykerk, V.P. (2008) Adalimumab for early rheumatoid arthritis. *Exp. Rev. Clin. Immunol.* **4:** 157–163.

Chang, H., Qin, W., Li, Y., *et al.* (2007) A novel human scFv fragment against TNF-alpha from de novo design method. *Mol. Immunol.* **44:** 3789–3796.

Jorritsma, A., Bins, A.D., Schumacher, T.N. and Haanen, J.B. (2008) Skewing the T-cell repertoire by combined DNA vaccination, host conditioning, and adoptive transfer. *Cancer Res.* **68:** 2455–2462.

Ranganathan, P. (2008) Pharmacogenomics in rheumatoid arthritis. *Methods Mol. Biol.* **448:** 413–435.

Rosenberg, S.A., Restifo, N.P., Yang, J.C., Morgan, R.A. and Dudley, M.E. (2008) Adoptive cell transfer: a clinical path to effective cancer immunotherapy. *Nature Rev. Cancer,* **8:** 299–308.

Stüve, O., Cravens, P.D. and Eagar, T.N. (2008) DNA-based vaccines: the future of multiple sclerosis therapy? *Exp. Rev. Neurother.* **8:** 351–360.

SELF-ASSESSMENT QUESTIONS

1. What does the term immunotherapy mean?
2. Is immunotherapy used only to target diseases such as autoimmunity?
3. Describe how an infectious agent could possibly be used as a therapeutic tool.
4. How does auto-vaccination work in the treatment of rheumatoid arthritis?
5. What fragments of antibody are used in immunotherapy and what are their advantages over whole antibody?
6. What is the key characteristic feature of the adaptive immune response which makes immunotherapy possible?
7. What is the drug methotrexate used for?
8. What is currently the most commonly used form of immunotherapy?
9. Give one potential risk associated with the use of an immunotherapy which targets the immune response.
10. Why have expectations for immunotherapy not been realized?

Answers to self-assessment questions

Chapter 1

1. Acute inflammation is quickly resolved and, despite the presence of temporary irritation and pain, is generally beneficial. The affected tissue returns to its original state. Chronic inflammation is long-lasting and may result in damage to the tissue in which it occurs.
2. Skin, stomach acid, lysozyme (an enzyme) in tears.
3. Innate immune responses are inborn, non-specific and similar on each encounter with a particular non-self. Adaptive (acquired) immune responses are specific for each different type of non-self and have memory such that they are permanently altered following each response that is mounted.
4. Immune responsiveness.
5. Phagocytosis.
6. Autoimmune diseases involve immune responses mounted against self.
7. HIV: human immunodeficiency virus; AIDS: acquired immune deficiency syndrome.
8. Edward Jenner was a pioneer of immunization who developed a vaccine against smallpox.
9. The immune system is everywhere in the body. There are of course specialized cells and molecules which are the only ones able to carry out particular functions, but the actions of these special cells cannot take place in isolation.
10. Any potential threat or harmful substance can be considered as non-self. In addition, during pregnancy the fetus can be considered non-self. On occasions, things will be introduced deliberately into the body, for example, transfused blood or transplanted tissues – these are also considered as non-self.

Chapter 2

1. Primary lymphoid tissues are generative tissues in which lymphocytes develop. In humans the primary lymphoid tissues are bone marrow and thymus. In the bone marrow B lymphocytes differentiate to the immature B cell stage. They leave the bone marrow and complete their maturation in the spleen. T lymphocytes develop in the thymus from pro-thymocytes that exit the bone marrow and migrate to the thymus.
2. Secondary lymphoid tissue includes the spleen and lymph nodes. Lymph nodes are situated along lymphatic vessels and allow foreign material present in tissues to be presented there for examination by lymphocytes. Mucosa-associated lymphoid tissues (MALT) are secondary lymphoid tissues adapted to acquire material at mucosal surfaces. The spleen is a highly vascular organ and is suited to filtering substances from the circulation.
3. Neutrophils. These are the first cells to arrive at sites of infection and are the predominant constituents of the acute inflammatory infiltrate. They engulf and destroy infectious agents via oxygen-dependent and -independent mechanisms. Eosinophils are also phagocytic and they are important for control of parasitic infections. Mast cells are important for regulating cellular infiltration at sites of inflammation and are referred to as the gatekeepers of the inflammatory response. Mononuclear cells consist of lymphocytes (T and B cells) the primary effector cells of adaptive immunity. B cells are responsible for secretion of antibodies. CD4$^+$ T cells are crucial for providing help to B cells and for regulating the immune response and they are

rich sources of cytokines, the proteins that help cells of the immune system communicate. Monocytes are precursors of tissue macrophages and dendritic cells and they infiltrate the tissue at sites of infection, helping to eliminate debris and senescent neutrophils. NK cells are cytotoxic cells and are important for the elimination of tumours and certain viral infections.

4. An epitope is a discrete portion of an antigen that is recognized by a given immune cell. Antigens usually contain many epitopes.

5. Cells secrete proteins which play key roles in communication within the immune system. They act like the mobile phones of the immune system, sending text messages and signals to surrounding cells. They allow the vital cross-talk and signalling to occur between all the cells of the immune system and also between the immune cells and other cells of the body. Such signals are essential for communication of instructions and to facilitate the movement of cells and regulation of the proteins cells express. Communication through these secreted factors results in a successful immune response.

6. Immunoglobulins are protein molecules that are secreted by cells of the B lymphocyte lineage. A B cell differentiates into a plasma cell and becomes a high-level immunoglobulin secreting factory. Immunoglobulins can also be called antibodies and in humans five different classes of immunoglobulin exist called: IgM, IgA, IgD, IgG and IgE. Each type carries out different biological functions; however, they all have a similar structure. Immunoglobulins can bind to antigens and facilitate their elimination.

7. The immune system can be divided into three stages of response to an invading agent. Each appears to be of increasing complexity and all three have the ultimate aim of protecting the integrity of the body. The first strategy is to prevent harmful material from even gaining access to the body. These include physical and chemical barriers. The second stage is a rapid, albeit relatively non-specific, innate immune attack that is primarily mediated by neutrophils. The third and most sophisticated approach is a highly specific adaptive immune response designed to eliminate the invaders without damaging host tissues.

8. Low zone tolerance describes the phenomenon of how antigen, when it is present below a threshold level, does not induce an immune response. At that low level the antigen could be described as non-immunogenic as it does not activate the immune system.

9. Acute phase proteins (APPs) play important roles in immune responses and are crucial for controlling the immune response against antigens. They are a group of soluble mediators made by hepatocytes and macrophages and their production is induced by cytokines IL-1, IL-6 and TNF-α. Plasma concentrations of APPs are elevated within two days of infection, a reaction that is called the acute phase response. APPs include: complement proteins; haemostatic proteins which induce blood clotting; C-reactive protein (CRP) and mannan-binding lectin which can activate the complement system; protease inhibitors such as α_1-proteinase inhibitor which inhibits neutrophil elastase to prevent tissue damage; and metal-binding proteins which have antibacterial properties.

10. Blood cells are made in the bone marrow of the pelvis and sternum by a process called haematopoiesis. Haematopoietically active bone marrow contains stem cells, termed pluripotent or totipotent haematopoietic stem cells (HSC). These HSCs are necessary for the production of blood cells of all types and they have a self-maintenance and self-renewal capacity that allows them to persist throughout adult life. HSCs are quite rare and constitute approximately 1 in 10^5 normal bone marrow cells. They in turn produce other progenitor cells, each of which can give rise to a more restricted range of blood cells which lose their capacity for self renewal. There are strict guidelines governing research into the self-renewal properties of HSCs. Many scientists hold great hope for the *in vitro* expansion of HSCs to reveal therapies for many diseases for which there are presently no successful treatments.

Chapter 3

1. During the adaptive immune response one cell, via its receptor (whether that is BCR or TCR), specifically recognizes one antigen. Due to this specificity it is essential that the immune response has a very large number of different receptors (TCRs and BCRs) to allow specific reactions against the wide and varied range of potential pathogens one could encounter.

Therefore immune cell receptor genes undergo the process of gene rearrangement to allow a great diversity of different antigens to be recognized.

2. For B cells, the variable regions of BCR heavy (H) and light (L) chains are encoded by gene segments: V, D and J segments for H chains, V and J gene segments for L chains. The gene segments are cut, rearranged randomly and joined imprecisely to form the wide array of genes to be expressed. The possible number of antigen-binding sites may be greater than 10^{11}. The process of TCR gene rearrangement follows the same processes as for BCR gene rearrangement.

3. When an immature B cell, developing in the bone marrow, binds to cell surface-associated self antigen on bone marrow stromal cells, a signal is transmitted into the immature B cell, which causes it to die. This binding to self antigen is taken as a potential reaction with self, so to protect the body from immune reactions to self antigen by this B cell, the cell receives a signal which induces death by apoptosis. If the BCR binds to soluble self antigen, a signal causes the B cell to become non-responsive. Signalling via a self-recognizing BCR may also cause further rearrangement of gene segments.

4. The thymus.

5. Mature T cells express TCR, CD3, and CD4 or CD8. In addition, they express a variety of receptors that control proliferation, differentiation and cell migration.

6. The Aire (autoimmune regulator) gene product in the thymic medullary epithelial cells (MECs) allows the process of testing thymocytes to see if their TCRs bind to an antigen that may, for example, normally only be present in the pancreas. The Aire gene product is a transcriptional activator that allows ectopic gene expression in MECs. This means that it induces the transcription, in the MECs, of genes that are not normally expressed there. Therefore, the presence of *Aire* allows expression in the thymus of proteins that are normally only expressed in other tissues. This function of *Aire* is essential for negative selection. The rare multi-organ autoimmune disease autoimmune polyendocrinopathy–candidiasis–ectodermal dystrophy (APECED) is a result of a mutated *Aire* gene.

7. Both: during the process of gene rearrangement, developing lymphocytes alter their genomic DNA by moving gene segments around *and* deleting DNA sequences.

8. We each have the capacity to generate more than 10^{15} different BCRs and TCRs. This would greatly exceed the coding capacity of our genome if each of these antigen receptors needed to be encoded by a separate gene. The process of gene rearrangement facilitates this diversity.

9. An immature B cell, which does not have an autoreactive BCR, will leave the bone marrow as a transitional B cell and migrate to secondary lymphoid tissues, predominantly the spleen, where it will again be tested for self-reactivity. If BCR is not autoreactive, the B cell will survive and undergo alternative splicing of the rearranged heavy chain RNA. This will allow the co-expression of IgM and IgD on the cell surface. At this stage of development the B cell is referred to as a mature B cell. The mature B cell will either remain in the spleen as a marginal zone B cell or localize to B cell areas of secondary lymphoid tissues as a follicular B cell. These mature B cells are now ready to respond to foreign antigen.

10. The processes whereby self-reactive T cells and B cells are eliminated during development in primary lymphoid tissues are collectively termed central tolerance.

Chapter 4

1. The five characteristic signs of acute inflammation are: swelling (oedema); redness (erythema); pain; heat (fever) and loss of function.

2. Immunological processes such as cytokine secretion, endothelial gene regulation, leukocyte adherence, phagocytosis, and fibroblast activation are responsible for systemic effects of inflammation such as loss of appetite and increased heart rate. The local increase in cytokines IL-1 and TNF-α cause heat, swelling, redness and pain. The dilation of blood vessels by histamine, eicosanoids and bradykinin increases the flow of blood to the affected tissue and leads to the redness associated with acute inflammation. Increased vascular permeability increases fluid entry into tissue, known as the inflammatory exudate, and leads to swelling. The exudate contains bradykinin, which can act on local nerve endings to cause pain. Loss of function can result.

3. Phagocytosis is a relatively non-specific mechanism of the immune system to defend against pathogens. Phagocytic cells such as neutrophils encounter pathogen and send out pseudopodia to surround the pathogen and engulf and eliminate it. This process is made much more efficient if the pathogen is opsonized with complement or antibody. Neutrophils destroy ingested pathogens by activation of the respiratory burst and destruction of the pathogen by oxidative attack with hydrogen peroxide and hypochlorite ions and through digestion with lysosomal enzymes.

4. The process of extravasation of leukocytes into tissues is a four-step process: rolling, tethering, arrest and diapedesis. Rolling is when the leukocyte rolls along the wall of the blood vessel, while tethering is a firmer adhesive contact with the endothelial cells, resulting in arrest when the leukocyte stops due to activation of integrin molecules prior to diapedesis across the endothelial monolayer. These steps allow inflammatory cells, predominantly neutrophils, to enter the infected tissue during an acute inflammatory response.

5. NK cell-deficient individuals are severely compromised in their ability to control infections with certain herpes viruses. NK cells destroy virally infected or tumour cells with reduced MHC class I expression using a perforin and granzyme-dependent killing mechanism. Type I interferon stimulates the cytocidal activity of NK cells. Cells devoid of surface MHC class I molecules evade CD8$^+$ T cell recognition. Killer inhibitory receptors (KIRs) and killer activator receptors (KARs) on NK cells bind to ligands on target cells and regulate signals for the NK cell to kill the target cell. KIRs bind to MHC class I, therefore reduced MHC I expression results in a KAR signal alone and targeted cell death. Therefore an individual devoid of NK cells would have no specific mechanism to target and eliminate virus-infected cells or cells with low MHC I levels.

6. Immunopathology is pathology or damage caused to the body by the immune system. It is a consequence of the immune response attempting to eliminate pathogens. Tuberculosis is an example of a disease with pathological consequences that are a result of the macrophages doing exactly what they are supposed to do: engulf invading pathogens. The bacterium *Mycobacterium tuberculosis*, when engulfed by a macrophage, resists destruction by lysosomal chemicals within the phagosome, escapes into the cytoplasm and resides there. It multiplies, bursts open the cell to release more bacteria and the macrophage, which dies by necrosis, initiates another inflammatory response. Cytokines produce hyperactivated macrophages within the lung, resulting in a chronic inflammatory state, which damages the lung.

7. For a successful immune response to a bacterial infection, recruitment of immune cells to the site of infection is essential. Certain bacteria secrete a tripeptide called FMLP (formylmethionyl-leucyl-phenylalanine), a highly potent chemo-attractant for neutrophils. Production of chemoattractants at the site of infection is an important early warning system that alerts the immune system to the location of the invading pathogens.

8. Complement activation can proceed by three distinct pathways: the classical pathway; the alternative pathway and the lectin pathway.

9. The functions of complement are to kill target cells and to regulate inflammatory responses by enhancing phagocytosis and increasing leukocyte recruitment from the circulation.

10. Cells attracted to a site of infection arrive via the circulation, but infection in the tissue requires movement of immune cells from the bloodstream into the tissue. Release of granules in the cytoplasm of mast cells that contain a variety of biologically active mediators (including cytokines, chemokines, eicosanoids, vasoactive amines such as histamine, prostaglandins (e.g. PGE$_2$) and leukotrienes (e.g. LTB$_4$)), aids such movement. C3a and C5a, generated following activation of complement, stimulate mast cells and trigger mast cell degranulation. Histamine, prostaglandins and leukotrienes (e.g. LTB$_4$) released by the activated mast cells bind to arteriolar smooth muscle cells and cause them to relax and vasodilate. Histamine binding to endothelial cells lining the adjacent venules causes them to contract. This brief increase in vascular permeability allows fluid to seep from the circulation into the tissues with resultant movement of cells to the site of infection.

Chapter 5

1. Antigen-presenting cells (APCs) acquire, process

and present antigens, with MHC molecules, to T cells.

2. Dendritic cells, monocyte/macrophages and B cells.

3. The first signal (signal 1) comes through binding of the TCR–CD3 complex MHC + peptide on the APC surface. The second signal (signal 2) is transmitted via CD28 on the T cell when it binds to its counter-receptor on the APC. The counter-receptor for CD28 belongs to a family of molecules called the B7 family.

4. Anergic T cells are incapable of responding to a particular antigen because a naïve T cell has received signal 1 without signal 2.

5. When a DC encounters a potentially harmful antigen it differentiates into a mature DC that has high levels of MHC class II, B7 and adhesion molecules on its surface. The mature DC loses active phagocytic activity and has altered responsiveness to particular chemokines.

6. MHC genes are also called immune response genes because they determine what it is that T cells will respond to.

7. T cells carrying a particular TCR can only respond to antigen presented in association with a particular MHC molecule.

8. Multiple MHC alleles in the population, each capable of binding different antigen peptides, ensures that some members of the population are likely to be able to present an antigen from a given pathogen. This minimizes the chances of the whole population succumbing to a particular infection.

9. Endogenous and exogenous pathways.

10. The invariant chain blocks the peptide-binding groove of MHC class II molecules so that endogenous peptides in the ER cannot bind to it. It also directs class II molecules to the endocytic compartment where they can bind peptides.

Chapter 6

1. IL-4 promotes B cell proliferation, stimulates Th2 cell proliferation and induces class switch recombination to IgE.

2. The interaction between CD154 on the T cell and CD40 on the B cell is essential for initiation of CSR. Other important signals for induction of CSR are delivered by the T cell surface molecule ICOS binding to B7-H2 on the B cells, as well as by BAFF on the T cell binding to BAFF-R and TACI on the B cell.

3. Subcapsular sinus macrophages capture antigen from the lymph and transfer the antigen, bound on the surfaces of their long cellular appendages, to the follicles where it binds to the complement receptors CR1 and CR2 on the surfaces of follicular B cells. The follicular B cells carry the antigen through the follicle to follicular dendritic cells (FDCs) and deposit the antigen on the surface of the FDCs.

4. Follicular B cells express the chemokine receptor CXCR5 and, therefore, migrate in response to CXCL13, the ligand for CXCR5. As CXCL13 is produced by follicular stromal cells, follicular B cells localize to follicles.

5. Primary immune responses are usually maximal by 8–10 days after exposure to antigen, whereas secondary responses are typically maximal within 3–4 days. The antibody produced in primary immune responses is usually IgM, whereas the antibody produced in secondary responses is normally IgG (or IgA or IgE). The magnitude of the secondary immune response is usually much greater than that of the primary response.

6. Somatic hypermutation and class switch recombination.

7. When the TCR of the CTL recognizes viral antigen presented on MHC class I of the infected cell, the CTL will bind tightly to the cell and degranulate in the direction of the infected cell. The released perforin inserts into the membrane of the infected cell and forms polyperforin pores. These pores allow granzymes to enter the infected cell where they initiate a cascade of events leading to apoptosis of the infected cell.

8. Th0 cells differentiate into: (a) Th1 cells in the presence of IL-12; (b) Th2 cells in the presence of IL-4; (c) iT$_{REG}$ cells in the presence of TGF-β; and (d) Th17 cells in the presence of TGF-β and IL-6.

9. The lymph node conduit system is a three-dimensional network of channels arising from the subcapsular sinus. The conduits are produced by fibroblast-like reticular cells and comprise a central core of collagen fibres surrounded by extracellular matrix proteins. The conduits ensure that material entering via the afferent lymphatic vessels is distributed throughout the paracortex. Interdigitating DCs settle along the conduits and constantly sample their contents for foreign antigen.

10. Marginal zone B cells, marginal zone macrophages, marginal zone metallophilic macrophages, dendritic cells and reticular cells.

Chapter 7

1. When an antigen has been eliminated the immune system must shut down the inflammatory response in order to avoid unnecessary damage to the host. An effective response to antigen rapidly generates increased numbers of antigen-specific T cells and B cells to counteract the threat. Once the threat is dealt with, regulation is essential to eliminate the majority of these antigen-specific cells and restore the numbers of lymphocytes to normal levels.

2. In a normal healthy immune system, without stimulation by antigen, there is no response. Antigen is the switch for turning the adaptive immune response on and off. The nature, dose and location of the antigen all have an effect on the type of immune response that is generated. Once antigen has been successfully removed from the body, the antigen-specific immune responses start to diminish. Insufficient quantities of antigen are no longer capable of stimulating T cells and B cells. Removal of antigen also results in decreased levels of the cytokines that are required for maintaining the proliferation of antigen-specific lymphocytes. This cytokine deprivation leads to death of the cells and the end result is a return to the situation as it was prior to the presence of the antigen.

3. Binding of CTLA-4 on activated T cells to B7 on APCs, or PD-1 to BTLA, transmits an inhibitory signal into the T cell and induces anergy. This results in the cell not responding to antigenic stimulus. Apoptosis, i.e. cell death, can remove antigen-specific lymphocytes. This can occur by two major pathways: activation-induced cell death (AICD) or activated cell autonomous cell death (ACAD). ACID involves Fas, on the surface of activated lymphocytes, interacting with Fas ligand and subsequent induction of apoptosis. Cytokine deprivation results in ACAD, an alternative apoptotic pathway that is independent of antigen receptor stimulation. B cell production of antibody may be modulated by feedback inhibition resulting from antibody binding to Fc receptors on the B cell surface. T cell responsiveness to cytokines can be inhibited by suppressor of cytokine signalling (SOCS) family members. T cell responses may also be inhibited by regulatory T cells.

4. Regulatory T cells include: nT_{REG} cells, iT_{REG} cells and Tr1 cells.

5. The three types of regulatory T cells differ in a number of ways. nT_{REG} cells develop in the thymus whereas iT_{REG} and Tr1 cells develop in the periphery from Th0 cells. nT_{REG} cells are thought to exert their immunosuppressive activity via cell–cell interaction via CTLA-4 or via membrane-associated TGF-β. By contrast, the immunosuppressive activities of iT_{REG} cells are believed to be mediated via release of the immunosuppressive cytokines TGF-β and IL-10. nT_{REG} and iT_{REG} cells also compete with effector T cells for binding of IL-2, leading to cytokine deprivation and death of the effector T cells. The suppressor activity of Tr1 cells is believed to be due to production of IL-10.

6. Immunoregulatory mechanisms operate during the recognition, activation and effector phases of an immune response.

7. Anergy, also known as non-responsiveness, is an important mechanism of down-regulating adaptive immune responses, and it renders the antigen-specific cells inactive in response to antigen. Activation of lymphocytes is mediated by positive signals transmitted via their antigen receptors and co-stimulatory molecules. By contrast, anergy is frequently induced through the delivery of inhibitory signals via co-receptor molecules. Negative signalling co-receptors transmit signals into cells that attenuate their responses and are important in maintenance of self-tolerance.

8. Feedback inhibition is a key regulatory mechanism used by the immune system. Examples include antibody binding to CD32 on B cells. CD32 is a low affinity receptor for IgG (FcγRII) sending a signal into B cells that leads to down-regulation of antibody production. As CD32 is a low affinity receptor for IgG this negative signalling will normally only occur when the levels of IgG-containing immune complexes are high. Thus, antibody production is inhibited under conditions where antibody levels are high. A similar mechanism of feedback inhibition controls IgE production through IgE binding to CD23 on B cells, resulting in inhibition of IgE production when IgE levels are high. Suppressor of cytokine signalling (SOCS) proteins inhibit JAK–Stat signalling pathways, renders cells less

susceptible to cytokine-mediated stimulation and down-regulates cell function or proliferation in a manner similar to that seen following cytokine deprivation.

9. If regulation of an immune response does not occur and reactions continue beyond elimination of the invading antigen, autoimmunity may result as a reaction to self. On the other hand, if immunoregulation is too severe and an immune response is not allowed to clear antigen from the body, there is always the risk of severe infections.

10. Complement has long been recognized as a regulator of B cell activity and more recently it has been recognized to regulate T cell activity. Binding of C3d to CD21, a B cell co-receptor, augments antigen-specific B cell responses and antibody production. Binding of C3b to CD46 on T cells during T cell activation promotes the development of Tr1 cells which down-regulate immune responses via the secretion of the immunosuppressive cytokine IL-10.

Chapter 8

Answers to Box 8.3 Case study

1. George is likely to be infected with Epstein–Barr virus (EBV). This is characterized by CD8$^+$ lymphocytosis. The massive expansion of CD8$^+$ T cells causes fever and general malaise. George's sore throat is due to inflammation caused by EBV infection of orthopharyngeal cells. This diagnosis can be confirmed by ELISA to detect EBV-specific antibody and by PCR to detect EBV genomic DNA in B cells.

2. The CD8$^+$ lymphocytosis, together with proliferation of infected B cells, leads to enlargement of lymphoid tissue.

3. EBV is a transforming virus of B cells and can cause lymphomas if cell-mediated immune responses are compromised. George's sister will be on immunosuppressive drugs to prevent rejection of her bone marrow transplant. It is crucial that her condition be closely monitored to ensure that she does not succumb to complications related to EBV infection.

1. Intracellular infections are inaccessible to antibody-dependent clearance mechanisms. Control of intracellular infections relies on cell-mediated immune responses such as CTL, NK and macrophage-mediated killing.

2. The capsule of *S. pneumoniae* is resistant to phagocytosis.

3. An attenuated vaccine consists of a live organism that has been 'weakened' by *in vitro* manipulation so that it causes only a mild illness compared to the parental organism. Inactivated vaccines consist of organisms that have been killed. In general, attenuated vaccines induce stronger immune responses than do inactivated vaccines.

4. *S. aureus* produces protein A which binds to the Fc portion of IgG molecules. This prevents the Fc portion binding to Fcγ receptors on phagocytes and therefore inhibits phagocytosis of opsonized material. The *S. aureus*-encoded CHIPS gene product inhibits neutrophil chemotaxis by preventing the chemoattractants FMLP and C5a binding to their receptors on neutrophils. In addition, *S. aureus* produces a protein called SCIN that prevents opsonization by C3b.

5. The schistosomal tegument absorbs proteins from the host and so 'tricks' the host into thinking it is 'self'. In addition, absorption of DAF by the tegument prevents complement-mediated attack on the adult worm.

6. Influenza can alter its surface proteins by antigenic shift and antigenic drift. Antigenic shift results from the reassortment of genomic RNA segments, whereas antigenic drift results from accumulation of mutations in genes encoding the viral surface antigens. As the surface antigens contain the main antibody epitopes of influenza, any time these epitopes are altered then the flu vaccine must be modified.

7. An opportunistic pathogen is a pathogen that will normally only cause disease in an individual whose immune system is compromised; for example, in a patient who is taking immunosuppressive medications.

8. Chagas' disease, also called American trypanosomiasis, is caused by the extracellular protozoan parasite *Trypanosoma cruzi*.

9. *P. falciparum* encodes a protein called erythrocyte membrane protein 1 (EMP1) which is expressed on the surface of infected RBCs. EMP1 binds to cell adhesion molecules (CAMs) such as ICAM-1, VCAM-1 and E-selectin. As a result of the EMP1–CAM interactions, infected RBCs localize to microvascular beds in tissues and avoid elimination by the spleen.

10. Control of cryptococcal infections is highly dependent on intact cell-mediated immune responses. The decline in CD4$^+$ T cell numbers

during AIDS leads to a loss of cell-mediated immunity and, consequently, dissemination of cryptococcal infections.

Chapter 9

Answers to Box 9.3 Case study

1. David presents with all the signs of a child with an allergy and he is likely to have allergic asthma, which is a Type I hypersensitivity reaction involving IgE and the associated exuberant Th2 response against the allergen. The raised eosinophil level would also be in line with a Type I hypersensitivity reaction. The initial allergen was most likely cat dander. Initial encounters with the neighbour's cat when he was under 3 years of age may have caused sensitization of mast cells, priming them for activation following subsequent encounters with cats. This would be typical of sensitization for a Type I hypersensitivity reaction whereby pre-exposure to the antigen triggers the hypersensitivity reaction. During this sensitization phase, David developed the type of immune response that leads to a hypersensitivity reaction upon subsequent re-exposure to the antigen, which occurred with his grandparents' cat. Like any allergic child, David now appears to be allergic to more than just cat dander and possibly house dust mite. His hypersensitivity disease appears to have progressed, so that now his airways are hyper-responsive to a variety of non-allergenic stimuli, e.g. cold air.

2. Known potential triggers for David's allergy would appear to be house dust mite allergen (Der p 1) on bed linen, cat dander (Fel p 1) and pollen. He may well be allergic to other allergens if exposed to them. Serum levels of allergen-specific IgE could be determined. Testing by skin prick test (with epinephrine/adrenaline available) for the specific allergens listed above should result in a wheal and flare reaction. The skin prick test involves injection of a diluted extract of potential allergens under the patient's skin or application to a small puncture wound made on the arm or back. A positive reaction consists of a small, raised, pale area with a surrounding flush and is called a wheal and flare reaction. The wheal is due to fluid build-up in the papillary body in the dermis and is an important clue in the diagnosis of an allergy. The flare is redness of the skin due to dilation of blood vessels. This wheal and flare response should be maximal within 30 minutes and will then diminish. Some doctors may suggest that the cleanliness of the home environment contributed to development of the allergy (the hygiene hypothesis).

3. The primary encounter with the allergen induces an allergen-specific Th2 response. The IL-4 and IL-13 produced cause class switching to IgE. Allergen-specific IgE sensitizes the mast cells in respiratory submucosa. Triggering of these mast cells following re-exposure to allergen causes release of their mediators, resulting in bronchoconstriction (histamine, leukotrienes) and vasodilation (histamine, prostaglandins). Th2 cells infiltrate the lungs in response to mast cell-derived PGD_2 and release CCL11 to attract eosinophils. Eosinophils recruit more Th2 cells, and Th2 cell-derived IL-5 promotes proliferation and survival of eosinophils, explaining the eosinophilia. LTC_4, LTD_4 and LTE_4 exacerbate bronchoconstriction. Goblet cell proliferation and mucus secretion is induced by IL-4, IL-9 and IL-13. Mast cell tryptase and chymase, and eosinophil-derived peroxidase and major basic protein cause local tissue damage resulting in airway remodelling. The chronic inflammatory response causes respiratory cells to become hyper-reactive to stimuli.

4. Cromolyn® inhaler, steroids and antihistamines would be prescribed for use as needed. David's mother should be advised to carry an EpiPen® (adrenaline) in case of severe anaphylactic reaction. The possibility of immunotherapy to treat house dust mite, pollen and cat dander allergy could be discussed for David. This would involve desensitization, also known as hyposensitization or allergy immunization, which attempts to reduce the patient's allergy symptoms in the long term. Patients receive subcutaneous injections of increasing concentrations of the allergen(s) into the back of the upper arm. Initially, very low doses of allergen are injected which are gradually increased over a period of 6–12 months. This generates a competing Th1 or T_{REG} response to inhibit the allergen-specific Th2 response. This, in turn, would reduce the amount of IgE produced and in the case of a Th1 response, promote production of IgG.

1. The Fc portion of IgE molecules differs from other isotypes in that it contains an additional C_H domain that binds to FcεRI.

2. Type I hypersensitivity is also called immediate hypersensitivity and this is appropriate as the symptoms can appear within minutes. It is also frequently referred to as allergy and affected individuals are said to be allergic.

3. Histamine, prostaglandins, leukotrienes and proteases are important mast cell-derived mediators involved in early phase allergic responses. Histamine binds H1 and H2 receptors leading to an increase in vascular permeability, transient muscle contraction, stimulation of mucus secretion or dilation of small blood vessels and stimulation of nerve endings. Mast cell-derived prostaglandins cause vasodilation and leukotrienes cause prolonged contraction of smooth muscle. The activity of mast cell-derived proteases (mast cell tryptases and chymase) can activate matrix metalloproteinases leading to tissue damage. Collectively, these mediators can cause the characteristic early phase responses including itching, sneezing, increased mucus secretion (rhinorrhoea), and bronchospasm.

4. Anaphylactic shock involves rapid vasodilation within the periphery. Significant volumes of blood drain from the central organs into the opened capillaries leading to consequences such as loss of consciousness. Injection of adrenaline induces the characteristic 'fight or flight' response in which blood is rapidly returned from the periphery and back to the vital organs.

5. The administered anti-D, plus complement, destroys any of the baby's RBCs that may have entered the mother's circulation. She does not then mount an immune response and the small amount of anti-D is rapidly cleared from her circulation.

6. Hyperacute rejection occurs when antibodies specific for the transplanted cells already exist in the recipient due to previous transplant(s) or transfusion(s). It usually occurs within the first 24 hours post-transplantation.

7. Persistent exposure to low dose antigen, low affinity antibody and complement deficiencies predispose to Type III hypersensitivity.

8. Type III hypersensitivity is frequently referred to as immune complex disease and involves antibodies, predominantly IgG and IgM. The sensitization phase of the type III response involves the production of antibodies against particular soluble antigens. The antibodies involved in type III responses usually bind to their specific antigens with low affinity. Consequently, the antibody–antigen complexes (immune complexes) formed tend to be small and, therefore, are not efficiently eliminated by phagocytes in the spleen and liver. The small immune complexes persist in the circulation and are ultimately deposited at susceptible sites in the body, including the renal glomeruli, choroid plexus, the skin, lungs, heart, small blood vessels and joints. Binding of immune complexes to Fc receptors, in particular to the FcγRIII receptor in tissues can trigger the release of inflammatory mediators that will enhance the inflammatory response (see *Figure 10.4*).

9. The granulomatous reaction is a type of DTH with severe consequences due to extensive tissue damage. There are two types of granuloma: immune granuloma and foreign body granuloma. An immune granuloma usually results from the persistence of micro-organisms within macrophages, while a foreign body granuloma results from the persistence of other particles that are unable to be eliminated, e.g. silica. Immune granulomata consist of epithelioid cells and macrophages surrounded by lymphocytes. Lymphocytes are absent from foreign body granulomata.

10. Benadryl® is an H1 receptor antagonist and blocks the action of histamine on H1 receptors. It is effective against the early phase symptoms of allergy.

Chapter 10

Answers to Box 10.2 Case study

1. A likely diagnosis is systemic lupus erythematosus (SLE). This presents with characteristic malar rash that is frequently induced by exposure to sunlight. Affected individuals develop anti-nuclear antibodies which are frequently directed against dsDNA.

2. In SLE, circulating immune complexes deposit in susceptible sites like the joints. A Type III hypersensitivity response then ensues. The deposited immune complexes activate complement. C5a is released and attracts neutrophils to the site. The neutrophils release reactive oxygen species and lysosomal enzymes, causing joint damage.

3. Low serum albumin together with protein-uria suggests that Mary has lupus nephritis. This is caused by the deposition of immune complexes in the glomeruli. The ensuing inflammatory response (see *Answer 2* above) damages the glomerular basement membrane. This compromises the filtration function of the kidney so that large molecules like albumin which are normally retained pass through the glomerular filter.

4. Activation of the complement cascade by the deposited immune complexes depletes C3 levels in the circulation.

1. Immunological tolerance can be defined as the lack of an immunological reaction to an antigen. It usually applies to lack of reaction to self. It is maintained through the processes known as central tolerance and peripheral tolerance. Central tolerance occurs during lymphocyte development in the primary lymphoid tissues when autoreactive thymocytes are deleted. Autoreactive immature B cells may be deleted, rendered non-responsive, or may alter their antigen receptor so that it is no longer self-reactive. During peripheral tolerance, self-reactive T cells and B cells may be deleted or may be rendered non-responsive to antigen, either via anergy or via active suppression.

2. Most autoimmune diseases are polygenic diseases, which means that they require contributions from multiple genes to confer disease susceptibility; the disease is not just as a result of one gene (monogenic). In addition, not all individuals with a susceptible genetic make-up will develop autoimmune disease. Progression from susceptibility to overt autoimmune disease requires an environmental trigger. Likely environmental factors that may trigger autoimmune disease include infectious agents and environmental pollutants.

3. Tissue damage in autoimmune diseases can be cell-mediated or predominantly antibody-mediated, or both. Cell-mediated damage may be dependent on Th17 cells which may play a role in the pathogenesis of rheumatoid arthritis, multiple sclerosis and type 1 diabetes. Antibody-mediated damage normally proceeds via a Type II hypersensitivity mechanism, following binding of autoantibody to a tissue, or via a Type III hypersensitivity mechanism, following deposi-

tion of autoantibody + self antigen complexes in tissues.

4. Autoimmunity is due to a breakdown in tolerance and a resultant reaction against self. Unlike a desirable immunological reaction to foreign antigen when the foreign antigen is eliminated, with autoimmunity the self antigens cannot be eliminated and so autoimmune reactions can develop into chronic inflammatory responses.

5. Deletion, receptor editing, non-responsiveness or immunological ignorance are all mechanisms which may result in tolerance. Immunological tolerance is essentially a lack of response of lymphocytes to specific antigens. Deletion is one mechanism through which this can occur and it is a result of lymphocytes receiving a signal to die after exposure to antigen. When immature B cells react with self antigen, this can result in reactivation of V(D)J recombinase activity, with replacement of an autoreactive immunoglobulin gene rearrangement with an alternative rearrangement which is non autoreactive. This mechanism is known as receptor editing. Exposure to antigen could render the lymphocyte non-responsive, or the antigen may not be immunogenic, or may not be accessible to the immune system, and therefore would not stimulate a lymphocyte response. This mechanism of tolerance induction is termed immunological ignorance.

6. HLA alleles.

7. The most commonly proposed environmental triggers of autoimmune disease are infections, environmental pollutants, or toxins. For infections, one hypothesis known as molecular mimicry proposes that an immune response generated against a pathogen may result in the expansion of lymphocytes that cross-react with a self antigen. Following elimination of the pathogen, the immune response targets the cross-reactive self antigen.

8. A diagnosis of autoimmune disease based on clinical and laboratory findings can be strengthened by any of the following criteria:
   - another autoimmune disease having been diagnosed in the same individual or the same family
   - the patient expresses an MHC haplotype for which there is a statistical association with an autoimmune disease
   - there is a favourable response to treatment by immunosuppression

9. Rheumatoid arthritis, multiple sclerosis, type 1 diabetes, systemic lupus erythematosus (SLE), myasthenia gravis, Goodpasture's syndrome, Graves' disease, and autoimmune thrombocytopaenic purpura (AITP).

10. The three major goals in the treatment of rheumatoid arthritis are:

- reduction of inflammation and pain
- maintenance of joint function
- prevention of future joint destruction and deformity

Chapter 11

Answers to Box 11.4 Case study

1. Renal transplant rejection is often classified according to the time at which rejection occurs, i.e. hyperacute, acute or chronic. Acute rejection usually occurs 1 week to 6 months following transplantation and can account for up to 80–90% of rejections. The grading depends on the severity of the rejection in terms of vascular changes – grade II is moderate.

2. The ABO blood group and the human leukocyte antigens (HLAs) represent antigens which need to be matched between donor and recipient to try to avoid rejection of the transplanted organ. With Mrs Graham, a kidney transplant requires most importantly that the donor has compatible ABO antigens. As with blood, if a donor was group O the kidney would be compatible with any recipient. If the correct ABO match is obtained and a graft is required urgently, HLA mismatching may be controlled by immunosuppressive therapy. The HLA class I genes encode MHC class I antigens while HLA class II genes encode MHC class II antigens. A microlymphocytotoxicity test assesses compatibility by incubation of donor lymphocytes with recipient serum. The presence of antibodies in recipient serum against MHC class I and II molecules causes cell death. The presence of antibodies reactive against MHC I antigen would mean that the donor tissue could not be used. Transplantation between individuals with perfect cross matching, such as HLA identical siblings, is the most successful.

3. Cyclosporine is a drug used to suppress the immune system. It is used to treat rejection reactions that occur when the donor organ is attacked by the recipient's immune system. Cyclosporine is a fungal peptide, isolated from *Tolypocladium inflatum Gams*. It selectively suppresses T cell-mediated immunity. It is thought to inhibit clonal expansion of T cells by inhibiting the activity of the transcription factor NFAT that regulates the synthesis of IL-2. It is often used in organ transplantation to prevent graft rejection in kidney, liver, heart, lung, combined heart–lung transplants, bone marrow transplantation, and in the prophylaxis of graft-versus-host disease.

4. The biopsy of the kidney indicated the presence of immune cells and suggested transplant rejection was occurring and that Mrs Graham's immune response was mounting an attack on the donor kidney. The use of antibodies against CD3 present on T cells would allow the T cells to be eliminated from the circulation and hinder the attack on the transplanted organ. This treatment can significantly reduce the number of T cells present.

1. Hyperacute rejection is caused by the presence in the transplant recipient of antibodies against the transplant. The antibodies are frequently formed during a previous encounter with antigens expressed on donor cells, e.g. on leukocytes in a blood transfusion.

2. Tissue typing.

3. The vast majority of transplant recipients receive immunosuppressive therapies and so have a diminished ability to respond to infectious micro-organisms.

4. Most transplants occur between individuals who have matching MHC alleles at some loci, but not all – usually at least four out of six loci are the same. The remaining differences, i.e. mismatches, can be overcome by treating recipients with immunosuppressants that decrease the likelihood of responses against the mismatches.

5. Whole body radiation destroys the patient's own bone marrow cells, allowing the transplanted cells to colonize primary lymphoid tissues without significant rejection responses.

6. Graft-versus-host disease (GvHD) is an immune response mounted by immune cells from a donor that is transferred to a recipient in a bone marrow transplant. The donor's cells recognize the recipient as being non-self and cause damage to a range of organs either in an acute or chronic process.

7. Tumour cells arise from a host's own cells and may not express tumour-specific antigens; tumour cells have a weak expression of MHC antigens; tumour cells frequently shed antigens and may re-express slightly different antigens; tumours may secrete substances, e.g. cytokines, that down-regulate immune responses.

8. Leukocytes are frequently visible on histological sections of tumours; however, they do not always indicate a beneficial immune response. It is likely that cytokines and other proteins, e.g. growth factors, secreted by the leukocytes can assist tumour growth and the development of a blood supply to the tumour (angiogenesis).

9. Tumour-associated antigens (TAA) are cell surface molecules expressed at high levels by tumour cells though they may be present at lower levels on other normal cells.

10. Myeloma proteins are immunoglobulin light chains that are secreted by plasma cells that have originated from a single malignant plasma cell.

Chapter 12

Answers to Box 12.8 Case study

1. No, Bill does not have selective IgA deficiency. Serum IgA concentrations of less than 0.05 mg ml^{-1} are characteristic of IgA deficiency. In addition, Bill also has abnormally low serum levels of IgM and IgG. IgM and IgG levels are not depressed in IgA deficiency. Bill's age as well as his low serum immunoglobulins, despite a normal number of lymphocytes, are suggestive of common variable immunodeficiency (CVID). Recurrent sinopulmonary infections with encapsulated bacteria and intestinal giardiasis are also common features of this disorder. Bill's earlier diagnosis of anaemia is consistent with CVID, as up to 20% of CVID patients present with autoimmune haemolytic anaemia or autoimmune thrombocytopaenia.

A low serum level of one or more of the immunoglobulin isotypes characterizes CVID. Affected individuals have normal numbers of lymphocytes but B cells are unable to differentiate into high level antibody-secreting plasma cells. It is not unusual for CVID patients to have siblings with IgA deficiency.

2. X-linked agammaglobulinaemia (XLA) results from a block early in B cell development. Consequently, XLA patients are severely deficient in mature B cells. In addition, XLA will always present in infancy.

3. Bill will require antibiotic treatment to eliminate his bacterial infections. Metronidazole should also be given to control his giardiasis. The most appropriate treatment for the underlying immunodeficiency is injection of intravenous immunoglobulin.

1. Primary immunodeficiencies arise from defects that are intrinsic to the immune system, often due to mutations in signalling or effector molecules critical for the function of the immune system. Secondary immunodeficiencies usually arise as a consequence of other conditions such as malnutrition or medical treatment, e.g. chemotherapy. With the exception of selective IgA deficiency, primary immunodeficiencies are rare disorders, whereas secondary immunodeficiencies are a major cause of morbidity and mortality worldwide.

2. Autosomal recessive SCID, probably due to JAK3 deficiency. X-SCID is ruled out as her father would have to have had this disorder to pass on the defective gene to her. Other autosomal recessive forms of SCID are possible, but the only one that presents with the T$^+$B$^+$NK$^+$ phenotype is JAK3 deficiency.

3. Selective IgA deficiency.

4. *Neisseria* infections.

5. DiGeorge syndrome.

6. For approximately the first 6 months of life the newborn infant is protected from infection by maternal antibodies, i.e. antibodies and associated immunity transferred from the mother.

7. X-linked CGD patients have a defect in the gene encoding the gp91^{phox} subunit of cytochrome b$_{245}$, a component of NADPH oxidase. This defect prevents effective killing of ingested organisms by phagocytes following phagocytosis.

8. CTL-mediated killing of infected CD4$^+$ T cells, cytopathic effect of virus production, gp120-anti-gp120 dependent ADCC.

9. HAART is highly active antiretroviral therapy. The antiretroviral drugs inhibit the activities of reverse transcriptase (RT) and HIV protease, activities required for replication of HIV. There are two types of RT inhibitors in current use, nucleoside analogue RT inhibitors (NRTI), e.g.

azidothymidine (AZT), and non-nucleoside RT inhibitors (NNRTI), e.g. nevirapine. HIV protease inhibitors include ritonavir and fosamprenavir. Due to the high rate of mutation of HIV, the virus can rapidly acquire mutations in RT or HIV protease that render it resistant to these drugs. Consequently, current treatment regimens consist of combinations of three drugs selected from at least two of the classes of antiretroviral drugs indicated above. This treatment is referred to as highly active antiretroviral therapy (HAART) and it can increase survival of people living with HIV to more than 20 years.

10. Immunosenescence refers to diminishing immune response associated with ageing, resulting in increased infections such as herpes zoster, or increased risk of mortality due to influenza in the elderly. Many factors can contribute to immunosenescence, such as ageing-associated thinning of the skin and drying of skin and mucous membranes, rendering them more susceptible to injury or invasion by bacteria. Production of mature T cells may decrease as a result of the thymic involution that accompanies ageing. The number of mature CD8$^+$ T cells declines with age while CD4$^+$ T cells show little change in absolute number. Studies in mice and humans have found that there is an accumulation of memory T cells in aged individuals and a concomitant decrease in the numbers of naïve T cells. The most prominent change in immune function associated with ageing is the decrease in lymphocyte proliferative responses. This results from the progressive shortening of telomeres during cell division.

Chapter 13

1. ELISA, immunohistochemistry, flow cytometry and real-time PCR.
2. Immunological reagents also play important roles in clinical biochemistry, haematology, histology and virology diagnostic laboratories. Research laboratories also take advantage of immunological molecules through the use of immunoassays.
3. In a research or diagnostic setting the most frequently used immunological molecule is antibody.
4. The indirect method may take longer to perform as both a primary and secondary antibody need

to be applied and incubated to allow binding, but the indirect method has a number of significant advantages over the direct method. Binding of the antibody to target antigen results in a signal and the indirect method can amplify this signal because several molecules of the labelled secondary antibody can bind to each bound molecule of primary antibody. With the direct method the label is attached to the primary antibody, therefore this amplification step cannot occur.

5. ELISA stands for enzyme-linked immunosorbent assay, and it exploits the specific interactions of antibodies with antigens. They are used to detect and quantify soluble molecules through the use of labelled antibodies. Microtitre plate ELISA uses very small quantities both of reagents and of samples, and many of the steps in the assay can be automated through the use of automatic place washers, reagent dispensers and plate readers. High throughput of samples for a wide range of different tests has been made possible through the widespread availability and use of ELISA. Robotic ELISA is used in most routine immunology diagnostic laboratories for the testing of patient blood for the presence of antibodies to allergens.

6. Specificity.

7. Flow cytometry does not play a role in diagnosis of HIV infection or AIDS, but it is used to monitor the blood of patients with HIV infection or AIDS to ensure rapid detection of decreased numbers of CD4$^+$ T cells – an early indicator of disease progression towards immune deficiency and AIDS. It can also dictate treatment regimens through the measurement of the ratio of CD4$^+$ cells : CD8$^+$ cells, as an indicator of T helper cell numbers in the blood. The number of T helper cells present dictates drug therapy.

8. FITC is fluorescein isothiocyanate. It is the isothiocyanate derivative of fluorescein dye. It is widely used for immunohistochemical techniques and the resultant staining technique is termed immunofluorescence. It forms strong permanent covalent binding with amino acids on antibody. Visualization requires the use of a specific fluorescence microscope with the ability to excite this fluorochrome with light at the appropriate wavelength (488 nm).

9. FACS is fluorescence-activated cell sorting. A FACS machine is a modified flow cytometer which allows fluorescently labelled cell populations to be separated into individual populations.

10. The peroxidase–anti-peroxidase method; alkaline phosphatase–anti-alkaline phosphatase method; glucose oxidase–anti-glucose oxidase method.

Chapter 14

Answers to Box 14.1 Case study

1. Taken together, all elements of Jessica's medical history would indicate she suffers from an inflammatory type arthritis, and most probably rheumatoid arthritis. The pattern of symptoms alleviating and increasing pre and post pregnancy would be in keeping with that expected with rheumatoid arthritis, and the initial onset post pregnancy is also indicative of rheumatoid arthritis.

2. When Jessica presented to her GP at 28, it was possible that if this was the initial onset, the disease would not have progressed and actual erosions and joint damage would be minimal. In addition, a range of severities of rheumatoid arthritis exist and Jessica may fortunately have a relatively non-aggressive form. The GP tested her blood for rheumatoid factor and it was not detected, therefore she is what is known as sero-negative. This cannot be taken as an indication of no rheumatoid arthritis, but the lack of rheumatoid factor is often indicative of a less severe form.

3. Jessica most likely declined treatment if she was considering a further pregnancy. Initial treatment involves NSAIDs, analgesics and corticosteroids to reduce joint pain and swelling and improve function, but they play no role in controlling the disease, and merely treat the symptoms. Additional drugs known as DMARDs are required to address the disease process, including the anti-cancer drugs methotrexate, sulphalazine, and leflunomide, and TNF inhibitors such as etanercept and infliximab. In some instances these drugs alone or in combination can help reduce joint damage and preserve joint integrity and function. Currently the first attempt at treatment would involve methotrexate, which is a cytotoxic drug with anti-metabolite function; methotrexate specifically targets folic acid uptake, and there are concerns surrounding its use during pregnancy or in females of childbearing age.

4. Many suffers of rheumatoid arthritis are known as non-responders and often a number of different treatment regimens need to be tested to find the one most suitable for any given individual. Initial treatment most likely involved NSAIDs and a DMARD such as methotrexate. Following on from this a number of the anti-cytokine therapies available such as etanercept, infliximab, adalimumab, or rituximab would be used alone, or in combination with methotrexate.

5. Jessica was most likely immunocompromised due to the treatment she was receiving for her rheumatoid arthritis or due to the disease itself, and was possibly suffering from pneumonia. As with any therapy which reduces the immune response and host defence mechanisms, complications can occur due to severe infections. Approximately 5% of rheumatoid arthritis patients undergoing active immunotherapy can be vulnerable to severe infections. As with any immunocompromised individual, precautionary measures such as having the flu vaccine are advised. Additionally, individuals taking methotrexate require full blood count monitoring as this drug may alter red blood cell growth and division, with resultant anaemia. Cell-mediated immunity is often reduced with rheumatoid arthritis and this would also reduce the patient's ability to fight infection.

1. Immunotherapy is the use of immunological reagents to manipulate the immune response or target specific proteins or molecules known to be involved in disease processes such as cancers or inflammatory disorders.

2. Immunotherapy can be used to target a wide range of disorders and diseases and it is limited only by the identification of a suitable target. It is by no means limited to autoimmune disease.

3. Injection of a bladder tumour with the tuberculosis BCG vaccine results in an immune response to the live but weakened form of *Mycobacterium bovis*, causing tumour shrinkage. Use of a genetically modified *Listeria monocytogenes* allows it to secrete a molecule found on the surface of cervical cancer cells, HPV-E7. Thus, upon entering the body this modified *Listeria* enters monocytes and HPV-E7 is expressed on the cell surface. The monocyte is an antigen-presenting cell and an immune response against HPV-E7-expressing cells results in tumour shrinkage.

4. Auto-vaccination for treatment of rheumatoid arthritis selectively stimulates a patient's immune response against pathogenic, self-reactive T lymphocytes. Patient blood lymphocytes are cultured *ex vivo* in the presence of cartilage-associated antigens (autoantigen known to be involved in the disease process) followed by vaccinotherapy of the patient with the prepared T lymphocytes. Successful vaccination results in immune-mediated, selective inactivation of the self-reactive T lymphocytes with resultant inhibition of disease progression.

5. Single or poly-chain antibody fragments are now commonly used in immunodiagnostics and immunotherapy. An scFv is a single chain variable fragment while a Fab fragment also contains a constant region linked through a disulphide bond. They have many advantages over traditional monoclonal antibodies as carrier of drugs or radionuclei to tumours. Due to their smaller size, Fab fragments can achieve better tumour penetration and quicker blood clearance with a much lower immune response. Fab fragments can be used in both a clinical or research setting.

6. Specificity.

7. Methotrexate is an anti-cancer drug which is commonly used in combination with anti-cytokine immunotherapies to target cells of the immune system and halt the inflammation associated with rheumatoid arthritis.

8. The chimeric monoclonal antibody rituximab, also known as Ritual® and MabtheraV, specifically targets and depletes CD20-positive B cells and is therefore used to treat diseases characterized by having too many B cells or dysfunctional or overactive B cells, such as in non-Hodgkin's lymphoma and rheumatoid arthritis. This B cell immunotherapy has been approved for the treatment of numerous malignancies, rheumatoid arthritis and a range of other autoimmune diseases, and to prevent transplant rejection. It has been administered to more than a million patients worldwide and it is the most successful immunotherapeutic agent used to date.

9. Any given individual undertaking an immunotherapy that targets the immune response is potentially at risk of becoming immunocompromised and hence is at risk of serious infection such as pneumonia.

10. The use of single cytokines for therapy has been shown in numerous studies to be unlikely to be beneficial. The development of effective multiple component regimens appears necessary to further develop truly effective immunotherapy.

Appendices

TABLE OF HUMAN CD ANTIGENS[a,b]

CD antigen	Synonym(s)	Cellular expression	Function(s)	Molecular weight (kDa)	Family
CD1a	R4, Leu 6	Cortical thymocytes, DCs, Langerhans cells	MHC class I-like, β_2-microglobulin-associated molecule; involved in non-peptide antigen presentation	49	IgSF
CD1b	R1	Cortical thymocytes, DCs, Langerhans cells	MHC class I-like, β_2-microglobulin-associated molecule; involved in non-peptide antigen presentation	45	IgSF
CD1c	R7	Cortical thymocytes, DCs, Langerhans cells, B cells	MHC class I-like, β_2-microglobulin-associated molecule; involved in non-peptide antigen presentation	43	IgSF
CD1d	R3	Cortical thymocytes, DCs, Langerhans cells, intestinal epithelial cells	MHC class I-like, β_2-microglobulin-associated molecule; involved in non-peptide antigen presentation	43	IgSF
CD1e	R2	Cortical thymocytes, DCs, Langerhans cells	MHC class I-like, β_2-microglobulin-associated molecule; involved in non-peptide antigen presentation	36	IgSF
CD2	T11, LFA-2	T cells, thymocytes, NK cells	Adhesion molecule, binds to CD58; can activate T cells	50	IgSF
CD2R	T11-3	Activated T cells	Activation-induced conformational variant of CD2	50	IgSF
CD3γ	T3	Thymocytes, T cells	Associates with TCR; required for TCR-mediated signal transduction	25–28	IgSF
CD3δ	T3	Thymocytes, T cells	Associates with TCR; required for TCR-mediated signal transduction	20	IgSF
CD3ε	T3	Thymocytes, T cells	Associates with TCR; required for TCR-mediated signal transduction	20	IgSF
CD4	T4, L3T4	Thymocyte subsets, ~65% of peripheral T cells, monocytes, macrophages	Binds to MHC class II molecules; binds lck tyrosine kinase; receptor for HIV	55	IgSF

Table of human CD antigens[a,b] *contd*

CD antigen	Synonym(s)	Cellular expression	Function(s)	Molecular weight (kDa)	Family
CD5	T1, Ly1	Thymocytes, T cells, subset of B cells	Binds to CD72; possible role in signal transduction	67	Scavenger receptor
CD6	T12	Thymocytes, T cells, B cell CLL	Binds to CD166; role in T cell co-stimulation and adhesion	100–130	Scavenger receptor
CD7	Leu 9	Haematopoietic cells, T cells, thymocytes	Possible role in T cell activation; marker for T cell ALL and pluripotential stem cell leukaemias	40	IgSF
CD8α	Lyt2	Thymocyte subsets, ~35% of peripheral T cells, DC subset	Forms homodimers or heterdimerizes with CD8β; dimer binds to MHC class I molecules and lck tyrosine kinase	32–34	IgSF
CD8β	Lyt3	Thymocyte subsets, ~35% of peripheral T cells	Forms heterodimers with CD8α; dimer binds to MHC class I molecules and lck tyrosine kinase	32–34	IgSF
CD9	p24	Widely expressed	Signal transduction; possible role in platelet aggregation and activation	22–27	TM4SF
CD10	CALLA	B and T cell precursors, bone marrow stromal cells	Zinc metalloproteinase, marker for pre-B ALL	100	ZMP
CD11a	LFA-1	Leukocytes	α_L subunit of integrin LFA-1 (associated with CD18) which binds to CD50, CD54 and CD102	180	Integrin α
CD11b	Mac-1	Myeloid cells, T cells, B cells, NK cells, DC subset	α_M subunit of integrin CR3 (associated with CD18) which binds CD54, CD102, complement component iC3b and extracellular matrix proteins	170 Integrin	α
CD11c	CR4	Myeloid cells, T cells, B cells, NK cells, DC subset	α_X subunit of integrin CR4 (associated with CD18) which binds CD54, complement component iC3b and fibrinogen	150	Integrin α
CDw12	p90–120	Monocytes, granulocytes, NK cells, platelets	Function unknown	90–120	
CD13	Aminopeptidase N	Myeloid cells, epithelial cells, endothelial cells	Forms homodimers; involved in processing of bioactive molecules including CCL3; trims peptides for binding to MHC class II molecules; a receptor for coronaviruses	150–170	ZMP
CD14	LPS receptor	Myeloid cells, epithelial cells	Associates with CD284; binds complex of LPS and LPS-binding protein	53–55	LPS receptor family
CD15	Lewis[x]	Leukocytes, epithelial cells	Trisaccharide expressed on glycolipids and many cell surface glycoproteins		Carbohydrate epitope
CD15s	Sialyl–Lewis[x]	Leukocytes, endothelial cells	Adhesion molecule; binds CD62E (strongly) and CD62P		Carbohydrate epitope

Table of human CD antigens[a,b] *contd*

CD antigen	Synonym(s)	Cellular expression	Function(s)	Molecular weight (kDa)	Family
CD15u	Sulphated CD15	Leukocytes, endothelial cells	Adhesion molecule; binds CD62P		Carbohydrate epitope
CD16a	FcγRIIIA	Neutrophils, macrophages, NK cells, mast cells, T cells	Component of low affinity receptor for aggregated IgG2 and IgG3; mediates ADCC	50–60	IgSF
CD16b	FcγRIIIB	Neutrophils, macrophages, NK cells, mast cells, T cells	GPI-anchored form of CD16a	50–60	IgSF
CD17	Lactosylceramide	Myeloid cells, T cells, B cell, DCs	Cell surface glycosphingolipid; binds to bacteria and may have role in phagocytosis		Carbohydrate epitope
CD18		Leukocytes	Integrin β_2 subunit which associates with CD11a, CD11b and CD11c	95	Integrin β
CD19	B4	B cells	Together with CD21 and CD81 forms a co-receptor on B cells	95	IgSF
CD20	B1	B cells	Possible role in B cell proliferation and differentiation into plasma cells	35–37	TM4SF
CD21	CR2, C3d receptor	B cells, follicular DCs	Receptor for C3d; EBV receptor; together with CD19 and CD81 forms a co-receptor on B cells	145	CCP superfamily
CD22	BL–CAM	B cells	Two forms generated by alternative splicing; role in adhesion and signalling	140 (major form) 130 (minor form)	IgSF
CD23	FcεRII	Activated B cells, activated macrophages, granulocytes, follicular DCs, platelets	Low affinity IgE receptor; role in regulation of IgE production	45	C-type lectin
CD24	HSA	Granulocytes, B cells	Function unknown	35–45	PI-linked HSA family
CD25	Tac, IL-2Rα chain	Activated T cells, B cells and macrophages	Together with CD122 and CD132 forms the high affinity IL-2 receptor which mediates the effects of IL-2	55	CCP
CD26	Dipeptidyl peptidase IV	Widely expressed, upregulated on activated memory T cells	Possible role in T cell signalling; binds HIV Tat protein	110	Type II membrane protein
CD27	TNFRSF7	Medullary thymocytes, T cells, NK cells, memory B cells	Homodimer; binds CD70 on B cells; role in B cell and T cell co-stimulation	50–55	TNFRSF
CD28	Tp44	Most T cells except for a subset of CD8$^+$ cells	Homodimer; binds CD80 and CD86 and provides signal 2 for T cell activation	44	IgSF
CD29	Platelet GPIIa	Leukocytes	Integrin β1 subunit, forms heterodimers with many integrin α chains; β chain of VLA integrins	130	Integrin β
CD30	Ki-1, TNFRSF7	Activated T and B cells, NK cells, monocytes	Binds CD153; co-stimulator of T cell proliferation; may inhibit autoreactive T cell proliferation	105–120	TNFRSF

Table of human CD antigens^{a,b} *contd*

CD antigen	Synonym(s)	Cellular expression	Function(s)	Molecular weight (kDa)	Family
CD31	PECAM-1	Endothelial cells, platelets, leukocytes	Adhesion molecule involved in leukocyte extravasation into tissues	130–140	IgSF
CD32	FcγRIIA FcγRIIB FcγRIIC	Monocytes, macrophages, Langerhans cells, granulocytes, B cells, DCs, platelets	Low affinity Fc receptor for aggregated IgG and immune complexes which participates in phagocytosis and ADCC; three forms generated by alternative splicing: A and C forms contain ITAM whereas B form contains ITIM; inhibitory receptor on B cells	40	IgSF
CD33	Gp67, SIGLEC-3	Myeloid progenitor cells, monocytes	Binds sialic acid; ITIM in cytoplasmic tail inhibits signal transduction	67	IgSF
CD34	Mucosialin	Haematopoietic progenitor cells, bone marrow stromal cells, small-vessel endothelial cells	Adhesion molecule, binds CD62L	116	Mucin
CD35	CR1	Erythrocytes, B cells, monocytes, neutrophils, eosinophils, follicular DCs, T cell subset	Complement receptor which binds C3b and C4b and promotes phagocytosis	190–285 (four alleles)	CCP superfamily
CD36	Platelet GPIIIb, GPIV	Platelets, monocytes, macrophages, DC subset, microvascular endothelial cells	Role in phagocytosis of apoptotic cells by macrophages; scavenger receptor for oxidized LDL; role in platelet adhesion	85–90	Scavenger receptor family
CD37	Tspan-26	B cells, T cell and myeloid cell subsets	Associates with MHC class II/CD53/CD81/CD82; possible role in signal transduction	40–52	TM4SF
CD38	T10	Widely expressed	Multi-catalytic ectoenzyme, augments B cell proliferation	45	
CD39	ENTPD1	Activated lymphoid cells, endothelial cells, DCs, macrophages	Possible role in B cell adhesion	78	Ecto-apyrase family
CD40	TNFRSF5	B cells, activated monocytes, macrophages, follicular DCs, DCs	Homodimer; binds CD154 and provides signal 2 for B cells	48	TNFRSF
CD41	Platelet GPIIb	Platelets, megakaryocytes	α_{IIb} integrin; precursor protein cleaved into disulphide-linked dimer (α and β chains); associates with CD61 to form GPIIb/IIIa integrin; binds fibrinogen, fibronectin, von Willebrand factor and thrombospondin	125 (α) 22 (β)	Integrin α
CD42a	Platelet GPIX	Platelets, megakaryocytes	Forms complexes with CD42b, CD42c and CD42d; essential for platelet adhesion; binds thrombin and von Willebrand factor	23	Mucin

Table of human CD antigens[a,b] *contd*

CD antigen	Synonym(s)	Cellular expression	Function(s)	Molecular weight (kDa)	Family
CD42b	Platelet GPIbα	Platelets, megakaryocytes	Disulphide-linked dimer with CD42c; forms complexes with CD42a and CD42d; essential for platelet adhesion; binds thrombin and von Willebrand factor	145	Mucin
CD42c	Platelet GPIbβ	Platelets, megakaryocytes	Disulphide-linked dimer with CD42b; forms complexes with CD42a and CD42d; essential for platelet adhesion, binds thrombin and von Willebrand factor	25	Mucin
CD42d	Platelet GPV	Platelets, megakaryocytes	Forms complexes with CD42a, CD42b, and CD42c; essential for platelet adhesion, binds thrombin and von Willebrand factor	82	Mucin
CD43	Leukosialin, sialophorin	All leukocytes except resting B cells	Adhesion molecule; binds CD54	95–135	Mucin
CD44	Hermes antigen, Pgp-1	Leukocytes, erythrocytes	Binds hyaluronan; mediates adhesion of leukocytes to extracellular matrix and to endothelial cells	80–100	CLP
CD45	Leukocyte common antigen (LCA), T200, B220	Haematopoietic cells	PTP that augments signalling through BCR and TCR; multiple isoforms (see below) result from alternative splicing	180–240	PTP receptor family; fibronectin type III superfamily
CD45RA		B cells, naïve T cells, monocytes	CD45 isoforms that contain the A exon; see CD45	220	PTP receptor family; fibronectin type III superfamily
CD45RB	T200	T cell subsets, B cells, monocytes, macrophages, granulocytes, DCs	CD45 isoforms that contain the B exon; see CD45	190–220	PTP receptor family; fibronectin type III superfamily
CD45RC		B cells, NK cells, monocytes, DCs, T cell subset	CD45 isoform that contains the C exon; see CD45	220	PTP receptor family; fibronectin type III superfamily
CD45RO		Memory T cells, B cell subset, monocytes, macrophages	CD45 isoform that contains none of the A, B and C exons; see CD45	180	PTP receptor family; fibronectin type III superfamily
CD46	MCP	Leukocytes, platelets, fibroblasts, epithelial cells	Binds to C3b and C4b and promotes their degradation by Factor I; 16 isoforms due to alternative splicing	56–76	CCP superfamily

Table of human CD antigens[a,b] *contd*

CD antigen	Synonym(s)	Cellular expression	Function(s)	Molecular weight (kDa)	Family
CD47	Integrin-associated protein	Widely distributed	Associates with integrins containing CD61; binds thrombospondin; role in cell adhesion	50	IgSF
CD47R	CDw149	Lymphocytes, monocytes	Function unknown	120	IgSF
CD48	Blast-1	Leukocytes except neutrophils	Binds to CD244 and inhibits NK cell effector function	45	IgSF
CD49a	VLA-1	Activated T cells, monocytes	α_1 integrin; associates with CD29 to form VLA-1; involved in leukocyte adhesion to extracellular matrix; binds laminin and collagens	210	Integrin α
CD49b	VLA-2, platelet GPIa	Monocytes, platelets, megakaryocytes, activated T cells, B cells, epithelial cells, endothelial cells	α_2 integrin; associates with CD29 to form VLA-2; involved in leukocyte adhesion to extracellular matrix; binds laminin and collagens	165	Integrin α
CD49c	VLA-3	B cells	α_3 integrin; precursor protein cleaved into disulphide-linked dimer (α and β chains); associates with CD29 to form VLA-3; involved in leukocyte adhesion to extracellular matrix; binds laminin, fibronectin and collagens	130 (α) 25 (β)	Integrin α
CD49d	VLA-4	Widely distributed	α_4 integrin; associates with CD29 to form VLA-4 or with β_7 integrin to form $\alpha_4\beta_7$ integrin; involved in leukocyte adhesion to endothelium and to extracellular matrix; binds to VCAM-1, MAdCAM-1, fibronectin and collagens	150	Integrin α
CD49e	VLA-5	T cells, monocytes, platelets, NK cells, DCs	α_5 integrin; precursor protein cleaved into disulphide-linked dimer (α and β chains); associates with CD29 to form VLA-5; involved in leukocyte adhesion to extracellular matrix; binds fibronectin	135 (α) 25 (β)	Integrin α
CD49f	VLA-6	T lymphocytes, monocytes, platelets, megakaryocytes	α_6 integrin; precursor protein cleaved into disulphide-linked dimer (α and β chains); associates with CD29 to form VLA-6; involved in leukocyte adhesion to extracellular matrix; binds fibronectin	125 (α) 25 (β)	Integrin α
CD50	ICAM-3	Leukocytes, some endothelial cells	Adhesion molecule; binds CD11a/CD18	110–140	IgSF
CD51	Vitronectin receptor α chain	Widely distributed	α_v integrin, precursor protein cleaved into disulphide-linked dimer (α and β chains); can associate with multiple integrin β chains including CD61; CD51/CD61 binds vitronectin, von Willebrand factor, fibrinogen and thrombospondin	125 (α) 24 (β)	Integrin α

Table of human CD antigens^{a,b} *contd*

CD antigen	Synonym(s)	Cellular expression	Function(s)	Molecular weight (kDa)	Family
CD52	CAMPATH-1	Thymocytes, lymphocytes, monocytes, macrophages, male reproductive tract epithelial cells	Function unknown	25–29	PI-linked HSA family
CD53	MRC OX44	Leukocytes, osteoblasts, osteoclasts	Signal transduction	32–42	TM4SF
CD54	ICAM-1	Activated lymphocytes, monocytes and endothelial cells	Adhesion molecule; binds CD11a/CD18 and CD11b/CD18 integrins; rhinovirus receptor	75–115	IgSF
CD55	DAF	Widely expressed	Binds C3b and C4b; promotes disassembly of C3 and C5 convertases; receptor for Coxsackie virus and Echovirus strains	55–70	CCP superfamily
CD56	Leu 19	NK cells, lymphocyte subsets	Isoform of N-CAM; adhesion molecule	175–220	IgSF
CD57	Leu 7	NK cell subset, B and T cell subsets, monocytes	Oligosaccharide found on many surface glycolipids and glycoproteins; role in cell adhesion; binds CD62L, CD62P and laminin		Carbohydrate epitope
CD58	LFA-3	Widely expressed	Adhesion molecule; binds CD2; role in T cell co-stimulation	40–70	IgSF
CD59	Protectin	Widely expressed	Binds C8 and C9 components of complement and inhibits assembly of membrane attack complex	19–25	PI-linked; Ly-6 superfamily
CD60a	Disialyl ganglioside D3 (GD3)	Subset of T cells, platelets, epithelium, fibroblasts	May be involved in regulation of apoptosis		Carbohydrate epitope
CD60b	9-O-acetyl-GD3	Subset of T cells, activated B cells, epithelium	Function unknown		Carbohydrate epitope
CD60c	7-O-acetyl-GD3	T cells	Augments signalling via CD3		Carbohydrate epitope
CD61	Platelet GPIIIa	Platelets, megakaryocytes, leukocytes, endothelial cells	Integrin β_3 subunit; associates with CD41 and with CD51	105	Integrin β
CD62E	E-selectin	Endothelial cells	Adhesion molecule; binds CD15s and mediates rolling of leukocytes on endothelium	115	C-type lectin
CD62L	L-selectin	B cells, T cells, monocytes, granulocytes, NK cells	Adhesion molecule; binds CD34 and mediates rolling of leukocytes on endothelium; lymph node-homing receptor of naïve T cells	74–95	C-type lectin
CD62P	P-selectin	Platelets, megakaryocytes, endothelial cells	Adhesion molecule, binds CD162; mediates interaction of platelets with neutrophils and monocytes; mediates rolling of leukocytes on endothelium	140	C-type lectin
CD63	LAMP-3	Activated platelets, monocytes, macrophages, endothelial cells, neutrophils	Possible role in signal transduction	40–60	TM4SF

Table of human CD antigens[a,b] *contd*

CD antigen	Synonym(s)	Cellular expression	Function(s)	Molecular weight (kDa)	Family
CD64	FcγRI	Monocytes, macrophages, activated neutrophils, eosinophils, DCs	High affinity receptor for IgG, involved in phagocytosis, ADCC and macrophage activation	72	IgSF
CD65	Ceramide dodecasaccharide	Granulocytes, monocyte subset	Function unknown; may bind to CD62E and CD62L		Carbohydrate epitope
CD65s		Granulocytes, monocytes	A fucoganglioside; function unknown		Carbohydrate epitope
CD66a	Biliary glycoprotein-1	Granulocytes, epithelial cells	Member of CEA family; binds CD62E; mediates homotypic adhesion and heterotypic adhesion with other CD66 family members; receptor for *Neisseria gonorrhoeae* and *N. meningitidis*	140–180	IgSF
CD66b	Formerly CD67	Granulocytes	Member of CEA family; mediates homotypic adhesion and heterotypic adhesion with other CD66 family members; possible role in signal transduction	95–100	IgSF
CD66c	Non-specific cross-reacting antigen	Granulocytes, epithelial cells	Member of CEA family; binds CD62E; mediates homotypic adhesion and heterotypic adhesion with other CD66 family members; receptor for *Neisseria gonorrhoeae* and *N. meningitidis*	90	IgSF
CD66d		Granulocytes	Member of CEA family; mediates homotypic adhesion and heterotypic adhesion with other CD66 family members; possible role in signal transduction; receptor for *Neisseria gonorrhoeae* and *N. meningitidis*	35	IgSF
CD66e	CEA	Epithelial cells	Member of CEA family; mediates homotypic adhesion and heterotypic adhesion with other CD66 family members; receptor for *Neisseria gonorrhoeae*	180–200	IgSF
CD66f	Pregnancy-specific glycoprotein	Placental syncytiotrophoblasts	Member of CEA family; function unknown	54–72	IgSF
CD68	Macrosialin	Monocytes, macrophages, neutrophils, DCs, activated T cells	Scavenger receptor; promotes phagocytosis	110	Mucin
CD69	Activation inducer molecule (AIM)	Haematopoietic cells	Homodimer; early activation antigen; role in signal transduction	28–32	C-type lectin
CD70	Ki-24	Activated B cells, activated T cells, macrophages	Homotrimeric; binds CD27; co-stimulation of T cell and B cell activation	75, 95, 170	TNFSF
CD71	Transferrin receptor	All proliferating cells	Homodimer; receptor for transferrin	95	Transferrin receptor family

Table of human CD antigens[a,b] *contd*

CD antigen	Synonym(s)	Cellular expression	Function(s)	Molecular weight (kDa)	Family
CD72	Lyb-2	B cells	Homodimer; binds CD100 and CD5; possible role in signalling	39–43	C type lectin
CD73	Ecto-5'-nucleotidase	B and T cell subsets, follicular DCs	Dephosphorylation of nucleotides to allow nucleoside uptake	69–72	5'-nucleotidase family
CD74	li	MHC class II-positive cells	Several isoforms; MHC class II-associated invariant chain; involved in exogenous pathway of antigen presentation	33, 35, 41, 43, 45 (isoforms)	
CD75		Mature B cells, T cell subsets	Function unknown; may bind CD22		Carbohydrate epitope
CD75s	CDw76	Mature B cells, T cell subsets	Function unknown; may bind CD22		Carbohydrate epitope
CD77	Burkitt's lymphoma antigen	Germinal centre B cells	Function unknown; may bind CD19		Carbohydrate epitope
CD79a	Igα,	MB1 B cells	Component of BCR complex; together with CD79b is required for cell surface expression of BCR and BCR-dependent signal transduction	32–33	IgSF
CD79b	Igβ, B29	B cells	Component of BCR complex; together with CD79a is required for cell surface expression of BCR and BCR-dependent signal transduction	37–39	IgSF
CD80	B7-1	DCs, activated B cells and macrophages	Binds to CD28 and CTLA-4; delivers signal 2 to T cells via CD28	60	IgSF
CD81	TAPA-1	Widely expressed	Associates with CD19 and CD21 to form B cell co-receptor; role in signal transduction	26	TM4SF
CD82	R2, C33, 4F9	Neutrophils, monocytes, epithelial cells, endothelial cells	Possible role in signal transduction	45–90	TM4SF
CD83	HB15	Activated B and T cells, DCs	Function unknown	43	IgSF
CD84	GR6	Haematopoietic cells	Function unknown	72–86	IgSF
CD85a	ILT5	NK cells, monocytes, macrophages, DCs, T cell subset, granulocytes	Binds to MHC class I molecules and suppresses NK cell-mediated killing	110	IgSF
CD85b	ILT8	NK and T cell subsets, monocytes, macrophages, DCs, B cells	Activation of NK cell-mediated killing		IgSF
CD85c		NK cells, T cell subsets, monocytes, macrophages, DCs, B cells	Activation of NK cell-mediated killing		IgSF
CD85d	ILT4	NK and T cell subsets, monocytes, macrophages, DCs, B cells	Suppression of NK cell-mediated killing	110	IgSF

Table of human CD antigens^{a,b} *contd*

CD antigen	Synonym(s)	Cellular expression	Function(s)	Molecular weight (kDa)	Family
CD85e	ILT6	NK cells, B cells, monocytes	Activation of NK cell-mediated killing		IgSF
CD85f	ILT11	Peripheral blood leukocytes	Activation of NK cell-mediated killing		IgSF
CD85g	ILT7	NK and T cell subsets, monocytes, macrophages, DCs, B cells	Activation of NK cell-mediated killing		IgSF
CD85h	ILT1	NK and T cell subsets, monocytes, macrophages, DCs, B cells	Activation of NK cell-mediated killing		IgSF
CD85i			Activation of NK cell-mediated killing		IgSF
CD85j	ILT2	Myeloid and lymphoid cells	Binds HLA-A and HLA-B molecules as well as some HLA-C molecules and HLA-G1; suppression of NK cell-mediated killing	110	IgSF
CD85k	ILT3		Suppression of NK cell-mediated killing	60	IgSF
CD85l	ILT9	NK and T cell subsets, monocytes, macrophages, DCs, B cells			IgSF
CD85m	ILT10				IgSF
CD86	B7-2	DCs, activated B cells and macrophages	Binds to CD28 and CTLA-4; delivers signal 2 to T cells via CD28	80	IgSF
CD87	UPA-R	Widely expressed	Urokinase plasminogen activator receptor	35–59	PI-linked; Ly-6 superfamily
CD88	C5aR	Granulocytes, macrophages, mast cells, DCs	Receptor for complement component C5a	43	GPCR
CD89	FcαR	Myeloid cells, B and T cell subsets	Six isoforms generated by alternative splicing; IgA receptor	45–100	IgSF
CD90	Thy-1	Haematopoietic cells, neurons	Function in humans unknown	25–29	IgSF
CD91		Macrophages and monocytes	α_2 macroglobulin receptor; precursor protein cleaved into non-covalently associated dimer (α and β chains); uptake of low density lipoproteins	515 (α) 85 (β)	EGF receptor family
CD92	GR9	Monocytes, granulocytes, platelets,endothelial cells	Choline transporter	70	
CD93	GR11	Granulocytes, monocytes, endothelial cells, NK cells	Possible role in clearance of apoptotic cells	126	
CD94	KP43	NK cells, T cell subsets	CD94 associates covalently with other C-type lectins such as CD159a to form inhibitory or activating NK cell receptors	30–43	C-type lectin
CD95	Apo-1, Fas	Widely distributed	Homotrimer; binds FasL leading to apoptosis	45	TNFRSF
CD96		Activated T cells, NK cells	Binds CD155; promotes T cell and NK cell adhesion to target cells	160	IgSF

Table of human CD antigens[a,b] *contd*

CD antigen	Synonym(s)	Cellular expression	Function(s)	Molecular weight (kDa)	Family
CD97	GR1	Activated T and B cells, monocytes, macrophages, granulocytes	Precursor protein cleaved into dimer (α and β chains); potential role in cell adhesion	75–85 (α) 28 (β)	GPCR
CD98	4F2	Widely distributed	Heterodimer; possible amino acid transporter	80 40	
CD99	MIC2, E2	Haematopoietic cells	Adhesion molecule	32	Mucin
CD99R		T cells, myeloid cells, NK cells, thymocytes	Modulates T cell adhesion	32	Mucin
CD100	GR3	Broad expression on haematopoietic cells	Roles in monocyte migration, T and B cell activation and T cell–B cell and T cell–DC interaction	150	Semaphorin; IgSF
CD101	V7, P126	Granulocytes, DCs, monocytes, activated T cells	Disulphide-linked homodimer; may co-stimulate T cell activation	120	IgSF
CD102	ICAM-2	Vascular endothelial cells, monocytes, some lymphocytes	Cell adhesion; binds CD11a/CD18	55–65	IgSF
CD103	HML-1, α_6 integrin, α_E integrin	Intraepithelial lymphocytes, colon, testis, breast	α_E integrin; precursor proteins cleaved into disulphide-linked dimer; binds to E-cadherin and promotes homing of mucosal T cells	150 25 (dimer)	Integrin α
CD104	β_4 integrin	Epithelial cells, Schwann cells	Associates with CD49f to form $\alpha_6\beta_4$ integrin; important for adhesion of epithelia to basement membranes; binds laminin	205–220	Integrin β
CD105	Endoglin	Endothelial cells, stromal cells	Homodimer; binds TGF-β	95	
CD106	VCAM-1	Endothelial cells, follicular DCs, macrophages	Adhesion molecule; ligand for CD49d/CD29 (VLA-4)	100–110	IgSF
CD107a	LAMP-1	Activated platelets, T cells, neutrophils, endothelium and epithelium	Maintenance and adhesion of lysosomes	100–120	LAMP family
CD107b	LAMP-2	Activated platelets, T cells, neutrophils, endothelium and epithelium	Maintenance and adhesion of lysosomes	100–120	LAMP family
CD108	GR2	Erythrocytes, lymphocytes, myeloid cells, stromal cells	Binds CD232; function unknown	76–80	Semaphorin
CD109	Platelet activation factor, GR56	Activated T cells and platelets, endothelial cells	Function unknown	175	
CD110	TPO-R	Platelets, megakaryocytes, haematopoietic progenitor cells	Thrombopoietin receptor; main regulator of megakaryocyte and platelet formation	85–92	Type I cytokine receptor family
CD111	Nectin1	Haematopoietic cells, epithelial cells	Adhesion molecule; receptor for herpes simplex virus-1	75	IgSF
CD112	Nectin-2	Widely distributed	Adhesion molecule; receptor for herpes simplex virus-1	64–72	IgSF

Table of human CD antigens[a,b] *contd*

CD antigen	Synonym(s)	Cellular expression	Function(s)	Molecular weight (kDa)	Family
CD113	Nectin-3	Epithelial cells, testis, gut, kidney, brain, liver, placenta	Adhesion molecule	60	IgSF
CD114	G-CSF receptor	Granulocytes, monocytes, platelets, endothelial cells	Binds to and mediates effects of granulocyte colony stimulating factor (G-CSF)	150	Type I cytokine receptor family
CD115	M-CSFR, c-fms	Monocytes, macrophages, osteoclasts, DCs	Binds to and mediates effects of macrophage colony stimulating factor (M-CSF)	150	IgSF; TKR
CD116	GM-CSFRα	Monocytes, neutrophils, eosinophils, endothelium	α chain of the granulocyte–macrophage colony stimulating factor (GM-CSF) receptor; associates with CD131 to bind to and mediate effects of GM-CSF	70–85	Type I cytokine receptor family
CD117	c-kit	Haematopoietic progenitor cells, mast cells, melanocytes	Binds to and mediates effects of stem cell factor (SCF)	145	IgSF; TKR
CD118	LIFR-α	Embryonic stem cells, epithelial cells, monocytes, fibroblasts	Associates with CD130 to form high affinity LIFR which binds LIF and OSM and mediates the effects of these cytokines	190	Type I cytokine receptor family
CD119	IFN-γRα	Macrophages, T cells, B cells, NK cells, neutrophils	Interferon-γ receptor; binds IFN-γ and associates with IFN-γAF to mediate the effects of this cytokine	90–100	Type II cytokine receptor family
CD120a	TNFR-I	Widely expressed, especially on epithelial cells	TNF receptor, binds both TNF-α and LT-α and mediates effects of these cytokines including apoptosis, anorexia, fever, and cytokine induction	50–60	TNFRSF
CD120b	TNFR-II	Widely expressed, especially on myeloid cells	TNF receptor, binds both TNF-α and LT-α and mediates effects of these cytokines including pro-inflammatory cellular responses, apoptosis and anti-viral activity; cleaved by CD156b into soluble receptor which may modulate activities of TNF-α and LT-α.	75–85	TNFRSF
CD121a	IL-1R type I	Widely expressed	Binds IL-1α and IL-1β and mediates the effects of these cytokines	80	IgSF
CD121b	IL-1R type II	B cells, macrophages, monocytes	Decoy receptor for IL-1; binds IL-1α (low affinity) and IL-1β (high affinity)	60–70	IgSF
CD122	IL-2Rβ, IL-15Rβ	NK cells, resting T cell subpopulation, some B cell lines	β chain of the IL-2 and IL-15 receptors; associates with CD25 and CD132 to bind to and mediate the effects of IL-2; associates with the IL-15Rα chain and CD132 to bind to and mediate the effects of IL-15	75	Type I cytokine receptor family

Table of human CD antigens[a,b] *contd*

CD antigen	Synonym(s)	Cellular expression	Function(s)	Molecular weight (kDa)	Family
CD123	IL-3Rα	Bone marrow stem cells, granulocytes, monocytes, megakaryocytes	IL-3 receptor α chain; associates with CD131 to bind to and mediate the effects of IL-3	70	Type I cytokine receptor family
CD124	IL-4Rα	B cells Th2 cells, haematopoietic precursor cells	IL-4 receptor α chain associates with CD132 to form high affinity IL-4R which binds to and mediates the effects of IL-4; associates with CD 213a1 to form the type II IL-4R and the high affinity IL-13 receptor which binds to and mediates the effects of IL-13	130–150	Type I cytokine receptor family
CD125	IL-5Rα	Eosinophils, basophils, B cells, mast cells	IL-5 receptor α chain which associates with CD131 to bind to and mediate the effects of IL-5	55–60	Type I cytokine receptor family
CD126	IL-6R	Plasma cells, activated B cells, T cells, monocytes	IL-6 receptor α subunit which binds IL-6 and associates with CD130 to mediate the effects of this cytokine	80	Type I cytokine receptor family
CD127	IL-7Rα	Lymphoid precursor cells, pro-B cells, T cells, monocytes	IL-7 receptor α chain which associates with CD132 to mediate the effects of IL-7	68–79, possibly forms homodimers	Type I cytokine receptor family
CD129	IL-9Rα	B cells, T cells, myeloid cells	IL-9 receptor α chain which associates with CD132 to mediate effects of IL-9	64	Type I cytokine receptor family
CD130	IL-6Rβ, IL-11Rβ, OSMRβ, LIFRβ	Activated B cells and plasma cells; weak on most leukocytes; endothelial cells	Common β chain of receptors for IL-6, IL-11, OSM and LIF	130	Type I cytokine receptor family
CD131	IL-3R common β chain	Monocytes, B cells, granulocytes, eosinophils	Associates with CD116 to bind to and mediate effects of GM-CSF; associates with CD123 to bind to and mediate the effects of IL-3; associates with CD125 to bind to and mediate the effects of IL-5	95–120	Type I cytokine receptor family
CD132	Common gamma chain, γc	T and B cells, NK cells, monocytes, macrophages, neutrophils, fibroblasts, haematopoietic precursor cells	Forms part of the receptors for the cytokines IL-2, IL-4, IL-7, IL-9, IL-15 and IL-21 and is required for signalling following cytokine binding to these receptors	64	Type I cytokine receptor family
CD133	AC133	Stem/progenitor cells	Function unknown	120	
CD134	OX-40	Activated T cells, fibroblasts, haematopoietic precursor cells	Binds CD252 and co-stimulates T cell activation, proliferation and cytokine production	48–50	TNFRSF
CD135	FLT3/FLK2	Haematopoietic stem cells	Growth factor receptor for early haematopoietic progenitor cells; binds FLT3 ligand	130–150	TKR

Table of human CD antigens[a,b] *contd*

CD antigen	Synonym(s)	Cellular expression	Function(s)	Molecular weight (kDa)	Family
CDw136	Macrophage-stimulating protein receptor	Epithelial cells, monocytes, macrophages, granulocytes	Binds macrophage-stimulating protein and induces cell migration and proliferation; role in development of epithelial tissues	150	TKR
CD137	TNFRSF9, 4-1BB	T cells, B cells, follicular DCs, monocytes	Binds to CD137L and co-stimulates T cell activation	30	TNFRSF
CD138	Syndecan-1	Plasma cells; immature B cells, epithelial cells	Bind collagen types I, III and V	85–92	HSP
CD139		Granulocytes, monocytes, B cells	Function unknown	209–228	
CD140a	PDGFRα	Widely distributed	Binds to CD140b to mediate effects of PDGF	180	TKR
CD140b	PDGFRβ	Widely distributed	Binds to CD140a to mediate effects of PDGF	180	TKR
CD141	Thrombomodulin	Endothelial cells, smooth muscle cells, platelets	Regulator of coagulation	105	C-type lectin
CD142	Tissue factor	Epithelial cells, stromal cells, activated endothelial cells	Binds clotting factor VIIa to initiate clotting	45–47	Type II cytokine receptor family
CD143	Angiotensin converting enzyme	Endothelial cells, epithelial cells, neurons, fibroblasts, macrophages	Peptidyl-hydrolase involved in metabolism of vasoactive peptides	170	Metallo-peptidase
CD144	Vascular endothelial cadherin, cadherin-5	Endothelial cells	Adhesion molecule; mediates homotypic adhesion	135	Cadherin
CD146	MUC18	Widely expressed	Potential adhesion molecule	118	IgSF
CD147	Neurothelin, basiglin	Endothelial cells, myeloid cells, lymphocytes	Potential adhesion molecule	55–65	IgSF
CD148	HPTP-η	Granulocytes, monocytes, T cells, DCs, nerve cells, haematopoietic cells	Unknown	240–260	PTP
CD150	SLAM	Activated lymphocytes, DCs, endothelial cells	Signalling molecule in B and T cell interactions	75–95	IgSF
CD151	PETA-3	Platelets, epithelial cells, endothelium	Cell adhesion; possible role in platelet aggregation	32	TM4SF
CD152	CTLA-4	Activated T cells	Inhibitory signal for T cells; binds to CD80 and CD86	44	IgSF
CD153	CD30L	Activated T cells, neutrophils, macrophages, monocytes	Binds CD30 on T cells to deliver co-stimulatory signal; may also inhibit autoreactive T cell proliferation	40	TNFSF
CD154	CD40L, TNFSF5	Activated T cells, DCs, macrophages	Co-stimulatory molecule; ligand for CD40	32–39	TNFSF
CD155	Polio virus receptor (PVR)	Monocytes, macrophages, thymocytes neurons	Adhesion molecule	80–90	IgSF

Table of human CD antigens[a,b] *contd*

CD antigen	Synonym(s)	Cellular expression	Function(s)	Molecular weight (kDa)	Family
CD156a	ADAM8	Myeloid cells, B cells	May be involved in leukocyte extravasation	69	ZMP
CD156b	ADAM17	Widely distributed	Proteolysis and release of TNF and TGF-α from cells	100	ZMP
CD156c	ADAM10	Widely distributed	Broad specificity endopeptidase involved in release of several cell surface molecules including TNF-α	70	ZMP
CD157	BST-1	Widely distributed	ADP ribosyl cyclase; promotes B cell growth	42–50	PI-linked
CD158a	p58.1, KIR2DL1	NK cells, T cells	Inhibits NK killing; binds HLA-C molecules	50/58	IgSF
CD158b1	p58.2, KIR2DL2	NK cells, T cells	Inhibits NK killing; binds HLA-C molecules	50/58	IgSF
CD158b2	KIR2DL3	NK cells, T cells	Inhibits NK killing; binds HLA-C molecules	50/58	IgSF
CD158d	KIR2DL4	NK cells, T cells	Inhibits NK killing; binds HLA-G molecules	41	IgSF
CD158e1	KIR3DL1	NK cells, T cells	Inhibits NK killing; binds HLA-B molecules	70	IgSF
CD158e2		NK cells, T cells	Activation of NK cell killing; binds to HLA-B molecules		IgSF
CD158f	KIR2DL5A	NK cells, T cells	Inhibits NK killing; binds HLA-B molecules		IgSF
CD158g	KIR2DS5	NK cells, T cells	Activates NK cell killing		IgSF
CD158h	KIR2DS1	NK cells, T cells	Activation of NK cell killing; binds to HLA-C molecules	50	IgSF
CD158i	KIR2DS4	NK cells, T cells	Activation of NK cell killing; binds to HLA-C molecules	35/58	IgSF
CD158j	KIR2DS2	NK cells, T cells	Activation of NK cell killing; binds to HLA-C molecules	50	IgSF
CD158k	KIR3DL2	NK cells, T cells	Inhibits NK killing; possibly binds to HLA-A molecules	70	IgSF
CD158z	KIR3DL3	NK cells, T cells	Inhibits NK killing		IgSF
CD159a	KLR-C1	NK cells, T cells	Associates with CD94 to form NK cell receptor; binds to MHC class I molecules and inhibits NK-mediated killing	26 (NK cell) 43 (T cell)	Lectin
CD159c	KLR-C2	NK cells, T cells	Associates with CD94 to form NK cell receptor; stimulates NK-mediated killing	26 (NK cell) 36 (T cell)	Lectin
CD160	BY55	T cells, NK cells	Binds to classical and non-classical MHC class I molecules	27	IgSF
CD161	NKR-P1A	NK cells, T cell subset	Regulation of NK cell-mediated killing	60 (homo-dimer)	Lectin

Table of human CD antigens[a,b] *contd*

CD antigen	Synonym(s)	Cellular expression	Function(s)	Molecular weight (kDa)	Family
CD162	PSGL-1	Granulocytes, monocytes, T cells, subset of B cells	Binds the selectins CD62E, CD62L and CD62P; leukocyte adhesion to endothelium	120 (homo-dimer)	Mucin
CD162R	PEN5	NK cells, lymphocytes, myeloid cells	Post-translational modification of CD162		Carbohydrate epitope
CD163	M130, GHI/61	Monocytes, macrophages, spleen, bone marrow	Binds haemoglobin; uptake and recycling of iron	110–130	Scavenger receptor family
CD164	MGC-24	Haematopoietic progenitors	Adhesion molecule	80–90	Mucin
CD165	AD2, gp37	T cells, NK cells, platelets, thymocytes, thymic epithelium	Adhesion molecule	37–42	
CD166	ALCAM	Activated B and T cells, fibroblasts, epithelial cells, neurons	Adhesion molecule; ligand for CD6	100	IgSF
CD167a	DDR1	Epithelial cells, tumour cells	Binds collagen	105	TKR
CD167b	DDR2	Skeletal muscle, cardiac muscle, skin, lung	Binds collagen	101	TKR
CD168	HMMR	Thymocytes, haematopoietic progenitors, malignancies	Binds hyaluronan; cell adhesion molecule	80–88	
CD169	Sialoadhesin, SIGLEC-1	Macrophages	Cell adhesion molecule	180–200	IgSF
CD170	SIGLEC-5	Neutrophils, monocytes	Cell adhesion molecule	67	IgSF
CD171	N-CAM L1	Neurons, Schwann cells, lymphocytes	Cell adhesion molecule	200–230	IgSF
CD172a	SIRPα	Haematopoietic progenitor cells, myeloid cells	Binds CD47; signal transduction	85–90	IgSF
CD172b	SIRPβ1	Myeloid cells, neural cells	Associates with DAP-12; signal transduction	110–120	IgSF
CD172g	SIRPγ, SIRPβ2	B cell, T cell, NK cell	Binds to CD47 with lower affinity than does CD172a; possible role in signalling	55	IgSF
CD173	Blood group H type 2	Widely expressed	Blood group antigen		Carbohydrate epitope
CD174	Lewis y	Widely expressed	Blood group antigen		Carbohydrate epitope
CD175	TN antigen	Widely expressed	Blood group antigen		Carbohydrate epitope
CD175s	Sialyl-TN	Widely expressed	Blood group antigen		Carbohydrate epitope
CD176	Thomsen–Friedrenreich antigen	Widely expressed	Blood group antigen		Carbohydrate epitope
CD177	NB1	Myeloid cells	Function unknown	56–64	Ly-6 superfamily
CD178	FasL, CD95L, TNFSF6	T cells, NK cells, tumour cells, endothelial cells	Binds CD95 and induces apoptosis; forms homotrimers	40	TNFSF

Table of human CD antigens^{a,b} *contd*

CD antigen	Synonym(s)	Cellular expression	Function(s)	Molecular weight (kDa)	Family
CD179a	VpreB	Pro-B cells, early pre-B cells	Associates with CD179b to form surrogate light chain component of pre-BCR	16–18	IgSF
CD179b	λ5	Pro-B cells, early pre-B cells	Associates with CD179a to form surrogate light chain component of pre-BCR	22	IgSF
CD180	RP105	B cells, DCs, monocytes	Associates with MD-1 and works in concert with TLR-4 in LPS signalling	95–105	TLR
CD181	CXCR1, IL8RA	Neutrophils, basophils, T cells	High affinity receptor for CXCL8 (IL-8); low affinity receptor for CXCL1	58–67	CRF/GPCR
CD182	CXCR2, IL8RB	Neutrophils, basophils, T cells	Receptor for CXCL1, CXCL2, CXCL3, CXCL5, CXCL7; low affinity receptor for CXCL8 (IL-8)	58–67	CRF/GPCR
CD183	CXCR3	T cells, NK cells, B cell subset	Receptor for CXCL9, CXCL10 and CXCL11	41	CRF/GPCR
CD184	CXCR4	Widely expressed	Receptor for CXCL12; co-receptor for lymphotropic HIV-1 strains	45	CRF/GPCR
CD185	CXCR5	B cells, T cell subset, monocytes, Burkitt's lymphoma cells	Receptor for CXCL13	42	CRF/GPCR
CD186	CXCR6	B cells, Th1 cells, NK cells	Binds CXCL16; co-receptor for strains of HIV-1, HIV-2 and SIV	39	CRF/GPCR
CD191	CCR1	T cells, monocytes, NK cells, DCs	Receptor for CCL3, CCL5, CCL7	41	CRF/GPCR
CD192	CCR2	Monocytes, basophils, subset of B, T and DCs	Receptor for CCL2	42	CRF/GPCR
CD193	CCR3	Eosinophils, basophils, T cells, DCs	Receptor for CCL5, CCL7, CCL11, CCL13, CCL26	41	CRF/GPCR
CD194	CCR4	Leukocytes, endothelial cells, brain	Receptor for CCL17, CCL22	41	CRF/GPCR
CD195	CCR5	Leukocytes, promyeloid cells	Receptor for CCL3, CCL4, CCL5; co-receptor for M-tropic strains of HIV-1	40	CRF/GPCR
CD197	CCR7	B cells, T cells, DCs, macrophages, NK cells	Receptor for CCL19 and CCL21	45	CRF/GPCR
CD200	OX-2	Brain cells, B cells, thymocytes	Unknown	41–47	IgSF
CD201	EPCR	Endothelial cells, liver	Binds protein C; endothelial cell activation	49	
CD202b	Tie2/Tek	Endothelial cells, haematopoietic cells	Vascular remodelling	140	IgSF
CD203c	ENPP3	Basophils, mast cells, haematopoietic progenitors	Ectonucleotidase	130	Type II membrane protein

Table of human CD antigens[a,b] *contd*

CD antigen	Synonym(s)	Cellular expression	Function(s)	Molecular weight (kDa)	Family
CD204	Macrophage scavenger receptor	Myeloid cells	Antigen capture	220	Scavenger receptor family
CD205	DEC205	DCs, B cells, T cell subsets	Antigen capture	205	C-type lectin
CD206	Macrophage mannose receptor	Macrophages, immature DCs	PRR, binds high mannose moieties on microbes	162–175	C-type lectin
CD207	Langerin	Langerhans cells	Antigen capture	40	C-type lectin
CD208	DC-LAMP	DCs	Sorting of peptide MHC class II molecules to DC surface	70-90	LAMP family
CD209	DC-SIGN	DCs	Binds ICAM-3; stabilizes DC-T cell interaction	44	C-type lectin
CDw210a	IL-10Rα	Haematopoietic cells, B cells, T cell subsets	CDw210a associates with CDw210b to bind to and mediate the effects of IL-10; the functional IL-10R is thought to consist of two molecules of CDw210a and two molecules of CDw210b	90–110	Type II cytokine receptor family
CDw210b	IL-10Rβ	Haematopoietic cells, B cells, T cell subsets	See CDw210a; CDw210b associates with IL-22R1 to form a high affinity receptor for IL-22; CDw210b also associates with IL-28R2 to form a high affinity receptor for both IL-28 and IL-29		Type II cytokine receptor family
CD212	IL-12Rβ1	Haematopoietic cells, activated T cells and NK cells	Associates with the IL-12β2 subunit to form the functional IL-12 receptor which binds to and mediates the effects of IL-12	130	Type I cytokine receptor family
CD213a1	IL-13Rα1	Widely distributed	Associates with CD124 to form the type II IL-4 receptor and also the functional IL-13 receptor	60–70	IgSF
CD213a2	IL-13Rα2, IL-13BP	Widely distributed	Non-signalling IL-13 decoy receptor	56	Type I cytokine receptor family
CD217	IL-17R	Widely expressed	Binds IL-17 with low affinity; functional IL-17 receptor is thought to be a heteromeric complex consisting at least of CD217 and IL-17RC	120	IL-17 receptor family
CD218a	IL-18Rα	Lymphocytes, neutrophils, NK cells, monocytes, granulocytes, endothelial, DCs	Ligand-binding portion of the IL-18R; associates with CD218b to bind to and mediate the effects of IL-18	62	IgSF
CD218b	IL-18Rβ	Activated T cells	Associates with CD218a to bind to and mediate the effects of IL-18	68	IgSF
CD220	Insulin receptor	Widely distributed	Signal transduction following insulin binding	α, 130 β, 90	TKR
CD221	IGF1R	Widely distributed	Signal transduction following insulin or IGF1 binding	α, 135 β, 90	IRTK

Table of human CD antigens[a,b] *contd*

CD antigen	Synonym(s)	Cellular expression	Function(s)	Molecular weight (kDa)	Family
CD222	M6PR, IGF2 receptor	Widely distributed	Binding of IGF2, intracellular sorting of M6P containing proteins	250	Lectin family
CD223	LAG-3	Activated T cells, NK cells	Binds to MHC class II; downregulation of response	70	IgSF
CD224	γ-glutmyl transpeptidase, GGT1	Widely expressed	Two polypeptide chains cleaved from single precursor, glutathione metabolism	62–68 22	GGT superfamily
CD225	Leu 13	Leukocytes, endothelial cells, B cells	Associates with CD19/CD21/CD81 complex; possible role in signalling	16–17	
CD226	DNAM-1	NK cells, platelets, monocytes, T and B subsets	Role in cell adhesion and activation; binds CD112 and CD155	65	IgSF
CD227	Muc1, Mucin 1	Activated T cells, monocytes and DCs, glandular and ductal epithelial cells, adenocarcinomas	Role in cytoprotection; potential adhesion molecule; binds to CD54 and CD169	300–700	Mucin
CD228	Melanotransferrin	Melanomas, brain cells	Iron uptake	97	Transferrin superfamily
CD229	Ly-9	Lymphocytes	Cell adhesion and activation	90–120	IgSF
CD230	Prion protein, PrP, PrPc	Widely expressed	Isoform is causative agent of spongiform encephalopathies	27–30	Prion
CD231	TALLA-1/A15	Neurons, T-ALL, neuroblastomas	Function unknown	150	TMS4F
CD232	VESPR, Plexin C1	Neurons	Regulates cell dissociation, receptor for virally encoded semaphorins	200	Plexin
CD233	Band 3	Erythroid and renal tubular epithelial cells	Membrane transport	93–110	Anion exchanger
CD234	Duffy antigen	Erythroid and non-erythroid cells	Non-signalling receptor for various cytokines; receptor for *Plasmodium vivax* and *P. knowlesi*	35	CRF
CD235a	Glycophorin A	Erythroid cells	Prevention of RBC aggregation; MN and Ss blood group antigens	31	Glycophorin A family
CD235b	Glycophorin B	Erythroid cells	MN and Ss blood group antigens	24	Glycophorin A
CD236	Glycophorin C/D	Erythroid cells	*Plasmodium falciparum* receptor; Webb and Dutch blood group antigens	24	Type III membrane protein
CD236R	Glycophorin C	Erythroid cells	Regulates RBC shape; Gerbich blood group antigens	32	Type III membrane protein
CD238	Kell	Erythroid cells	Kell blood group antigens	93	ZMP
CD239	B-CAM	Widely expressed	Lutheran blood group antigens	78	IgSF
CD240CE	Rh30CE	Erythroid cells	Membrane transport; blood group antigen	30	Rh
CD240D	RhD, Rh30D	Erythroid cells	Membrane transport; RhD antigen	30	Rh
CD240DCE		Erythroid cells	Membrane transport; blood group antigen	30	Rh

Table of human CD antigens[a,b] *contd*

CD antigen	Synonym(s)	Cellular expression	Function(s)	Molecular weight (kDa)	Family
CD241	RhAg, RH50A	Erythroid cells	Assembly and transport of Rhesus complex to RBC membrane	50	Rh
CD242	ICAM-4	Erythroid cells	Adhesion molecule	42	IgSF
CD243	MDR-1, P-glycoprotein	Stem cells, progenitor cells	Pumps toxic drugs out of cells and confers multidrug resistance	1170	ABC
CD244	2B4, NAIL	NK cells	Regulation of NK function; CD48 receptor	66	IgSF
CD245	p220/240	T cells	Possible role in cell cycle progression	220–240	
CD246	ALK	Small intestine, testis, brain	Oncogenesis following chromosomal translocation	177–200	IRTK
CD247	ζ chain, CD3ζ	T cells, NK cells	Signal transduction following antigen binding to TCR	21–23	IgSF
CD248	Endosialin	Fibroblasts, endothelial cells	Function unknown; possible role in cell–cell interactions	175	C-type lectin
CD249	Aminopeptidase A	B cell precursors, thymic cortical epithelial cells	Metallopeptidase involved in rennin–angiotensin catabolism	160	ZMP
CD252	TNFSF4, CD134L	B cells, DCs, monocytes, mast cells, endothelial cells	Binds to CD134; co-stimulates T cell activation, proliferation, and cytokine production	34	TNFSF
CD253	TNFSF10, TRAIL	DCs, NK cells, activated B and T cells, monocytes	Binds to CD261, CD262 and induces apoptosis; binds decoy receptors CD263 and CD264;	33	TNFSF
CD254	TNFSF11, RANKL	Osteoblasts, osteoclasts, stromal cells, activated T cells, lymph nodes	Binds to CD265; promotes osteoclast differentiation and activation; promotes bone development and lymph node development	35	TNFSF
CD255	TNFSF12	Widely expressed	Soluble and transmembrane forms; binds to CD266, weak inducer of apoptosis; promotes angiogenesis	18 (soluble) 35 (membrane)	TNFSF
CD256	TNFSF13, APRIL	Myeloid cells, leukocytes	Secreted after intracellular proteolysis; binds to CD267 and CD269; promotes B cell development and T and B cell proliferation	28	TNFSF
CD257	TNFSF13b, BAFF	Leukocytes, lymphoid and non-lymphoid tissues	Binds to CD267, CD268 and CD269; promotes B cell survival, activation and proliferation	31	TNFSF
CD258	TNFSF14, HVEML	DCs, T cells, monocytes, spleen, brain	Binds to CD270 and the LT-β receptor; promotes DC activation and Th1 cell proliferation and cytokine secretion	29	TNFSF
CD259	Nerve growth factor-β		Homodimerizes and forms part of a larger complex; has nerve growth stimulating activity	14	TNFSF
CD261	TNFRSF10a	Widely expressed	Binds to CD253; transduces cell death signal	50	TNFRSF

Table of human CD antigens[a,b] *contd*

CD antigen	Synonym(s)	Cellular expression	Function(s)	Molecular weight (kDa)	Family
CD262	TNFRSF10a	Widely expressed	Binds to CD253; transduces cell death signal	48	TNFRSF
CD263	TNFRSF10c	Widely expressed	Decoy receptor for CD253	65	TNFRSF
CD264	TNFRSF10d	Widely expressed	Decoy receptor for CD253	35	TNFRSF
CD265	TNFRSF11a, RANK	Widely expressed	Binds to CD254; promotes osteoclast differentiation and activation; promotes bone development and lymph node development	97	TNFRSF
CD266	TNFRSF12a	Widely expressed	Binds to and mediates activities of CD255	14	TNFRSF
CD267	TNFRSF13b, TACI	B cells, activated T cells	Binds to CD256 and CD257; role in B cell homeostasis; augments T cell function	32	TNFRSF
CD268	TNFRSF13b, BAFF-R	Peripheral blood lymphocytes, leukocytes, lymphoid tissues	Two isoforms generated by alternative splicing; binds to CD257; promotes B cell survival	19 25	TNFRSF
CD269	TNFRSF17	B cells, plasma cells	Binds to CD256 with high affinity and CD257 with low affinity; promotes survival, proliferation and differentiation of B cells	27	TNFRSF
CD270	TNFRSF14, HVEM	T cells, monocytes, immature DCs	Binds LT-α; binds to CD258, CD272 and glycoprotein D of HSV-1 and HSV-2	30	TNFRSF
CD271	TNFRSF16, nerve growth factor receptor	Neurons, stromal cells, follicular DCs, B cells	Binds all neurotrophins including CD259; promotes survival as well as death of neural cells	75	TNFRSF
CD272	BTLA	Th1 cells, B cells, DCs, macrophages	Binds to CD270 and suppresses lymphocyte responses	33	IgSF
CD273	B7-DC	DCs, macrophages, T cells, activated monocytes	Binds CD279; inhibits T cell proliferation	25	IgSF
CD274	B7-H1	Macrophages, DCs, activated T cells, B cells and monocytes	Binds to CD279; inhibits T cell proliferation	40	IgSF
CD275	ICOS-L	Widely expressed	Two isoforms generated by alternative splicing; binds to CD278; promotes T cell and B cell proliferation and differentiation	40 60	IgSF
CD276	B7-H3	Epithelial cells, NK cells, B cells, T cells, activated monocytes, DC subsets	Two isoforms generated by alternative splicing; inhibitor of T cell function	40 110	IgSF
CD277		B cells, T cells, NK cells, DCs, monocytes, endothelial cells	Function unknown; may play a role in regulation of the immune response	56	IgSF
CD278	ICOS	T cells (especially Th2 cells), B cells	Binds to CD275; promotes T cell proliferation and Th2 cytokine production	55	IgSF
CD279	PD-1	T cells, B cells, macrophages	Binds to CD273 and CD274; inhibits T cell and B cell responses; promotes cell death	55	IgSF

Table of human CD antigens[a,b] *contd*

CD antigen	Synonym(s)	Cellular expression	Function(s)	Molecular weight (kDa)	Family
CD280	Mannose receptor 2	Myeloid precursor cells, osteoclasts, fibroblasts, osteocytes, chondrocytes	Binds extracellular matrix proteins and mediates their uptake and degradation	160–170	C-type lectin
CD281	TLR-1	DCs, keratinocytes, macrophages, monocytes, neutrophils	Associates with CD282; binds bacterial lipoproteins and lipopeptides; induces pro-inflammatory cytokine production	90	TLR family
CD282	TLR-2	Macrophages, granulocytes, keratinocytes, DCs	Associates with CD281 or CD286; binds bacterial lipopeptides, lipoproteins and glycans; induces production of pro-inflammatory cytokines	85	TLR family
CD283	TLR-3	Myeloid DCs, fibroblasts, epithelial cells	Binds double-stranded RNA; induces pro-inflammatory cytokine production	100	TLR family
CD284	TLR-4	Monocytes, activated T cells, DCs, macrophages, granulocytes, endothelial cells	CD284 homodimers associate with CD14; binds LPS; induces production of pro-inflammatory cytokines	85	TLR family
CD285	TLR-5	Leukocytes	Binds flagellin; induces production of pro-inflammatory cytokines	120	TLR family
CD286	TLR-6	Leukocytes, endothelial cells	Associates with CD282; binds bacterial lipopeptides and lipoproteins; induces production of pro-inflammatory cytokines	85	TLR family
CD287	TLR-7	DCs, B cells, macrophages	Binds single-stranded RNA; induces pro-inflammatory cytokine production	118	TLR family
CD288	TLR-8	Macrophages, DCs, leukocytes	Binds single-stranded GU-rich RNA; induces pro-inflammatory cytokine production	83	TLR family
CD289	TLR-9	DCs, B cells, monocytes	Binds unmethylated CpG DNA; induces pro-inflammatory cytokine production; promotes Th1 cell differentiation	115–120	TLR family
CD290	TLR-10	B cells, Langerhans cells, DCs	Ligands for CD290 have not yet been defined	91–100	TLR family
CD291	TLR-11	Macrophages, epithelial cells	Role for CD291 in humans has not yet been defined	97	TLR family
CD292		Bone progenitor cells, chondrocytes, epithelial cells	Binds to bone morphogenetic protein (BMP)-2 and BMP-4; role in embryonic development	50–58	TMSTK
CD294	CRTH2	Th2 cells, eosinophils, basophils, widely expressed outside the immune system	Binds to PGD_2; chemo-attractant receptor	43	GPCR
CD295	Leptin receptor	Widely expressed	Binds to and mediates the effects of the hormone leptin	130–150	IgSF

Table of human CD antigens[a,b] *contd*

CD antigen	Synonym(s)	Cellular expression	Function(s)	Molecular weight (kDa)	Family
CD296	ADP-ribosyltransferase-1	T cells, NK cells, neutrophils, epithelial cells	Modifies function of proteins such as CD11a and CD18 by transferring ADP-ribose group on to arginine residue of protein	37	ART family
CD297	ADP-ribosyltransferase-4	T cells, erythrocyte lineage, epithelial cells, monocytes	Modifies protein function by transferring ADP-ribose group on to arginine residue of protein	38	ART family
CD298	Na/K ATPase β3-subunit	All leukocytes and many tissues	Dimerizes with ATPase α subunit; transport of Na^+ and K^+ across cell membrane	32	
CD299	DC-SIGN2	Endothelial cells	Binds CD50 and high mannose carbohydrate structures; involved in pathogen uptake	40	C-type lectin
CD300a		Granulocytes, DCs, NK cells. T cells, B cells	Potential inhibitory receptor	60	IgSF
CD300c		Granulocytes, DCs, NK cells. Subset of T and B cells, monocytes	Potential inhibitory receptor	23	IgSF
CD300e		Macrophages, monocytes, neutrophils	Potential activating receptor		IgSF
CD301		Macrophages, immature DCs	Binds to carbohydrates with terminal galactose and N-acetylgalactosamine moieties; uptake of glycosylated antigens	38	C-type lectin
CD302		Macrophages, granulocytes, monocytes, DCs, B cells	Role in endocytosis of glycosylated antigens	30	C-type lectin
CD303		DCs, neutrophils, macrophages	Role in endocytosis of glycosylated antigens	38	C-type lectin
CD304	Neuropilin-1	DCs, neurons, T cells, endothelial cells	Promotes angiogenesis	140	Neuropilin family
CD305	LAIR-1	Widely expressed on cells of the immune system	Inhibits T cell and NK cell function	32–42	IgSF
CD306	LAIR-2	T cells, monocytes	Function unknown; may inhibit cell activation	16	IgSF
CD307	Fc receptor-like 5	B cells, centroblasts	Binds aggregated IgG	100	IgSF
CD308	Fms-related tyrosine kinase 1	Vascular endothelial cells, monocytes	Binds vascular-endothelial growth factor and placental growth factor; role in vascular development	152	TKR
CD309		Vascular endothelial cells, megakaryocytes, platelets	Binds vascular-endothelial growth factor; role in vascular development	230	TKR
CD310		Placenta, lung, heart, kidney, lymphatic endothelium	Binds vascular-endothelial growth factor; critical for embryonic angiogenesis; role in angiogenesis and lymphangiogenesis in adults	146	TKR
CD311		Peripheral blood mononuclear cells	Function unknown	98	GPCR

Table of human CD antigens[a,b] *contd*

CD antigen	Synonym(s)	Cellular expression	Function(s)	Molecular weight (kDa)	Family
CD312		DC subsets, neutrophils, activated monocytes and lymphocytes	Binds chondroitin sulphate, glycosaminoglycan and dermatan sulphate; possible role in cell adhesion	90	GPCR
CD313		Neutrophils, monocytes, macrophages	Function unknown		GPCR
CD314	NKG2D	NK cells, CD8+ T cells, CD4+ T cell subset	Binds MHC class I-related ligands; activation of NK cell killing; co-stimulation of T cell proliferation	42	C-type lectin
CD315		B cell subsets, activated monocytes, endothelial cells, epithelial cells	Possible role in regulation of cell motility	135	IgSF
CD316	IgSF8	T cells, B cells, NK cells	Associates with CD9 and CD81	63	IgSF
CD317		B cells, plasma cells, T cells, monocytes, stromal cells, NK cells	Function unknown	29–33	
CD318		Haematopoietic precursor cells, epithelial cells	Function unknown	140	
CD319	SLAM family member-7	NK cells, cytotoxic T cells, B cells, DCs	Regulation of T cell and NK cell functions	66	IgSF
CD320	8D6	Follicular DCs	Augments proliferation of plasma cell precursors in germinal centres	29	
CD321	Junctional adhesion molecule-1	Endothelial cells, epithelial cells, erythrocytes, leukocytes	Adhesion molecule with role in leukocyte extravasation; associates with CD322 and CD323 and is involved in the formation and maintenance of tight junctions	32–35	IgSF
CD322	Junctional adhesion molecule-2	Endothelial cells, monocytes, B cells, T cell subsets	Adhesion molecule with role in cell–cell interactions; associates with CD321 and CD323 and is involved in the formation and maintenance of tight junctions	45	IgSF
CD323	Junctional adhesion molecule-3	Widely expressed	Adhesion molecule with role in leukocyte extravasation; associates with CD322 and CD323 and is involved in the formation and maintenance of tight junctions	43	IgSF
CD324	Cadherin-1	Non-neural epithelial cells, stem cells, platelets	Crucial role in cell–cell adhesion	120	Cadherin
CD325	Cadherin-2	Expressed mainly on CD234− cells	Important for cell–cell adhesion and formation of neural synapses	140	Cadherin
CD326		Expressed on most epithelial cells, carcinoma-associated antigen	Adhesion molecule; associates with CD305 and CD306; may contribute to formation of immunological barrier in gut	40	
CD327	SIGLEC-6	Placental syncytiotrophoblastic cells, splenic B cells	Adhesion molecule	49	IgSF
CD328	SIGLEC-7	NK cells, T cell subsets	Adhesion molecule; inhibits T cell and NK cell activation	51	IgSF

Table of human CD antigens^{a,b} *contd*

CD antigen	Synonym(s)	Cellular expression	Function(s)	Molecular weight (kDa)	Family
CD329	SIGLEC-9	Neutrophils, monocytes, NK cells, T cells, B cells	Adhesion molecule; suppresses TCR-dependent signalling	50	IgSF
CD330	SIGLEC-10	Widely expressed	Multiple isoforms generated by alternative splicing; function unknown; possible inhibitory receptor	90–120	IgSF
CD331	FGFR-1	Fibroblasts, epithelial cells, endothelial cells	Multiple isoforms generated by alternative splicing; high affinity receptor for acidic and basic FGFs	130	TKR
CD332	FGFR-2	Fibroblasts, epithelial cells, mesenchymal cells	Multiple isoforms generated by alternative splicing; high affinity receptor for acidic and basic FGFs	115–135	TKR
CD333	FGFR-3	Fibroblasts, epithelial cells	Three isoforms generated by alternative splicing; high affinity receptor for acidic and basic FGFs	115–135	TKR
CD334	FGFR-4	Fibroblasts, epithelial cells, lymphocytes, macrophages	High affinity receptor for acidic FGFs	110	TKR
CD335	NKp46, LY94	NK cells	Activates NK cell-mediated killing; binds Sendai virus and influenza virus haemagglutinins	46	IgSF
CD336	NKp44, LY95	IL-2-activated NK cells, γ/δ T cell subset	Activates NK cell-mediated killing; binds Sendai virus and influenza virus haemagglutinins	44	IgSF
CD337	NKp30, LY117	NK cells	Activates NK cell-mediated killing	30	IgSF
CD338	ABC-G2	Subset of haematopoietic and tissue stem cells, epithelial cells, endothelial cells	ATP-dependent extrusion of drugs and toxic chemicals across cell membranes	72	ABC
CD339	Jagged 1	Bone marrow stromal cells, epithelial cells	Binds to Notch 1, Notch 2 and Notch 3 and triggers Notch signalling; role in regulation of cell-fate decisions during haematopoiesis	150	*Drosophila* Jagged ligands family
CD340	HER-2/neu	Epithelial cells, bone marrow mesenchymal cells, many cancers	Activates MAPK, phospholipase-Cγ and PI-3K signalling pathways	185	TKR
CD344	Frizzled-4	Lung, brain, liver, kidney	Receptor for Wnt proteins; essential for embryonic development and for regulation of tissue and cell polarity and of cell proliferation	60	GPCR
CD349	Frizzled-9	Bone marrow and placental mesenchymal stem cells, adult and fetal brain, testis, eye, skeletal muscle, kidney	Receptor for Wnt proteins; important for development of the nervous system, B cell development and plasma cell homeostasis	65	GPCR
CD350	Frizzled-10	Placental syncytiotrophoblasts, fetal brain, kidney and lung	Receptor for Wnt proteins; essential for embryonic development and for regulation of tissue and cell polarity and of cell proliferation	65	GPCR

^a 'w' indicates that the CD molecule has been assigned a workshop designation.

ᵇ **Abbreviations**: ABC, ATP-binding cassette; ADAM, a disintegrin and metalloprotease; ADCC, antibody-dependent cell-mediated cytotoxicity; ALCAM, activated leukocyte CAM; ALK, anaplastic lymphoma kinase; ALL, acute lymphocytic leukaemia; APRIL, a proliferation-inducing ligand; ART, ADP-ribosyltransferase; BAFF(-R), B cell activating factor (-receptor); B-CAM, B cell adhesion molecule; BST1, bone marrow stromal cell antigen 1; BTLA, B and T lymphocyte attenuator; CALLA, common acute lymphocytic leukaemia antigen; CAM, cell adhesion molecule; CCL, CC chemokine ligand; CCP, complement control protein superfamily; CCR, CC chemokine receptor; CEA, carcinoembryonic antigen; CLP, cartilage link protein family; CR, complement receptor; CRF, chemokine receptor family; CRTH2, chemo-attractant receptor homologous molecule expressed by Th2 cells; CTLA, cytotoxic T lymphocyte antigen; CXCL, CXC chemokine ligand; CXCR, CXC chemokine receptor; DAF, decay accelerating factor; DC, dendritic cell; DC-SIGN, dendritic cell-specific ICAM-3-grabbing non-integrin; DDR, discoidin domain receptor; EGF, epidermal growth factor; ENPP3, ecto-nucleotide pyrophosphatase phosphodiesterase; ENTPD, ectonucleoside triphosphate diphosphohydrolase; EPCR, endothelial cell protein C receptor; FGF(R), fibroblast growth factor (receptor); GGT, γ-glutamyl transpeptidase; GPCR, G-protein coupled receptor; HMMR, hyaluronan-mediated motility receptor; HPTP, high density PTP; HSA, heat stable antigen; HSP, heparin sulphate proteoglycan; HSV, herpes simplex virus; HVEM(L), herpes virus entry mediator (ligand); ICAM, intercellular adhesion molecule; ICOS(-L), inducible costimulator (-ligand); IFN-γ(AF), interferon-γ (associated factor); IGF(1/2), insulin-like growth factor (1/2); IgSF, immunoglobulin gene superfamily; ILT, immunoglobulin-like transcript; IRTK, insulin receptor tyrosine kinase; ITAM, immunoreceptor tyrosine-based activation motif; ITIM, immunoreceptor tyrosine-based inhibition motif; KIR(n)D(L/S), killer cell immunoglobulin-like receptor with n domains and long/short cytoplasmic tail; KLR, killer cell lectin-like receptor; LAG, lymphocyte activation gene; LAIR, leukocyte-associated immunoglobulin-like receptor; LAMP, lysosome-associated membrane protein; LDL, low-density lipoprotein; LFA, leukocyte function-associated antigen; LIF, leukaemia inhibitory factor; LPS, lipopolysaccharide; LT, lymphotoxin; M6P(R), mannose-6-phosphate (receptor); MAdCAM, mucosal addressin CAM; MAPK, mitogen-activated protein kinase; MDR, multidrug resistance; MGC, multi-glycosylated core protein; NAIL, NK cell activation-inducing ligand; NB1, neutrophil-specific antigen B1; N-CAM, neural CAM; NKR, NK cell receptor; OSM, oncostatin M; PDGF(R), platelet-derived growth factor (receptor); PETA, platelet-endothelial tetra-span antigen; PI, phosphatidylinositol; PI-3K, phosphatidylinositol-3-kinase; PSGL, P selectin glycoprotein ligand; PTP, protein tyrosine phosphatase; RANK(L), receptor activator of NF B (ligand); Rh, Rhesus; SIGLEC, sialic-acid binding Ig-like lectin; SIRP, signal regulatory protein; SLAM, surface lymphocyte activation antigen; TACI, transmembrane activator and CAML interactor; T-ALL, T cell acute lymphoblastic leukaemia; TAPA-1, target for antiproliferative antigen-1; TCR, T cell receptor; Tie, tyrosine kinase with immunoglobulin-like and EGF-like domains; TKR, tyrosine kinase receptor; TLR; toll-like receptor; TM4SF, transmembrane 4 superfamily/tetraspannins; TMSTK, transmembrane serine/threonine kinase; TNF(R)(SF), tumour necrosis factor-(receptor)(superfamily); TRAIL, TNF-related apoptosis-inducing ligand; VESPR, virally encoded semaphorin receptor; VLA, very late antigen; ZMP, zinc metalloproteinase.

SELECTED HUMAN CYTOKINES AND THEIR FUNCTIONS[a]

	Cytokine	Source	Receptor(s)	Selected function(s)
Interleukins (IL)	IL-1α	Macrophages, epithelial cells	CD121a/IL-1RAcP CD121b/IL-1RAcP	Induces macrophage activation; augments T cell activation; induces fever and acute phase protein synthesis Decoy receptor that binds IL-1α with low affinity
	IL-1β	Macrophages, epithelial cells	CD121a/IL-1RAcP CD121b/IL-1RAcP	Induces macrophage activation; augments T cell activation; induces fever and acute phase protein synthesis Decoy receptor that binds IL-1β with high affinity
	IL-1RA	Macrophages, monocytes, neutrophils, hepatocytes	CD121a/IL-1RAcP	Antagonist of IL-1 function
	IL-2	T cells	CD25/CD122/CD132	Induces T cell proliferation
	IL-3	T cells, mast cells, endothelial cells	CD123/CD131	Stimulates growth and differentiation of haematopoietic cells; potent mast cell growth factor
	IL-4	Th2 cells, mast cells	CD124/CD132 (Type I); CD124/CD213a1 (Type II)	Induces B cell and Th2 cell proliferation; promotes class switch to IgE
	IL-5	Th2 cells, mast cells, eosinophils	CD125/CD131	Promotes eosinophil survival and B cell differentiation
	IL-6	Macrophages, T cells, endothelial cells	CD126/CD130	Induces acute phase protein production; plasma cell development; antibody secretion
	IL-7	Bone marrow and thymic stromal cells	CD127/CD132	Promotes T and B cell development, survival and homeostasis
	IL-8	Macrophages, endothelial cells, lymphocytes	CXCR1 CXCR2	Induces neutrophil chemotaxis and activation
	IL-9	T cells	CD129/CD132	Promotes mast cell differentiation
	IL-10	Monocytes, Th2 cells, mast cells, B cell subset, T_{REG} cells	CDw210a/CDw210b; CDw210b	Inhibits pro-inflammatory cytokine production by macrophages; inhibition of antigen presentation; promotes survival and differentiation of B cells
	IL-11	Bone marrow stromal cells	IL-11Rα/CD130	Acute phase protein production; megakaryocyte maturation; osteoclast production; lymphopoiesis
	IL-12	Macrophages, DCs	CD212/IL-12Rβ2	Promotes Th1 cell differentiation and NK cell activation
	IL-13	T cells, mast cells	CD124/CD213a1/CD132 CD213a2 (decoy receptor)	Stimulates B cell growth and differentiation and IgE production; inhibits pro-inflammatory cytokine production by macrophages; inhibits Th1 cell responses; induces class switch to IgE (with IL-4)
	IL-14	T cells	IL-14R	Stimulates B cell proliferation; inhibits antibody secretion
	IL-15	Mononuclear phagocytes	IL-15Rα/CD122/CD132	Promotes growth of T cells and NK cells; promotes survival of memory CD8$^+$ cells
	IL-16	T cells, mast cells, eosinophils	CD4	Chemo-attractant for CD4$^+$ T cells, macrophages and eosinophils
	IL-17A[b]	Th17 cells	CD217/IL-17RC	Stimulates pro-inflammatory cytokine production by many cell types
	IL-18	Macrophages	CD218a/CD218b	Induces IFN-γ production by NK cells and T cells; promotes Th1 responses

Selected human cytokines and their functions[a] *contd*

	Cytokine	Source	Receptor(s)	Selected function(s)
	IL-19	Monocytes, B cells	IL-20Rα/IL-20Rβ	Induces pro-inflammatory cytokine production; possible role in endotoxic shock
	IL-20	Activated keratinocytes, monocytes	IL-20Rα/IL-20Rβ IL-22R/IL-20Rβ	Regulates keratinocyte proliferation and differentiation; role in psoriasis
	IL-21	Activated CD4$^+$ T cells, T$_{FH}$ cells, NK cells	IL-21Rα/CD132	Stimulates B cell differentiation into antibody secreting cells; enhances the cytoxicity of NK cells and CD8$^+$ T cells; inhibits T$_{REG}$ development
	IL-22	T cells, especially Th17 cells	CDw210b/IL-22R	Increases production of acute phase proteins; inhibits IL-4 production by Th2 cells
	IL-23	DCs, macrophages	CD212/IL-23R	Promotes expansion and function of Th17 cells; promotes angiogenesis; induces proliferation of CD4$^+$ memory T cells
	IL-24	Activated monocytes, macrophages and Th2 cells, keratinocytes	IL-20Rα/IL-20Rβ; IL-22R/IL-20Rβ	Exhibits anti-tumour activity ; induces production of IL-6 and TNF-α
	IL-25[b]	Th2 cells, mast cells	IL-25R	Induces production of IL-4, IL-5 and IL-13 which promote expansion of eosinophils
	IL-26	Th17 cells, NK cells	IL-20Rα/CDw210b	Induces IL-8 and IL-10 secretion; induces expression of CD54
	IL-27[c]	Monocytes, DCs, macrophages	IL-27Rα//CD130	Induces expression of IL-12 and promotes Th1 responses; inhibits Th17 development
	IL-28	Monocytes, DCs, many other cells	IL-28Rα/CDw210b	Induces antiviral state; induces Th1 cytokine production
	IL-29	Monocytes, DCs, many other cells	IL-28Rα/CDw210b	Induces antiviral state; stimulates production of IL-6, IL-8 and IL-10
	IL-31	Th2 cells	IL-31Rα/OSMRβ	Promotes skin inflammation; promotes allergic asthma
	IL-32	NK cells, epithelial cells, T cells, monocytes	Proteinase-3 (soluble receptor)[d]	Induces production of TNF-α, IL-1β and IL-6
	IL-33	Endothelial cells	ST2/IL-1RAcP[e]	Induces production of IL-4, IL-5 and IL-13; attracts Th2 cells
	IL-34	Spleen, kidney, brain	CD115	Regulates differentiation, proliferation and survival of myeloid lineage cells
	IL-35[d]	T$_{REG}$ cells	Unknown	Induces T$_{REG}$ cell proliferation; inhibits Th17 activity
Chemokines[e]	CCL1	Macrophages, T cells, NK cells, monocytes	CCR8	Attracts neutrophils and T cells
	CCL2	Leukocytes, osteoclasts, keratinocytes	CCR2	Attracts T cells, monocytes, basophils
	CCL3	Widely expressed	CCR1; CCR5	Attracts monocytes, macrophages, T cells, immature DCs, NK cells, basophils
	CCL4	Widely expressed	CCR5	Attracts monocytes, macrophages, T cells, immature DCs, NK cells, basophils
	CCL5	Leukocytes, epithelial cells, T cells	CCR1; CCR3; CCR5	Attracts monocytes, macrophages, T cells, immature DCs, NK cells, basophils, eosinophils

Selected human cytokines and their functions[a] *contd*

Cytokine	Source	Receptor(s)	Selected function(s)
CCL7	Widely expressed	CCR1; CCR2; CCR3	Attracts monocytes, T cells, DCs, eosinophils, basophils
CCL8	Widely expressed	CCR2; CCR3; CCR5	Attracts monocytes, T cells, eosinophils, basophils
CCL11	Widely expressed	CCR3	Attracts eosinophils
CCL13	Widely expressed	CCR2; CCR3	Attracts monocytes, T cells, DCs, eosinophils, basophils
CCL14	Widely expressed	CCR1; CCR5	Attracts monocytes
CCL15	Widely expressed	CCR1; CCR3	Attracts monocytes, T cells, DCs
CCL16	Leukocytes, bone marrow, hepatocytes	CCR1; CCR2	Attracts monocytes
CCL17	Widely expressed	CCR4	Attracts T cells, immature DCs, NK cells
CCL18	Widely expressed	Unknown	Attracts T cells
CCL19	Lymphoid tissue	CCR7	Attracts T cells, DCs, B cells
CCL20	Widely expressed	CCR6	Attracts T cells, DCs, B cells
CCL21	Lymphoid tissue	CCR7	Attracts T cells, B cells, mesangial cells
CCL22	Widely expressed	CCR4	Attracts immature DCs, NK cells, T cells
CCL23	Widely expressed	CCR1	Attracts monocytes, T cells
CCL24	Activated monocytes, T cells	CCR3	Attracts eosinophils, basophils, T cells
CCL25	Thymic DCs, small intestine	CCR9	Attracts macrophages, DCs
CCL26	Widely expressed	CCR3	Attracts eosinophils, basophils
CCL27	Skin, thymus, testis, ovary	CCR10	Attracts T cells
CCL28	Epithelial cells, leukocytes	CCR3; CCR10	Attracts T cells, eosinophils
CXCL1	Macrophages, epithelial cells, neutrophils	CXCR1; CXCR2	Attracts neutrophils
CXCL2	Monocytes, macrophages	CXCR1; CXCR2	Attracts neutrophils, haematopoietic progenitors
CXCL3	Monocytes, macrophages	CXCR1; CXCR2	Attracts neutrophils
CXCL4	Activated platelets	CXCR3B	Attracts fibroblasts, neutrophils, monocytes
CXCL5	Epithelial cells, eosinophils	CXCR1; CXCR2	Attracts neutrophils
CXCL6	Widely expressed	CXCR1; CXCR2	Attracts neutrophils
CXCL7	Activated platelets, monocytes	CXCR1; CXCR2	Attracts fibroblasts, neutrophils
CXCL8	Macrophages, mast cells, endothelial cells, epithelial cells	CXCR1; CXCR2	Attracts neutrophils, T cells

Selected human cytokines and their functions[a] *contd*

Cytokine	Source	Receptor(s)	Selected function(s)
CXCL9	Fibroblasts, endothelial cells, monocytes	CXCR3	Attracts activated T cells, DCs
CXCL10	Fibroblasts, endothelial cells, monocytes	CXCR3	Attracts activated T cells, DCs, NK cells, monocytes
CXCL11	Leukocytes, hepatocytes	CXCR3	Attracts activated T cells
CXCL12	Widely expressed	CXCR4	Attracts haematopoietic progenitor cells, T cells, B cells, DCs
CXCL13	DCs, follicular stromal cells	CXCR5	Attracts B cells, T cell subset, T_{FH} cells
CXCL14	Widely expressed	Unknown	Attracts T cells, monocytes, DCs
CXCL16	Interdigitating DCs	CXCR6	Attracts T cells, NK cells
CX3CL1	Endothelial cells	CX3CR1	Attracts T cells, monocytes
XCL1	Widely expressed	XCR1	Attracts T cells, NK cells
XCL2	T cells	XCR1	Attracts T cells, NK cells
Interferons (IFN) IFN-α	Leukocytes, DCs	IFNAR1/IFNAR2	Induces antiviral state; enhances expression of MHC class I
IFN-β	Fibroblasts, epithelial cells	IFNAR1/IFNAR2	Induces antiviral state; enhances expression of MHC class I
IFN-γ	T cells (specially Th1 cells), NK cells	CD119/IFN-γAF	Activates macrophages; enhances expression of MHC class I and class II; inhibits Th2 responses; induces class switch recombination
Tumour necrosis factor (TNF) TNF-α	T cells, macrophages, NK cells	CD120a; CD120b	Induces acute phase protein production; activates endothelial cells; promotes DTH responses
LT-α	T cells, B cells	CD120a; CD120b; CD270	Induces cell death; activates endothelial cells; promotes DTH responses
LT-α$_1$β$_2$	T cells, B cells	LTβR	Promotes lymphoneogenesis
BAFF	Monocytes, DCs, stromal cells	CD267; CD268; CD269	Promotes B cell survival, activation and proliferation
Transforming growth factors (TGF) TGF-α	Macrophages, keratinocytes, transformed cells	EGF-R	Promotes epithelial development; promotes anchorage-independent growth of fibroblasts
TGF-β	Monocytes, T_{REG} cells, transformed cells	TGF-βR	Inhibits T cell proliferation; promotes class switch to IgA

[a] **Abbreviations**: BAFF; B cell activating factor; IL-1RAcP, IL-1 receptor accessory protein; LT, lymphotoxin; T_{FH}, follicular helper T cell; T_{REG}, regulatory T cell.

[b] The IL-17 family of cytokines consists of 6 members, IL-17A–F. IL-17E is also known as IL-25.

[c] The IL-27α subunit of the IL-27 heterodimer was formerly called IL-30.

[d] IL-35 is a heterodimer consisting of the IL-12α chain and the IL-27β chain.

[e] There are no human orthologues of the murine CCL6, CCL9, CCL10, CCL12 and CXCL15 chemokines.

Glossary

Acquired immunodeficiency syndrome (AIDS): a disease caused by infection with human immunodeficiency virus (HIV), transmitted in blood and body secretions such as semen.

Active immunity: long-term immunity acquired after exposure to antigen.

Acute phase response: the production of substances called acute phase proteins within hours of exposure to a pathogen. Acute phase proteins, such as C-reactive protein and α_1-proteinase inhibitor, take part in the early response to infection.

Adaptive immune response: also referred to as acquired immune response, it involves immunity acquired after exposure to antigen. It takes over a week after the initial exposure to be fully active.

Adhesion molecules: molecules that allow cells to bind tightly to other cells or to the extracellular matrix.

Adjuvant: substance used to enhance the immune response against an antigen.

Agammaglobulinaemia: significantly reduced, or absent, levels of gammaglobulin (immunoglobulin, i.e. antibody).

Agglutination: the formation of antigen aggregates by antibodies.

AIDS (acquired immune deficiency syndrome): secondary immunodeficiency caused by human immunodeficiency virus and characterized by progressive loss of CD4$^+$ T cells.

Allelic exclusion: the mechanism whereby successful rearrangement at one immunoglobulin or TCR locus prevents rearrangement at that locus on the homologous chromosome.

Allergen: an antigen responsible for inducing allergic reactions that include IgE formation.

Allergy: immune reactions to non-pathogenic antigens or harmless foreign substances which result in inflammation and deleterious effects in the host. This is also referred to as hypersensitivity.

Allograft: a tissue transplant between two genetically non-identical members of a species.

Alternative pathway: a mechanism of complement activation which begins with the activation of C3.

Anaphylatoxin: a substance which can induce a rapid hypersensitivity reaction with the release of histamine from mast cells.

Anaphylaxis: a serious life-threatening immediate hypersensitivity response to antigenic challenge by an anaphylatoxin. It is mediated by IgE and mast cells.

Anergy: state of non-responsiveness of lymphocytes to specific antigen.

Antibody: a serum protein secreted in large amounts by B cells/plasma cells in response to antigen. The antigen can be a bacterium, virus, parasite or transplanted tissue. Antibodies neutralize the antigen by binding to it and often tagging it for destruction by phagocytes. An antibody is also referred to as immunoglobulin.

Antibody-dependent cell-mediated cytotoxicity (ADCC): a mechanism for killing cells in which antibody-coated target cells are destroyed by NK cells or macrophages, which express surface receptors that bind to the Fc portion of the coating antibody (Fc receptors).

Antigen: a substance (usually a protein or carbohydrate) to which specific antibodies bind. Antigens which are able to trigger an immune response are immunogens while those that do not trigger it, usually because they are too small, are haptens.

Antigen-presenting cell (APC): a specialized type of

cell with surface expression of MHC class II and co-stimulatory molecules, e.g. macrophage or dendritic cells. These cells are involved in processing and presentation of antigen to T cells.

Antigen processing and presentation: limited proteolysis of large antigens into peptides for presentation to T cells within the groove of an MHC molecule on the surface of an antigen-presenting cell.

Antigenic determinant: a single antigenic/immunogenic site or epitope on a complex antigenic molecule.

Atopy: a term used to describe IgE-mediated allergic reactions, usually involving skin rash.

Autograft: a tissue transplant from one area of an individual's body to another.

Autoimmune diseases: conditions in which the immune system can mount a reaction to self with pathological consequences.

Autoimmunity: an immune response to self antigens that may lead to autoimmune diseases.

Autoreactive: refers to immune cells which react against self antigens.

B cell: a type of lymphocyte that produces antibodies/immunoglobulins.

Basophil: a circulating polymorphonuclear leukocyte with granules containing heparin, histamine and other vasoactive amines.

BCR (B cell receptor): cell membrane bound immunoglobulin that allows B cells to respond to specific antigen.

Cancer: unlimited and unrestricted growth of cells resulting in a malignant tumour which expands locally by invasion and spreading in a process called metastasis.

CD4$^+$ helper T cells: T lymphocytes (T cells) with CD4 molecules on their surfaces. They respond to antigen by secreting cytokines that stimulate B cells and killer T cells.

Cell-mediated immunity: immune reaction mediated by T cells; in contrast to humoral immunity, which is antibody-mediated.

Chemoattractant: a molecule that induces cells to migrate.

Chemokine: member of a large family of low molecular weight chemoattractant cytokines.

Chemokinesis: random, non-directional migration of cells induced by a chemoattractant.

Chemotaxis: migration of cells along a concentration gradient of an attractant towards a stimulus.

Class II-associated invariant chain peptide (CLIP): portion of the invariant chain that inserts into the peptide binding groove of MHC class II molecules.

Classical pathway: the mechanism of complement activation initiated by antigen–antibody aggregates binding to C1.

Class-switch recombination: the mechanism a B cell uses to produce antibody of a different isotype but with the same V regions. For example, IgM to IgG class switch.

Clonal deletion: induce death of autoreactive lymphocytes due to contact with self.

Cluster of differentiation (CD): serologically defined cell surface antigen.

Complement: a series of serum proteins involved in innate and adaptive immune reactions.

Conduits: channels in lymph nodes and spleen that disperse material throughout the T cell area.

Constant region (C region): the invariant carboxyl-terminal portion of an antibody or TCR.

Co-stimulatory molecules: molecules such as CD28 that transduce signals into T cells and are required for activation of naïve T cells.

Cross-presentation: process whereby exogenous antigens are taken up by certain dendritic cells and are processed and presented on MHC class I molecules to CD8$^+$ T cells.

Cross-reactivity: the ability of an antibody or TCR, specific for one antigen, to react with a similar antigen.

Cytokine: a protein secreted by cells which acts as a messenger to regulate the function of other cells (paracrine or juxtacrine response) or of the cell secreting the cytokine (autocrine response). Examples of cytokines include interleukins, interferons and chemokines.

Cytotoxic (cytolytic) T lymphocyte (CTL): CD8$^+$ T cell which kills target cells carrying a specific antigen within the groove of an MHC class I molecule.

Danger theory: theory proposing that the immune system responds when damage to the host is detected, rather than by discriminating between self and non-self antigens.

Delayed type hypersensitivity (DTH): a Type IV hypersensitivity reaction mediated by T cells, which takes 24–48 hours to develop, with the release of lymphokines and recruitment of monocytes and macrophages.

Dendritic cell: a professional antigen-presenting cell which can activate lymphocytes and stimulate the secretion of cytokines.

Endogenous pathway: pathway whereby endogenously synthesized antigens are processed and presented on MHC class I molecules to CD8⁺ T cells.

Enzyme-linked immunosorbent assay (ELISA): an assay that uses specific antibodies to quantify soluble molecules. An enzyme is linked to an antibody and the enzyme produces a coloured product in proportion to the amount of antibody–enzyme that is bound.

Eosinophil: a granulocyte with large eosinophilic cytoplasmic granules. Eosinophils are important in asthma and in defence against metazoan parasites.

Epitope: a portion of an antigen (an antigenic determinant) that is recognized by a lymphocyte.

Exogenous pathway: pathway whereby exogenous antigens are taken up by an antigen-presenting cell, processed and presented on MHC class II molecules to CD4⁺ T cells.

Fab: a fragment of antibody containing the antigen-binding site, generated by cleavage of the antibody with the enzyme papain to generate two Fab fragments and one Fc fragment from one antibody molecule.

F(ab′)₂: a fragment of an antibody containing two antigen-binding sites generated by cleavage of the antibody molecule with the enzyme pepsin.

Fc: fragment of antibody without antigen-binding sites, generated by cleavage with papain; the Fc fragment contains the C-terminal domains of the heavy immunoglobulin chains.

Fc receptor (FcR): a cell surface receptor found on many cell types which binds specifically to the Fc portion of an antibody molecule.

Fluorescent antibody: an antibody tagged with a fluorescent dye which is often used to detect antigen in cells (immunocytochemistry) or tissues (immunohistochemistry).

Follicle: area of lymphoid tissue where B lymphocytes are concentrated.

Follicular dendritic cell: cell in follicle that displays antigen on its surface for selection of B cells after somatic hypermutation.

Follicular helper T cell: CD4⁺CXCR5⁺ T cell that provides help to B cells in germinal centres.

Gene rearrangement: the process whereby gene segments are recombined in the immunoglobulin and TCR loci to generate immunoglobulin and TCR genes, respectively.

Germinal centre: region of B cell follicle where somatic hypermutation and class-switch recombination occur.

Graft-versus-host disease (GvHD): the pathologic response initiated when immunocompetent T lymphocytes are transplanted into an allogeneic host who is unable to reject the grafted T cells. The T cells in the graft react against the host.

Heavy chain (H chain): the larger of the two types of chains (heavy and light) which comprise the immunoglobulin/antibody molecule.

Helper T cells: CD4⁺ T cells which help B cells to make antibody.

Herpes: inflammatory diseases of the skin caused by one of the DNA herpes simplex viruses and characterized by clusters of blisters.

High endothelial venule (HEV): a site where lymphocytes cross from the circulation into lymph nodes.

Histamine: a compound often released during allergic reactions that causes stretching of capillaries, contraction of smooth muscle, and stimulation of gastric acid secretions.

Histocompatibility: refers to the similarity or differences between tissues in terms of their expression of MHC antigens.

Human immunodeficiency virus (HIV): a retrovirus that infects CD4⁺ T cells. HIV is the virus that causes AIDS.

Humoral immunity: immune response involving specific antibody.

Hybridoma: a hybrid cell formed by fusion of an antibody-secreting cell with a malignant cell. They are used during the production of monoclonal antibodies and are capable of growing continuously.

Hygiene hypothesis: hypothesis stating that the lack of exposure to pathogens early in life predisposes to the development of allergic diseases.

Hypersensitivity: an exaggerated immune response to an antigen (an allergen) which has a deleterious outcome rather than a protective one.

Hypervariable regions: the antigen-binding site of an antibody molecule or TCR, which contain highly variable amino acid sequences.

Immune complex: antigen bound to antibody and, usually complement.

Immunogen: a substance (an antigen) capable of inducing an immune response.

Immunoglobulin (Ig): a general term for all

antibody molecules. Each Ig unit is made up of two protein heavy chains and two protein light chains and has two antigen-binding sites.

Immunological synapse: region of interaction between T cells and antigen-presenting cells.

Immunoproteasome: multicatalytic cytosolic protease complex that generates the majority of peptides that are presented by MHC class I molecules.

Inflammation: an early immune response which results in the movement of fluid and cells to fight infection.

Innate immune response: also known as natural immune response, it is a quickly mobilized immune system that is non-specific and has no memory.

Interferons: a family of cytokines that include interferon (IFN)-α and IFN-β, which are important in the innate response against viruses, as well as IFN-γ which is a key cytokine involved in adaptive immune responses.

Interleukins: glycoproteins secreted by a variety of cells which are important in regulation of the immune response.

Invariant chain: protein that associates with MHC class II molecules to prevent peptide binding in the endoplasmic reticulum.

Isograft: a tissue transplanted between two genetically identical individuals.

Isotype switch: see *Class-switch recombination*.

Isotypes: antibody isotypes differ in the constant region of the heavy chain and such differences also result in different biological activities of the antibodies.

Janus kinases (JAKs): enzymes involved in signal transduction via certain cytokine receptors. They activate members of the Stat (signal transducing and activators of transcription) family of transcription factors.

Latency: the state where a virus lies dormant within cells and is not actively multiplying and symptoms of the infection are not seen.

Lectin pathway: pathway of complement activation that is initiated by the binding of mannan-binding lectin or ficolins to microbial surfaces.

Light chain (L chain): the light chain of immunoglobulin is a structural feature that occurs in two forms: κ (kappa) and λ (lambda).

Lymph: extracellular fluid that accumulates in tissues and is collected by lymphatic vessels and returned to the circulation.

Lymph nodes: secondary lymphoid tissues interspersed along lymphatic vessels.

Lymphocyte: a type of white blood cell involved in the immune system and includes T cells and B cells. They are highly specific for antigenic material. Each lymphocyte has a single specificity and exposure to specific antigen results in clonal expansion.

Macrophage: a large mononuclear phagocytic cell with functions in immune response including removal of antigenic material through phagocytosis. Macrophages present antigen to T cells.

Major histocompatibility complex (MHC) molecules: a cluster of genes on chromosome 6 which encode, among others, molecules involved in presentation of antigen to T cells.

Marginal zone: area rich in macrophages and marginal zone B cells that separates the splenic white pulp from the perifollicular zone and the red pulp.

Mast cell: a tissue cell that is crucial for inflammatory responses, hypersensitivity responses, and wound healing. It expresses receptors that bind to the Fc portion of IgE.

MHC class I molecule: a molecule encoded in the MHC which binds peptides and presents them to cytotoxic (CD8$^+$) T cells.

MHC class II loading compartment (MIIC): modified endosomal compartment in which peptides are loaded on to MHC class II molecules.

MHC class II molecule: a molecule encoded in the MHC which binds peptides and presents them to helper (CD4$^+$) T cells.

MHC restriction: the ability of T lymphocytes to respond only when they 'see' the appropriate antigen in association with 'self' MHC class I or class II proteins on the surface of antigen-presenting cells.

Mitogen: a substance that stimulates the proliferation of many different clones of lymphocytes.

Molecular mimicry hypothesis: a hypothesis proposing that autoimmune diseases result from immune responses against foreign antigens that cross-react with self antigens.

Monoclonal antibodies: antibodies derived from a single clone of B cells that are highly specific for one antigen. They are the most common immunological reagent used in immunoassays.

Monocyte: a mononuclear leukocyte in the blood that becomes a macrophage when it moves into tissue.

Myeloma: a tumour of plasma cells, generally secreting immunoglobulin of a single specificity.

NK (natural killer) cells: naturally occurring, large, granular, lymphocyte-like cells that kill various tumour cells.

Opsonin: substances, e.g. antibody and C3b that coat an antigen such as a bacterium to enhance phagocytosis.

Opsonization: coating of a bacterium with an opsonin to promote phagocytosis.

Paracortex: the T cell area of lymph nodes.

Pathogen: any agent which has the potential to cause disease.

Pathogen-associated molecular patterns (PAMPs): molecular signatures or patterns such as nucleic acid sequences or surface molecules that are characteristic of particular pathogens. PAMPs are recognized by pattern recognition receptors.

Pattern recognition receptors (PRRs): receptors of the innate immune system that bind to pattern-associated molecular patterns and initiate inflammatory responses.

Peptide loading complex (PLC): complex containing TAP, tapasin, ERp57 and calreticulin that transfers peptides translocated by TAP into the peptide binding groove of MHC class I molecules.

Peri-arteriolar lymphoid sheath (PALS): the T cell area of the spleen.

Perifollicular zone: region of the human spleen between the marginal zone and red pulp. It is open to the splenic circulation and contains blood-filled spaces. It is the site through which cells enter the white pulp from the circulation.

Phagocyte: a cell which can engulf foreign material such as micro-organisms and eliminate them from the host.

Phagocytosis: the ingestion of a particle or a micro-organism and intracellular destruction.

Plasma cell: a high level antibody-secreting cell that develops from a B cell following stimulation with specific antigen.

Polymorphism: the existence of multiple variants of a gene or protein.

Primary lymphoid organs: organs in which T and B lymphocytes mature.

Primary response: this is the first response to an antigen. It is usually small with a long induction phase and involves IgM antibodies.

Protease: an enzyme that breaks proteins into smaller parts.

Receptor editing: process whereby an autoreactive B cell may alter the variable region of its BCR to generate a non-autoreactive BCR.

Recombination activating genes: genes whose products (RAG-1 and RAG-2) are required for immunoglobulin and TCR gene rearrangement.

Regulatory T cells (T$_{REG}$ cells): specialized T cells which regulate or suppress immune responses.

Respiratory burst: oxygen-dependent increase in metabolic activity of phagocytic cells stimulated by the ingestion of bacteria or parasites.

Rheumatoid factor: the IgM autoantibody present in some cases of rheumatoid arthritis. Often measured as an aid to diagnosis of rheumatoid arthritis though its concentration does not often correlate with disease progression.

Secondary lymphoid organs: organs where antigen-driven proliferation and differentiation of lymphocytes occur.

Secondary response: the immune response generated following the second and all subsequent exposures to antigen. It is more rapid in onset and greater in magnitude than the primary response. Secondary antibody responses are usually dominated by the production of isotypes other than IgM.

Severe combined immunodeficiency (SCID): serious disease resulting from a deficiency of T cells and B cells due to a block early in lymphocyte development.

Signal transducers and activators of transcription (Stat): Stat proteins are involved in transducing signals from certain cytokine receptors. Following phosphorylation by JAKs, Stat proteins dimerize and translocate to the nucleus to activate gene transcription.

Somatic hypermutation: high level mutation in germinal centres targeted at rearranged V(D)J regions of immunoglobulin genes.

Supramolecular activation cluster (SMAC): area of immunological synapse where recognition and signalling molecules are localized. The SMAC consists of a central cSMAC surrounded by a peripheral pSMAC.

T-dependent antigen: antigen that requires T cell help to induce antibody production.

T-independent antigen: antigen that does not require T cell help to induce antibody production.

T cell: a lymphocyte which completes its development in the thymus. It has highly specific cell surface antigen receptors which dictate cell type such as: CD4$^+$ helper T cells and CD8$^+$ cytotoxic T cells.

TAP: transporter associated with antigen presentation that pumps peptides from the cytosol into the lumen of the endoplasmic reticulum where they bind to MHC class I molecules.

TCR (T cell receptor): molecule expressed on the surface of T cells that allows them to respond to specific antigen.

T$_{FH}$: see *Follicular helper T cell.*

Th1 cell: CD4$^+$ T cell that secretes IFN-γ but not IL-4, IL-5, IL-10 or IL-13. Th1 cells promote cell-mediated immune responses and are important in defence against intracellular bacterial and viruses.

Th2 cell: CD4$^+$ T cell that secretes IL-4, IL-5, IL-10 and IL-13, but not IFN-γ. Th2 cells promote humoral immune responses and are important in defence against extracellular pathogens such as parasitic worms.

Th17: a pro-inflammatory CD4$^+$ T cell subset characterized by the production of IL-17.

T$_{REG}$: see *Regulatory T cell.*

Tolerance: state of non-responsiveness to an antigen.

Toll-like receptors (TLRs): family of pattern recognition receptors of the innate immune system.

Tuberculosis: a disease caused by *Mycobacterium tuberculosis* which is transmitted by inhalation; affects the lungs but may spread. It is characterized by fever, coughing, difficulty in breathing and inflammation.

Two-signal theory: activation of T cells and B cells requires two signals, one signal transmitted through the antigen receptor (TCR or BCR) and the other transmitted via CD28 on T cells and CD40 on B cells.

Xenograft: a tissue transplant from a member of another species.

X-linked agammaglobulinaemia (XLA): immunoglobulin deficiency characterized by the lack of mature B cells due to mutation or deletion of the gene encoding Bruton's tyrosine kinase (Btk).

X-linked hyper-IgM syndrome: immunoglobulin deficiency caused by the inability to undergo class-switch recombination predominantly due to mutations in CD154.

Index